Advancing the Science of Cancer in Latinos

Amelie G. Ramirez • Edward J. Trapido
Editors

Advancing the Science of Cancer in Latinos

Building Collaboration for Action

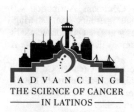

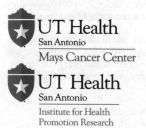

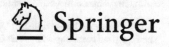

Editors
Amelie G. Ramirez
Department of Population Health Sciences
Institute for Health Promotion Research
UT Health San Antonio
San Antonio, TX, USA

Edward J. Trapido
Epidemiology Program
LSU Health Sciences Center
School of Public Health
New Orleans, LA, USA

This book is an open access publication.

ISBN 978-3-031-14438-7   ISBN 978-3-031-14436-3   (eBook)
https://doi.org/10.1007/978-3-031-14436-3

© The Editor(s) (if applicable) and The Author(s) 2023
Open Access This book is licensed under the terms of the Creative Commons Attribution 4.0 International License (http://creativecommons.org/licenses/by/4.0/), which permits use, sharing, adaptation, distribution and reproduction in any medium or format, as long as you give appropriate credit to the original author(s) and the source, provide a link to the Creative Commons license and indicate if changes were made.
The images or other third party material in this book are included in the book's Creative Commons license, unless indicated otherwise in a credit line to the material. If material is not included in the book's Creative Commons license and your intended use is not permitted by statutory regulation or exceeds the permitted use, you will need to obtain permission directly from the copyright holder.
The use of general descriptive names, registered names, trademarks, service marks, etc. in this publication does not imply, even in the absence of a specific statement, that such names are exempt from the relevant protective laws and regulations and therefore free for general use.
The publisher, the authors, and the editors are safe to assume that the advice and information in this book are believed to be true and accurate at the date of publication. Neither the publisher nor the authors or the editors give a warranty, expressed or implied, with respect to the material contained herein or for any errors or omissions that may have been made. The publisher remains neutral with regard to jurisdictional claims in published maps and institutional affiliations.

This Springer imprint is published by the registered company Springer Nature Switzerland AG
The registered company address is: Gewerbestrasse 11, 6330 Cham, Switzerland

Preface

The *Advancing the Science of Cancer in Latinos* national conference was a call to action for addressing cancer health disparities in Hispanic/Latino communities. It emerged from the need for Latino disparities researchers to seek solutions through multidisciplinary collaborations and to keep pace with the substantial advancement in cancer prevention, screening, diagnosis, treatment, and survivorship. Held in San Antonio from February 26 to 28, 2020, the conference was co-hosted by the Mays Cancer Center and the Institute for Health Promotion Research at UT Health San Antonio and sponsored by the National Institute on Minority Health and Health Disparities. The conference offered a robust platform that fostered discussion on the latest findings in Latino cancer disparities research.

While most conferences on cancer health disparities focus solely on policy and public health issues, this conference also focused on Latino-centric perspectives from basic scientists, clinicians, population health experts, and patient advocates to emphasize the need for timely translation of research. The conference assembled an international, multidisciplinary group of speakers and attendees who explored wide-ranging issues, including Latino cancer-related health disparities, survivorship, patient advocacy, and recent developments in research approaches. A primary aim of the conference was to promote collaboration to stimulate development of new transdisciplinary research in Latino cancer health disparities. By bridging research and disciplinary silos, the conference fostered interactions and collaborations that would not have occurred otherwise, allowing discussions of broader, systemic cross-cutting issues and promoting translation from one discipline to another.

This book documents conference outcomes and highlights recommendations and priority areas for future research in Latino cancer health disparities; it is a resource for physicians, researchers, scientists, patient advocates, and students at all levels. With the ongoing rise in the US Latino population and cancer burden, we believe these pages hold many key insights into actionable targets for basic science research, suggestions for clinical best practices and community interventions, as well as other novel strategies and advocacy opportunities to reduce Latino cancer health disparities.

As you explore the papers and posters from *Advancing the Science of Cancer in Latinos,* we hope that you will gain a fresh perspective on Latino cancer health disparities and that it will inform your own thinking, research, and practice at your program, institution, business, and nonprofit. We are optimistic that discussions and interactions at our scientific conference and the information in these proceedings will be a catalyst for more conferences, collaboration, research, and success in reducing Latino cancer health disparities in these challenging times.

Amelie G. Ramirez, DrPH, MPH
San Antonio, TX, USA

Edward J. Trapido, ScD, FACE
New Orleans, LA, USA

Acknowledgments

We would like to express our extreme gratitude to the 2020 *Advancing the Science of Cancer in Latinos* conference Scientific Planning Committee: Program Co-chair Edward J. Trapido, ScD, FACE, at Louisiana State University School of Public Health and the Stanley S. Scott Cancer Center; Anna M. Nápoles, MPH, PhD, at the National Institute on Minority Health and Health Disparities; Barbara Segarra Vasquez, MT, DHSc, University of Puerto Rico; Elena V. Rios, MD, MSPH, from the National Hispanic Medical Association; Filipa C. Lynce, MD, at the Lombardi Comprehensive Cancer Center, Georgetown University Medical Center; Frank J. Penedo, PhD, at the Sylvester Comprehensive Cancer Center, University of Miami; Laura Fejerman, PhD, University of California San Francisco; Laura Magana Valladares, PhD, Association of Schools and Programs of Public Health; Laura Tenner, MD, at the Mays Cancer Center, UT Health San Antonio; Marcia R. Cruz-Correa, MD, PhD, University of Puerto Rico; Mariana C. Stern, PhD, at the Norris Comprehensive Cancer Center, University of Southern California; Martin Mendoza, PhD, at the Food & Drug Administration; Matthew P. Banegas, PhD, MPH, Kaiser Permanente; Patricia I. Moreno, PhD, Northwestern University; and Sandi Stanford from the Alamo Breast Cancer Foundation. Gratitude is also expressed to our distinguished speakers: Sandro Galea, MD, MPH, DrPH, Boston University; Douglas R. Lowy, MD, National Cancer Institute; Eliseo Pérez-Stable, MD, Director of the National Institute on Minority Health and Health Disparities; Otis Brawley, MD, John Hopkins University; Robert Croyle, PhD, National Cancer Institute; and Edith Perez, MD, Professor of Medicine at the Mayo Clinic College of Medicine.

Our sincere appreciation to Nina Caris, PhD, for her editorial contributions to this publication. Finally, we are grateful to our lead program coordinator, Harriet Van Loggerenberg, MS, for her significant efforts in organizing the *Advancing the Science of Cancer in Latinos* conference from concept to completion.

Preparation of this book was supported (in part) by the Mays Cancer Center at UT Health San Antonio, Institute for Health Promotion Research at UT Health San Antonio, and the National Institute on Minority Health and Health Disparities (R13MD012457-01). The views expressed in this publication do not necessarily reflect the official policies of the Department of Health and Human Services, nor does mention by trade names, commercial practices, or organizations imply endorsement by the US Government.

Contents

About the Editors

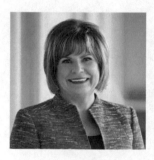

Amelie G. Ramirez, DrPH, MPH

Program Chair
Professor and Chair,
Department of Population Health Sciences
Director, Institute for Health Promotion Research
Dielmann Chair in Health Disparities Research &
Community Outreach
Max and Minnie Tomerlin Voelcker Endowed
Chair in Cancer Health Care Disparities

UT Health San Antonio
San Antonio, TX, USA

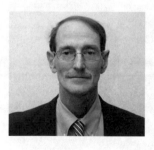

Edward J. Trapido, ScD, FACE

Program Co-Chair
Associate Dean for Research,
Professor and Wendell H. Gauthier Chair of Cancer
Epidemiology, LSU School of Public Health
Deputy Director, Stanley S. Scott Cancer Center
Professor of Medicine and Senior Liaison to the Dean
of the School of Medicine, LSU Health
Sciences Center

LSU Health Sciences Center
New Orleans, LA, USA

Contributors

Carolina Aristizabal USC Norris Comprehensive Cancer Center and Department of Preventive Medicine, Keck School of Medicine, University of Southern California, Los Angeles, CA, USA

Elva M. Arredondo Division of Health Promotion and Behavioral Science, School of Public Health, San Diego State University, San Diego, CA, USA

Lourdes Baezconde-Garbanati USC Norris Comprehensive Cancer Center and Department of Preventive Medicine, Keck School of Medicine, University of Southern California, Los Angeles, CA, USA

Sharon H. Baik Department of Medical Social Sciences, Northwestern University Feinberg School of Medicine, Chicago, IL, USA

Elisa V. Bandera Rutgers Cancer Institute of New Jersey, New Brunswick, NJ, USA

Rosa Barahona USC Norris Comprehensive Cancer Center and Department of Preventive Medicine, Keck School of Medicine, University of Southern California, Los Angeles, CA, USA

Austin L. Brown Baylor College of Medicine, Houston, TX, USA

Texas Children's Hospital, Houston, TX, USA

Diana Buitrago Department of Medical Social Sciences, Northwestern University Feinberg School of Medicine, Chicago, IL, USA

Joanna Buscemi Department of Psychology, DePaul University, Chicago, IL, USA

Institute for Health Research and Policy, University of Illinois at Chicago, Chicago, IL, USA

Mariana Chavez Mac Gregor Health Services Research Department, Breast Medical Oncology Department, The University of Texas MD Anderson Cancer Center, Houston, TX, USA

Elam Day-Friedland Albany High School, Albany, CA, USA

Randa El-Zein Houston Methodist Hospital, Houston, TX, USA

Laura Fejerman Department of Public Health Sciences, Division of Epidemiology, University of California, Davis, CA, USA

UC Davis Comprehensive Cancer Center, University of California, Davis, CA, USA

Anna R. Giuliano Center for Immunization and Infection Research in Cancer, Moffit Cancer Center, Tampa, FL, USA

Melissa Gonzales Genentech, San Francisco, CA, USA

Stefano Guerra University of Arizona, Tucson, AZ, USA

Dolores D. Guest University of New Mexico Comprehensive Cancer Center, Albuquerque, NM, USA

Department of Internal Medicine, University of New Mexico, Albuquerque, NM, USA

Judith Guitelman ALAS-WINGS, Latina Association for Breast Cancer, Chicago, IL, USA

Chi-Chen Hong Roswell Park Comprehensive Cancer Center, Buffalo, NY, USA

Darryl B. Hood Department of Environmental Health Sciences, College of Public Health, Ohio State University, Columbus, OH, USA

Francisco Iacobelli Department of Computer Science, Northeastern Illinois University, Chicago, IL, USA

Shoshana Adler Jaffe University of New Mexico Comprehensive Cancer Center, Albuquerque, NM, USA

Paul D. Juarez Department of Family and Community Medicine, Meharry Medical College, Nashville, TN, USA

Nanette V. Lopez Department of Health Sciences, Northern Arizona University, Flagstaff, AZ, USA

Philip J. Lupo Baylor College of Medicine, Houston, TX, USA

Texas Children's Hospital, Houston, TX, USA

Catalina Malinowski Health Services Research Department, The University of Texas MD Anderson Cancer Center, Houston, TX, USA

Katie M. Marker Human Medical Genetics and Genomics Program, School of Medicine, University of Colorado Anschutz Medical Campus, Aurora, CO, USA

Bibiana Martinez Division of Health Behavior, Institute for Prevention Research, Department of Preventive Medicine, Keck School of Medicine of USC, University of Southern California, Los Angeles, CA, USA

Dinorah Martinez Tyson College of Public Health, University of South Florida, Tampa, FL, USA

Jean A. McDougall University of New Mexico Comprehensive Cancer Center, Albuquerque, NM, USA

Department of Internal Medicine, University of New Mexico, Albuquerque, NM, USA

Angela L. W. Meisner University of New Mexico Comprehensive Cancer Center, Albuquerque, NM, USA

New Mexico Tumor Registry, Albuquerque, NM, USA

Sheila Murphy Annenberg School for Communication and Journalism, University of Southern California, Los Angeles, CA, USA

Gila Neta Division of Cancer Control and Population Sciences, National Cancer Institute, National Institutes of Health, Rockville, MD, USA

Carol Ochoa Division of Health Behavior, Institute for Prevention Research, Department of Preventive Medicine, Keck School of Medicine of USC, University of Southern California, Los Angeles, CA, USA

Alexander N. Ortega Department of Health Management and Policy, Center for Population Health and Community Impact, Drexel Dornsife School of Public Health, Drexel University, Philadelphia, PA, USA

Laura B. Oswald Department of Health Outcomes and Behavior, Moffitt Cancer Center, Tampa, FL, USA

V. Shane Pankratz University of New Mexico Comprehensive Cancer Center, Albuquerque, NM, USA

Department of Internal Medicine, University of New Mexico, Albuquerque, NM, USA

Frank J. Penedo Department of Psychology, University of Miami, Coral Gables, FL, USA

Bo Qin Rutgers Cancer Institute of New Jersey, New Brunswick, NJ, USA

Kimberly P. Raghubar Baylor College of Medicine, Houston, TX, USA

Texas Children's Hospital, Houston, TX, USA

Aramandla Ramesh Department of Biochemistry, Cancer Biology, Neuroscience and Pharmacology, Meharry Medical College, Nashville, TN, USA

Amelie G. Ramirez Department of Population Health Sciences, Institute for Health Promotion Research, UT Health San Antonio, San Antonio, TX, USA

Kenneth S. Ramos Texas A&M Health Science Center, Houston, TX, USA

Yaneth L. Rodriguez Division of Health Behavior, Institute for Prevention Research, Department of Preventive Medicine, Keck School of Medicine of USC, University of Southern California, Los Angeles, CA, USA

Erik L. Ruiz College of Public Health, University of South Florida, Tampa, FL, USA

Rogelio Sáenz University of Texas at San Antonio, San Antonio, TX, USA

Michael E. Scheurer Baylor College of Medicine, Houston, TX, USA

Texas Children's Hospital, Houston, TX, USA

Melissa A. Simon Department of Obstetrics and Gynecology, Northwestern University Feinberg School of Medicine, Chicago, IL, USA

Robert H. Lurie Comprehensive Cancer Center, Chicago, IL, USA

Min-ae Song Department of Environmental Health Sciences, College of Public Health, Ohio State University, Columbus, OH, USA

Sandra Soto School of Nursing, University of North Carolina at Chapel Hill, Chapel Hill, NC, USA

Andrew L. Sussman University of New Mexico Comprehensive Cancer Center, Albuquerque, NM, USA

Department of Community and Family Medicine, University of New Mexico, Albuquerque, NM, USA

Lizeth I. Tamayo Department of Public Health Sciences, The University of Chicago, Chicago, IL, USA

Marisa S. Torrez-Ruiz Division of Health Promotion and Behavioral Science, School of Public Health, San Diego State University, San Diego, CA, USA

School of Public Health, University of California, San Diego, CA, USA

Edward J. Trapido Epidemiology Program, LSU Health Sciences Center, School of Public Health, New Orleans, LA, USA

Charles L. Wiggins University of New Mexico Comprehensive Cancer Center, Albuquerque, NM, USA

Department of Internal Medicine, University of New Mexico, Albuquerque, NM, USA

New Mexico Tumor Registry, Albuquerque, NM, USA

Betina Yanez Department of Medical Social Sciences, Northwestern University Feinberg School of Medicine, Chicago, IL, USA

Robert H. Lurie Comprehensive Cancer Center, Chicago, IL, USA

Valentina A. Zavala Department of Public Health Sciences, Division of Epidemiology, University of California, Davis, CA, USA

Part I
Introduction

Chapter 1
Advancing the Science of Cancer in Latinos

Amelie G. Ramirez and Edward J. Trapido

Introduction

Cancer is the second leading cause of death among non-Hispanic white (NHW) men and women in the United States—but is the leading cause of death among Latinos [1]. The US Latino population was 60.6 million in 2019, as one of the largest, youngest, and fastest growing minority groups in the United States, its population will nearly double by 2060, making up 27.5% of the projected US population [2, 3]. Thus, advancing the science of cancer in Latinos has become an imperative for the nation, as Latinos will contribute a significant portion to its future cancer burden.

The good news is that age-adjusted cancer mortality rate in the US population has steadily declined, dropping 31% from 1991 to 2018 [4]. Later in the decade, Latino cancer mortality rate also declined and is now lower than most other groups in the United States. For example, the overall cancer mortality rate (per 100,000 population) during 2014–2018 for Hispanics was 110.8–30.8% lower than NHWs [5].

Despite this encouraging news, cancer health disparities stubbornly persist among the US Latino population. While Hispanics as a group have lower incidence rates than NHWs for most cancers including breast, colorectal, lung, and prostate, they experience higher incidences of gallbladder cancer and infection-related cancers of the stomach, liver, and uterine cervix [1]. For some cancers such as liver and stomach cancers and pediatric acute lymphoblastic leukemia, Hispanics are diagnosed with more aggressive or advanced disease and experience higher mortality

A. G. Ramirez (✉)
Department of Population Health Sciences, Institute for Health Promotion Research,
UT Health San Antonio, San Antonio, TX, USA
e-mail: ramirezag@uthscsa.edu

E. J. Trapido
Epidemiology Program, LSU Health Sciences Center, School of Public Health,
New Orleans, LA, USA

© The Author(s) 2023
A. G. Ramirez, E. J. Trapido (eds.), *Advancing the Science of Cancer in Latinos*, https://doi.org/10.1007/978-3-031-14436-3_1

rates than other groups [6]. Furthermore, compared to NHWs, Hispanics are more likely to be diagnosed with cancer at a later stage when it is more difficult to treat, and they are also more likely to experience longer delays from diagnosis to treatment leading to poorer treatment outcomes.

Why these disparities exist is the result of a complex interplay of many factors. One determinant is socioeconomic status (SES). Compared to NHWs, Hispanics are more likely to live in poverty, which also means they are less likely to have health insurance and access to health care, including cancer screening and preventive care. They are also more likely to have fewer cancer treatment options, more treatment delays, and lower treatment adherence rates [7]. Other important factors are in the cultural domain. Hispanic ethnic identity, values, and beliefs can influence healthy behavior, engagement with health providers, and how one copes with cancer diagnosis and treatment. Generational status, level of acculturation, and country of origin are also associated with varied cancer outcome. Paradoxically, low acculturation is associated with lower cancer burden despite being associated with lower income and less access to health care. As individuals become more acculturated to the United States, however, their cancer incidence rates rise and may even surpass that of NHWs [1]. Finally, differences in cancer burden and treatment outcomes may be a function of inherited genetic variation. Hispanics are not a homogeneous group, but rather comprise subgroups that differ by geographic regions of origin and varying degrees of genetic admixture from predominantly Indigenous American, African, and European ancestries.

Building Collaboration for Action

Because of the multifactorial nature of cancer disparity, finding solutions requires a collaborative and transdisciplinary approach. The second national conference—Advancing the Science of Cancer in Latinos—was designed to provide opportunities for collaboration to build implementation science to better address cancer health disparities and reduce the burden of cancer in Latino communities. Held in San Antonio on February 26–28, 2020, the conference was co-hosted by the Mays Cancer Center and the Institute for Health Promotion Research at UT Health San Antonio and was sponsored by the National Institute on Minority Health and Health Disparities. Bringing people together from across the cancer continuum, it included those with expertise in genetics, social determinants of health, early detection and screening, diagnosis, treatment, and survivorship. Furthermore, it brought the voice of the community, researchers, educators, and intervention specialists. Attending were people from academia, government, professional organizations, businesses, and non-governmental organizations. So, the breadth of expertise and experience was wide. There were opportunities for formal and informal discussions during the meeting, and the material presented reflected this diversity of backgrounds and interests. Joining people with these backgrounds was meant to serve as a stimulus for developing new joint research and interventions—particularly in implementation and dissemination science.

The following sections set some context and briefly describe the papers contributed by many of the conference presenters. Note that the terms Hispanic, Latino/a, and Latin(x) are used interchangeably and reflect the preferences of the authors or US federal designation.

Vulnerable Populations and Health Threats in the Latino Community

Vulnerable populations experience significant health disparities, suffering greater disease risk, morbidity, and mortality than the general population. The vulnerable among them includes racial/ethnic minorities, the poor, those with chronic health conditions or disabilities, the elderly and the young, those who are socially vulnerable such as members of the LGBTQ+ community, and those who are geographically isolated.

Acute Lymphoblastic Leukemia (ALL) in Latino Children Latino children are a vulnerable population who experience a higher incidence of acute lymphoblastic leukemia (ALL) and poorer treatment outcomes than non-Latino children. This cancer disparity, like many others, is cross-cutting along the cancer treatment continuum from heightened risk to less favorable treatment outcome and untoward treatment effects that last into survivorship. Brown et al. describe research that suggests Latino children with ALL may be more vulnerable to the adverse neurotoxic effects of CNS-directed therapy with methotrexate. From their own study of pediatric patients, they found a nearly 2.5-fold increased risk of neurotoxicity in Latino pediatric patients compared to non-Latino patients. In addition to these short-term adverse effects of therapy, they propose that Latino survivors may also be more vulnerable to long-term neurocognitive impairment that affects quality of life in survivorship. Why these disparities exist is unknown and may be related to inherited genetic variation and sociocultural differences such as acculturation and socioeconomic status.

Population Health Challenges and the Affordable Care Act The Patient Protection and Affordable Care Act (ACA) became the US law in 2010. Its purpose was to make health insurance more affordable and accessible by offering insurance plans through marketplaces, expanding Medicaid, and providing incentives to improve cost and quality of care. In Part II, Ortega describes how the ACA affects healthcare access and utilization among Latinos. His research confirms that, in general, Latino adults and youth overall have benefitted from the ACA; however, they still fared worse when compared to non-Latino whites. A subgroup comparison of Latino heritage groups (Puerto Rican, Mexican, Cuban, Central American, and other Latino) showed that most reductions in disparities were experienced between

Puerto Ricans and non-Latino whites; Mexicans and Central Americans experienced more pervasive inequities—especially non-citizens and those in states that have not expanded Medicaid as part of the ACA.

Financial Hardship and Food Insecurity For cancer patients and survivors, the high cost of cancer treatment and care can cause financial hardship such as inability to pay medical bills, debt, and bankruptcy. Such hardship may put cancer survivors at risk for food insecurity—the inability to access enough food for a healthy lifestyle because of insufficient money or other resources. McDougall et al. present results from a cross-sectional survey comparing financial hardship and food insecurity among population-based Hispanic and non-Hispanic cancer survivors in New Mexico. They found that Hispanic cancer survivors were more likely than non-Hispanic cancer survivors to be unable to cover the cost of medical bills and were more likely to reduce spending on food and clothing as a result of cancer treatment. The prevalence of food insecurity among Hispanic cancer survivors in the year after cancer diagnosis was about 47%—considerably higher than the 36% for the overall project and 11% for US adults. While there were no significant differences by ethnicity, new and persistent food insecurity for the project was strongly associated with forgoing, delaying, or having to make changes to cancer care. The results of the study point to the need for food-insecurity screening and interventions that specifically address financial hardship and food insecurity among cancer survivors.

Disparities Research Along the Cancer Control Continuum

Cancer Prevention and Screening

Strength-Based Approach to Cancer Prevention US Latinos overall have a lower cancer burden than other groups; however, as Latinos become acculturated to US culture, their risk for cancer rises [1]. Torrez-Ruiz et al. point out that less acculturated Latinos still retain the cultural and behavioral patterns of their home country, which influences the quality of diet and the level of physical activity—two lifestyle factors that contribute to cancer risk. They consume more nutrient dense foods such as fruits, vegetables, and whole grains and are more physically active than their more acculturated US counterparts. As Latinos become more exposed to US culture, they often become less active and adopt a less healthy diet. To lessen these effects of acculturation, the authors advocate using a strength-based approach that focuses on the positive aspects of Latino culture to inform intervention research. Specifically, they propose developing culturally appropriate interventions that leverage values such as collectivism, *personalismo*, and *familismo*—Latino cultural elements that can promote healthy protective behaviors and lower cancer risk.

Cervical Cancer Elimination Some viral and bacterial infections are linked to cancer; the four most common cancer-related infectious agents are human papilloma virus (HPV), hepatitis B virus (HBV), hepatitis C virus (HCV), and *Helicobacter pylori*. Fortunately, many of these infections can now be treated or prevented, making them potentially modifiable risk factors [8]. In her paper, Giuliano describes the goal and strategy for preventing HPV-related cancers (cervical, vulvar, vaginal, anal, oropharyngeal, and penile), the majority of which are preventable with the use of three readily available tools—HPV vaccine (e.g., Gardasil and Gardasil 9), cervical cancer screening, and treatment for pre-cancerous lesions. Despite the fact that these tools exist, the cervical cancer incidence in the US Hispanic population is higher than in other groups; Hispanic women are about 40% more likely than non-Hispanic white women to be diagnosed with cervical cancer [9]. Furthermore, among non-Hispanic white women, the incidence of cervical cancer declines after age 40, but among Hispanic women, the incidence of cervical cancer continues to increase with age. These disparities in incidence likely result from women either skipping screening or not receiving treatment. Compared to other groups in the United States, vaccine uptake is as high or higher in the adolescent Hispanic population, but to eliminate cervical cancer, we must promote all three prevention tools—vaccination, screening, and follow-up treatment for abnormal dysplasia.

Cancer Treatment

Treatment Delays among Latino Breast Cancer Patients Breast cancer incidence among Hispanic women is lower than that of non-Hispanic white women, yet Hispanic women are more likely to be diagnosed with more aggressive disease and to experience delays in treatment, contributing to worse outcomes. Malinowski and Chavez Mac Gregor describe some of the unique challenges in cancer care delivery that Hispanic breast cancer patients face including the detrimental effects of treatment delays. To determine whether biological factors alone can explain disparities in outcome, the authors evaluated breast cancer patients treated with similar neoadjuvant preoperative chemotherapy and found that race or ethnicity was not associated with the rates of pathological complete response. In another study, they analyzed patients taking part in phase II/III clinical trials and found that when Hispanic breast cancer patients received uniform treatment and follow-up in a highly controlled setting, their survival outcomes were similar to that of non-Hispanic women. The authors hypothesized that differences in outcomes between Hispanics and non-Hispanics may be less a function of biology and more the result of differences in social determinants of health such as lower economic stability, language differences, lower health literacy, lack of health insurance, and poorer access to regular medical services.

Compared to non-Hispanic white women, Hispanic women experience disparities along the entire cancer continuum, contributing to adverse breast cancer outcomes. These disparities run the gamut from lower mammography screening
prevalence and diagnostic delays to longer times from diagnosis to surgery and
delays in chemotherapy, radiation therapy, and endocrine therapy. To address this
issue, the authors are beginning a new qualitative study to identify why breast cancer patients experience delays in the start of chemotherapy. Using validated instruments, they will examine factors at the operational, medical, and personal/social
level including social support, health literacy, and trust in health providers.

Genetic Ancestry and Precision Medicine Approaches

Genetic Ancestry and Breast Cancer Subtypes Breast cancer is the most common cancer among Hispanic women. However, as a group, Hispanic women have a
lower incidence of this cancer than non-Hispanic white or black women. There are
intrinsic biological subtypes of breast cancer, each associated with different progno-
ses. In clinical practice, these subtypes are inferred by immunohistochemical markers for the estrogen receptor (ER), progesterone receptor (PR), and human epidermal
growth factor receptor 2 (HER2). Compared to the other subtypes, ER−/PR−
tumors [10] have fewer treatment options and poorer prognosis. Tamayo et al.
describe results of studies examining correlations between genetic ancestry and
breast cancer subtypes among US Hispanic or Latin American patients. According
to the authors, studies show that Hispanic women have a 20–40% higher risk than
non-Hispanic white women of developing ER−/PR− HER2+ and ER−/PR−
HER2− breast cancer. There is also an emerging body of research that suggests
there is an association between genetic ancestry of Hispanic women and breast cancer subtype. For example, evidence points to an association between the degree of
Indigenous American ancestry and HER2+ tumors and an association between
degree of African ancestry and ER− tumors. The authors conclude that more studies
are needed to improve understanding of tumor subtype etiology of breast cancer in
admixed minority populations.

Precision Medicine Approaches for Patients at Risk of Lung Cancer African
ancestry is associated with worse clinical outcomes for chronic obstructive pulmonary disease (COPD) and lung cancer, and the degree of African ancestry varies
among some Latinx subgroups. Thus, there is a need to develop risk stratification
strategies and targeted lung cancer therapies that consider genetic admixture among
Latinx populations. Lung cancers in all racial and ethnic groups are often diagnosed
too late for a surgical cure, so there is also a need for early biomarkers of disease.

Ramos et al. propose that the current precision medicine approaches for treating
lung cancer should be refined by improving risk stratification for patients with
COPD, who are at heightened risk for lung cancer. In their paper, Ramos and his

colleagues review their research on ORF1p—a protein encoded by the retroelement, Long Interspersed Element-1 (LINE-1). Overexpression of ORF1p is associated with genetic instability and poor prognosis in patients with non-small-cell lung cancer (NSCLC). Because it accumulates in lung cancer cells and is found in circulating exosomes, the authors hypothesized that circulating ORF1p may be used as a sensitive biomarker of genetic instability in patients with COPD and lung cancer. Further, the authors found that the cellular protein, nucleolin (NCL), regulates ORF1p expression and that using NCL antagonists can stop NSCLC growth in a mouse model of lung cancer.

Outcomes and Survivorship

Obesity and Breast Cancer Survivorship The number of Hispanic breast cancer survivors in the United States is increasing as the Hispanic population grows and breast cancer survival improves. Further, this growing population is more likely than non-Hispanic whites to experience increased obesity and related comorbidities into survivorship. To address these issues, Bandera, Hong, and Qin compared Hispanic and Black breast cancer survivors in a pilot study and found that the cohort of Hispanic breast cancer survivors had lower patient-reported health-related quality of life (QoL) scores, particularly those who were obese. Among breast cancer survivors, the association between obesity and patient-reported outcomes is poorly understood and not well studied among Hispanic women, emphasizing the need for more research on cancer survivorship in this vulnerable population.

Latino Men Cancer Survivors Compared to Hispanic women and other racial/ethnic groups, Hispanic men overall experience higher incidence of most cancers and higher cancer-related mortality. The number of Hispanic men cancer survivors (HMCS) continues to grow and their unique supportive care needs have not been adequately addressed. Based on evidence from recent preliminary research, Martinez Tyson and Ruiz describe unmet supportive care needs of Hispanic men cancer survivors. HMCS participants reported the need to overcome language barriers so that they not only can understand treatment information but also can ask clarifying questions; they prefer bilingual conversation and do not trust that interpreters accurately convey their concerns. These men want culturally competent care that includes, for example, the constructs of *confianza* and *personalismo* so that they can build better rapport with providers and speak more openly about their concerns. Many participants felt the need for more information about their treatment and its effects, a better understanding of post-treatment follow-up including screenings, and a more holistic approach that focuses on overall health and wellbeing. Along with the demands of cancer therapy or employment changes, many were troubled by changing gender role expectations within the family brought about by the financial and emotional burden placed on female family members. Furthermore, the authors found many HMCS want to connect with other survivors and discuss their shared experiences. How do HMCS cope with their cancer diagnosis? Many survivors believe that overall attitude is important in overcoming the disease process; they advocate maintaining a positive outlook through optimism, humor, and faith in God. For some, incorporating home remedies into the overall treatment plan and making lifestyle changes gave them a sense of agency and self-efficacy. They also reported their social support systems helped them feel less isolated and more able to contend with the logistics of attending appointments and going to treatments.

E-health Interventions in Cancer Control and Survivorship Now that cell phone use is becoming commonplace among US Hispanics, smartphone applications can be used to deliver scalable, evidence-based supportive care interventions, reaching out to those who may have logistical barriers to in-person cancer care. Hispanic breast cancer survivors (BCS) experience worse health-related quality of life (HRQOL) and symptom burden than non-Hispanic BCS. To reduce these disparities in psychosocial outcomes, Baik et al. used community-engaged research approaches to develop and evaluate two culturally informed, bilingual smartphone applications—*My Guide* (intervention) and *My Health* (control)—tailored to address the unique needs of Hispanic women. Even though the results were similar between the intervention and control groups, the researchers were able to demonstrate the feasibility and efficacy of these applications in improving cancer symptom burden and HRQOL. Participants of both groups said they would have liked to have also used these applications during breast cancer treatment, so the researchers expanded the scope of *My Guide* to address the needs of Hispanic women in active breast cancer treatment. *My Guide* and the newer *My Guide for Breast Cancer Treatment* are among the first bilingual, supportive-care smartphone applications, which have the potential to improve patient-reported outcomes among Hispanic women during both active cancer treatment and into survivorship.

Cross-cutting Research and the Future of Cancer Care

Optimizing Engagement of the Latino Community in Cancer Research Baezconde-Garbanati et al. describe signature initiatives designed to engage Latino communities in cancer research by reducing barriers toward inclusion. Two of their population-based studies in Los Angeles—*Es Tiempo* and *Tamale Lesson*—were designed using a community-based participatory research approach to optimize participation and retention of Latinos in cervical cancer and HPV trials. These model interventions included *promotores de salud* and community members who took part in all stages of research, from conceptualization, recruitment, translation, cultural adaptation, and information dissemination. The intent was to make the members of the participating communities feel they were an essential part of the research. A promising third exploratory study used virtual reality to better understand vaccine hesitancy and explore end-of-life improvements for immigrant Latinos. To influence attitudes and behaviors that place Latinos at risk for cancer, the researchers used bidirectional communication; educational information was broadcast out to the community while knowledge was received by academic researchers who learned about community issues and barriers to participation. Their strategies for increasing Latino participation in cancer research focused on three key areas: (1) information delivery or knowledge transfer; (2) consultation with Latino community stakeholders and partners, including community advisory boards, patient advocates, and citizen scientists; and (3) collaboration with community opinion leaders.

Advancing Inclusive Research Melissa Gonzales from Genentech describes how one biotechnology company is addressing clinical research disparities to achieve personalized healthcare for everyone, including the most vulnerable Hispanic communities. Their initiative—*Advancing Inclusive Research*—aims to expand inclusion of diverse patient populations into their clinical research. To accomplish this, they intend to imbed inclusive research principles so that clinical trial enrollment reflects real-world populations; expand site networks to include more diverse catchment areas; and identify and remove barriers to participation in clinical trials such as providing transportation and child care. Further, they will increase genomic data and scientific insights from underrepresented populations and will leverage relationships with external partners to develop strategies for increasing participation of underrepresented groups in clinical trials.

Exposome-wide Association Study Approach Because Latino cancer disparities are so persistent and their underlying causes so varied, Juarez et al. propose that we need a new way of conducting disparities research that accounts for environmental, endogenous, and social factors. They suggest using a research strategy based on the exposome—all of the external and internal exposures experienced by individuals across their lifespans from conception to death and how these exposures affect health. Applying an ExWAS approach can help identify how environmental exposures alter key biological pathways at the cellular, molecular, and system level, and help explain the increased risk for population-level cancer disparities among Latinos. Measured exposures can be linked to biochemical and molecular changes through the use of prognostic and diagnostic biomarkers based on "omics" technologies such as genomics, epigenomics, transcriptomics, metabolomics, proteomics, and lipidomics.

Implementation Science There is often an unacceptable lag time of years and even decades before new research evidence becomes part of broadly adopted medical practice, and many new, effective, health interventions are not reaching Latino populations to the same degree as the general public. Gila Neta from the National Cancer Institute (NCI) points out that to ensure new cancer discoveries reduce the cancer burden for Latinos, researchers must focus not only on what evidence-based interventions can improve outcomes but also on how those interventions can be adopted, implemented, and sustained. To bridge the gap between research and practice, NCI supports research in implementation science—the study of strategies to adopt and integrate evidence-based health interventions into clinical and community settings, improving individual outcomes and benefitting population health [11]. This science also includes studying strategies to de-implement practices that are ineffective, unproven, low value, or harmful. In her paper, the author describes the discipline and goals of implementation science and the role of the National Institutes of Health (NIH) in providing trans-NIH funding opportunities in this field. Neta further emphasizes that implementation science must consider the multilevel context and engage stakeholders in two-way communication so that strategies not only address critical barriers but are also workable and appropriate for the relevant settings and populations, and are likely to be integrated, sustained, and scaled.

The Changing Demography of Cancer   Even though Latinos have a lower cancer burden than other groups in the United States, their disproportionate growth will likely shift the demography of cancer in the future [12]. Sáenz examined this trend by analyzing recent cancer statistics from the CDC and population projections from the US Census Bureau. The analysis was based on two time periods—past (1999–2016) and future (2016–2060).

Sáenz found that compared to non-Latino whites and blacks during 1999–2016, US Latinos had the lowest age-adjusted cancer incidence and death rates, and they made up only a fraction of the nation's cancer cases (8.2%) and deaths (6.6%) in 2016. However, because of their growing population, Latinos contributed to nearly one-fifth (18.8%) of the increase in US cancer cases and two-fifths (39.5%) of the increase in cancer deaths between 1999 and 2016. Because the population growth of Latinos is expected to outpace that of non-Latinos, the percentage of Latino cancer cases and deaths will likely double from 2016 to 2060. Latinos will account for one-third of the US projected increase in cancer cases and one-fourth of the projected increase in cancer deaths during this time frame. By 2060, Latinos will still be a younger group, so they will make up a larger share (25%) of cancer cases and deaths among those less than 45 years.

The author points out that the growing presence of Latinos in the future has implications for public policy. For example, current inequities in access to affordable health care and lack of health insurance will increase the risk of Latinos having cancer and dying from the disease. In addition, public policy that discourages migration from Mexico to the United States could erode the Latino morbidity and mortality advantages they currently possess.

Conclusion

The Advancing the Science of Cancer in Latinos conference brought together a diverse group of health professionals to encourage collaboration and a free exchange of ideas from different perspectives; the papers in the following chapters show the breadth of their research across the cancer care continuum. Exploring this book, you will learn about vulnerable Latino populations, Latino lifestyles, and health threats in the Latino community; cancer prevention, cancer outcomes, and survivorship among Latinos; genetic ancestry and precision medicine; advances in cancer therapy, clinical trials, and engaging Latinos in cancer research; and implementation science and innovative technologies. The papers and posters presented here are part of an ongoing dialogue, providing new insights and solutions to the problem of cancer disparities among Latinos.

References

1. American Cancer Society. Cancer facts and figures for Hispanics/Latinos 2018–2020. Atlanta: American Cancer Society, Inc.; 2018.
2. Vespa J, Medina L, Armstrong DM. Demographic turning points for the United States: population projections for 2020 to 2060. Washington, DC: U.S. Census Bureau; 2020. Report No.: P25-1144. https://www.census.gov/library/publications/2020/demo/p25-1144.html. Accessed 25 Aug 2021.
3. Noe-Bustamante L, Lopez MH, Krogstad JM. U.S. Hispanic population surpassed 60 million in 2019, but growth has slowed. Pew Research Center; 2020. https://www.pewresearch.org/fact-tank/2020/07/07/u-s-hispanic-population-surpassed-60-million-in-2019-but-growth-has-slowed/. Accessed 28 Aug 2021.
4. Siegel RL, Miller KD, Fuchs HE, Jemal A. Cancer statistics, 2021. CA Cancer J Clin. 2021;71(1):7–33. https://doi.org/10.3322/caac.21654.
5. Islami F, Ward EM, Sung H, Cronin KA, Tangka FKL, Sherman RL, et al. Annual report to the nation on the status of cancer, part 1: national cancer statistics. J Natl Cancer Inst. 2021. https://doi.org/10.1093/jnci/djab131.
6. Pinheiro PS, Callahan KE, Siegel RL, Jin H, Morris CR, Trapido EJ, et al. Cancer mortality in Hispanic ethnic groups. Cancer Epidemiol Biomark Prev. 2017;26(3):376–82. https://doi.org/10.1158/1055-9965.EPI-16-0684.
7. Yanez B, McGinty HL, Buitrago D, Ramirez AG, Penedo FJ. Cancer outcomes in Hispanics/Latinos in the United States: an integrative review and conceptual model of determinants of health. J Lat Psychol. 2016;4(2):114–29. https://doi.org/10.1037/lat0000055.
8. de Martel C, Georges D, Bray F, Ferlay J, Clifford GM. Global burden of cancer attributable to infections in 2018: a worldwide incidence analysis. Lancet Glob Health. 2020;8(2):e180–e90. https://doi.org/10.1016/s2214-109x(19)30488-7.
9. Henley SJ, Ward EM, Scott S, Ma J, Anderson RN, Firth AU, et al. Annual report to the nation on the status of cancer, part I: national cancer statistics. Cancer. 2020;126(10):2225–49. https://doi.org/10.1002/cncr.32802.
10. Goldhirsch A, Wood WC, Coates AS, Gelber RD, Thürlimann B, Senn HJ. Strategies for subtypes--dealing with the diversity of breast cancer: highlights of the St. Gallen International Expert Consensus on the Primary Therapy of Early Breast Cancer 2011. Ann Oncol. 2011;22(8):1736–47. https://doi.org/10.1093/annonc/mdr304.
11. NIH. Dissemination and implementation research in health program announcement. 2019. https://grants.nih.gov/grants/guide/pa-files/PAR-19-274.html. Accessed 11 Aug 2020.
12. Miller K, Goding Sauer A, Ortiz A, Fedewa S, Pinheiro P, Tortolero-Luna G, et al. Cancer statistics for Hispanics/Latinos, 2018. CA Cancer J Clin. 2018;68(9):425–45. https://doi.org/10.3322/caac.21494.

Open Access   This chapter is licensed under the terms of the Creative Commons Attribution 4.0 International License (http://creativecommons.org/licenses/by/4.0/), which permits use, sharing, adaptation, distribution and reproduction in any medium or format, as long as you give appropriate credit to the original author(s) and the source, provide a link to the Creative Commons license and indicate if changes were made.

The images or other third party material in this chapter are included in the chapter's Creative Commons license, unless indicated otherwise in a credit line to the material. If material is not included in the chapter's Creative Commons license and your intended use is not permitted by statutory regulation or exceeds the permitted use, you will need to obtain permission directly from the copyright holder.

Part II
Health Threats in the Latino Community

Chapter 2
Applying an Exposome-wide Association Study (ExWAS) Approach to Latino Cancer Disparities

Paul D. Juarez, Darryl B. Hood, Min-ae Song, and Aramandla Ramesh

Introduction

Exposome

The exposome was introduced into the literature by Dr. Christopher Wild in 2005 [1] as all exposures a person has in one's lifetime and the biological mechanisms and processes through which those exposures affect health. Introduction of the exposome paradigm has challenged us to reconsider how we consider the causes of cancer and other chronic diseases; research methods and analytics we use to understand them; and the implications for clinical practice, health disparities, and public health policy. Key elements of the exposome include a real-world approach, inclusion of multiple environmental exposures and internal and external environments, and the ability to assess the effects of exposures at key developmental periods across the life course and trans-generationally. The main aim of exposomics is to provide an early warning system for understanding disease pathways, which will allow early targeting of prevention and early intervention strategies.

P. D. Juarez (✉)
Department of Family and Community Medicine, Meharry Medical College,
Nashville, TN, USA
e-mail: pjuarez@mmc.edu

D. B. Hood · M.-a. Song
Department of Environmental Health Sciences, College of Public Health, Ohio State
University, Columbus, OH, USA
e-mail: dhood@cph.osu.edu; song.991@osu.edu

A. Ramesh
Department of Biochemistry, Cancer Biology, Neuroscience and Pharmacology, Meharry
Medical College, Nashville, TN, USA
e-mail: aramesh@mmc.edu

© The Author(s) 2023
A. G. Ramirez, E. J. Trapido (eds.), *Advancing the Science of Cancer in Latinos*, https://doi.org/10.1007/978-3-031-14436-3_2

The exposome consists of one's internal and external environments. The external or eco-exposome has been operationalized by Juarez [2] as four broad domains: the natural, built, social, and policy environments. He later added health and healthcare as a fifth domain. Each domain consists of subdomains: natural (air, water, land), built (places you live, work, and play), social (demographic, social, economic, and political factors), and policy (federal, state, and local government policies and regulations). Each subdomain is further broken down into categories, subcategories, and variables. Juarez and colleagues have developed a national, public health exposome, relational-data repository with metadata, comprising over 55,000 variables covering the period 2003–2018 [3].

The internal or endo-exposome, on the other hand, has been described as the body's endogenous metabolic response to environmental influences, which modulate vulnerability to subsequent exposures [4]. Understanding the biological effects and responses to environmental exposures can shed light onto the mechanistic connections between exposures and health [5]. An exposome approach provides a dynamic risk profile of multiple risk and protective factors and thus is particularly applicable to chronic disease onset, progression, and outcomes.

Applying an exposome-wide association study (ExWAS) approach to cancer and cancer disparities provides a novel way for conceptualizing the relationships of multiple chemical and non-chemical exposures in the etiology and progression of cancer at key developmental periods, over the life course, and across generations. Understanding the biological effects of exposures provides new opportunities for measuring why populations with similar exposure profiles experience similar poor health outcomes [6].

Public Health Exposome

Juarez [2] created an ontology, called the public health exposome (PHE), to represent the vast array of external environmental exposures. In addition, he has curated a database, that to date, includes over 55,000 variables. The PHE data repository contains both annual and county measures of health and environmental exposures from the natural, built, social, and policy environments for 3141 counties and county equivalents over 15 years (2003–2018) (Fig. 2.1). The PHE is fully curated with metadata and a searchable data dictionary. Metadata include names and definitions of variables; units of measurement; date, time, and location of data collection; the identity of the individual who collected the data; and sampling design. The PHE data repository has been geocoded and harmonized at an annual and county level and provides spatial–temporal and contextual environmental data for understanding place-based health disparities. The data repository includes crosswalks that allow for the aggregation of data obtained in smaller geographic and temporal units upward to the county or annual levels. Other spatial resolutions included in the data repository are point, polygon, block groups, census tracts, zip codes, 3 km grids,

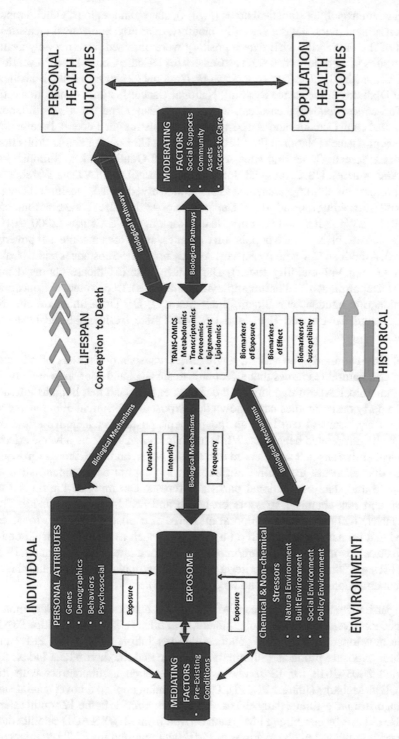

Fig. 2.1 ExWAS approach to Latino cancer disparities

1 km grids, metropolitan statistical areas (MSAs), states, and regions. Other temporal units included in the dataset are daily, monthly, quarterly, and annual measures.

Most of the data in the PHE data repository were obtained from publicly available web sites at no or low cost, such as Centers for Disease Control and Prevention (WONDER, BRFSS, CDC Tracking Network, National Center for Health Statistics, National Diabetes Surveillance System), National Cancer Institute (small area estimates for cancer-related measures), North American Land Data Assimilation System, National Oceanic and Atmospheric Administration, Federal Emergency Management Agency (National Flood Hazard Layer), US Environmental Protection Agency (EJ Screen, Superfund sites, Environmental Quality Index, National Air Toxics Assessment), US Geological Survey (water usage), HRSA Data Warehouse (health professions shortage areas, medically underserved areas), Health Indicators Warehouse (morbidity, mortality), US Department of Agriculture (Food Environment Atlas), Robert Wood Johnson (County Health Rankings), US Census (2000, 2010, decennial census, bridged race population estimates, small area income and poverty estimates), American Community Survey, Agency for Toxic Substances and Disease Registry (Social Vulnerability Index), Dartmouth Atlas (Medicare claims data), AIDSVU, Department of Labor (unemployment statistics), Department of Education (graduation rate, student enrollment, adult literacy), US Department of Interior (National Land Cover/Land Use), and US Post Office (residential and business vacancies).

Natural Environment The natural environment consists of datasets of climate, weather, and natural resources that affect human survival and economic activity. It includes chemical exposures found in the air, water, and land that humans interact with on a daily basis. Studies have shown that exposure to different components of the natural environment can have an independent, positive or negative effect on health and health-related behaviors. While much is known about the adverse effects of chemical emissions that are released into the air, water, and land, there is growing evidence that exposure to positive attributes of the natural environment, such as green space and state and national parks and forests, can mitigate the impact of chemical and non-chemical stressors on health and health-related behavior. The PHE database includes spatial–temporal measures of exposure from the air, water, and land that humans interact with on a daily basis such as meteorological conditions (particulate matter, minimum/maximum temperature, and maximum Heat Index); EPA Air Quality System (criteria pollutants, particulates, toxins); and chemicals from emissions, pesticides, and land cover/land use.

Fine particulate matter measures ($PM^{2.5}$) and heat metrics data were determined using models developed by Dr. Mohammad Al-Hamdan (USRA) for an EPA STAR grant; he developed algorithms to generate high resolution, daily, 3-km, $PM^{2.5}$ and 1-km, heat exposure products (minimum/maximum and maximum heat index) for the period 2003–2018 for 12 southern states. Through a subcontract with the HDRCOE at Meharry (Juarez, PD, PI), Dr. Al-Hamdan applied a novel spatial surfacing algorithm to estimate daily, 3-km, $PM^{2.5}$ surfaces/grids in the 12 southeastern states. He did this by combining $PM^{2.5}$ data derived from MODIS AOD satellite data (12 km grid) with ground observations of $PM^{2.5}$ data reported from EPA ambient air quality monitoring stations of the EPA Air Quality System (AQS). To generate high resolution daily exposure measures, Al-Hamdan first validated AOD-PM$^{2.5}$ regression models for 36 cities across the 12 southeastern states of the SCCS. These combined regional regression models then were integrated into a modified version of a spatial surfacing algorithm that merges the MODIS-derived and EPA/AQS PM$^{2.5}$ data to create daily, 3-km, PM$^{2.5}$ spatial surfaces/grids for the 12 southeastern states, geographic region of the SCCS. These data are available to center investigators [7].

Built Environment The built environment includes the physical characteristics of places we live, work, and play (e.g., homes, buildings, streets, open spaces, and infrastructure) as well as patterns and types of development, building location and design, and transportation infrastructure in communities that can have a direct or indirect impact on health. The degree to which the built environment is important to health may differ, depending on the broader social context. For instance, the location of supermarkets, fast-food restaurants, farmers' markets, liquor stores, pharmacies, and health-care facilities can have a significant effect on people's diets and their health. Likewise, inaccessible or nonexistent sidewalks and bicycle or walking paths may contribute to sedentary habits and a person's level of physical activity and can contribute to poor health outcomes such as obesity, cardiovascular disease, stroke, and diabetes. Measures of the built environment included in the public health exposome database include land use, TRI facilities, highways, neighborhood resources, health-care facilities, green space, parks, and occupational codes.

Social Environment The social environment (i.e., social determinants of health) constitutes the conditions in which people are born, grow, work, live, and age and are shaped by social/cultural norms, economic and employment policies and systems, the distribution of money, power, and resources, and political systems. Social determinants constitute the conditions of daily life and include factors like socioeconomic status, poverty, education, employment, crime, residential segregation, and social support networks, and provision of and access to culturally and linguistically appropriate health-care services. Social environmental stressors in the public health exposome database include population level measures of social, demographic, economic, and political variables derived principally from the US Census/American Community Survey, as well as measures of crime and social stress, such as GINI (measure of economic inequality), residential segregation, and multidimensional measures of social deprivation.

Applying an Exposome-wide Association Study (ExWAS) Approach to Latino Cancer Disparities

There is no single cause of Latino cancer disparities. First, cancer is not a single disease. Rather, cancer can start anywhere in the body; where it starts is how it is named (lung, breast, colorectal, etc.). The causes of cancer arise from genetic mutations, often caused by the body's response to chemical and non-chemical exposures in one's environment. Cancers are alike in some ways, but they are different in the ways they grow and spread. An ExWAS approach to Latino cancer disparities provides a framework for understanding how multiple environmental exposures lead to biological changes that produce certain health outcomes and lead to population-level disparities (Fig. 2.1).

Population-level cancer disparities may arise from common exposures experienced by subpopulations across a state or region or from place-based environmental exposures experienced by people who live in a neighborhood. While much attention has been given to the role of social determinants in Latino cancer disparities, to date, much remains unknown about how social determinants get under the skin to actually cause cancer and lead to disparate outcomes. The exposome provides a model for understanding the biological mechanisms and pathways through which non-chemical stressors, such as social factors, can lead to cancer.

Cancers in Latinos and Health Disparities

Cancer statistics compiled by the American Cancer Society [8] for the years 2018–2020 indicate that among Latinos, lung, liver, and colorectal cancer were expected to account for 16, 12, and 11%, respectively, of the deaths in men; while breast, lung, and colorectal were expected to contribute to 16, 13, and 9%, respectively, of the deaths in women. In regard to the emergence of new cases, prostate, colon, and lung cancers were expected to constitute 21, 12, and 8%, respectively, in men; while breast, thyroid, and uterine cancers amount to 29, 8, and 8%, respectively, in women. From a health disparities standpoint, the following are the predominant cancers in Latinos.

Lung Cancer

Even though lung cancer is one of the leading causes of deaths in Latinos, mortality due to this disease is low compared to other racial groups [9]. A study conducted in South Florida revealed that men of Cuban decent have higher mortality rates than their counterparts from Puerto Rico and South America [10]. It has been reported that 48% of Latino patients with metastatic lung adenocarcinomas have epidermal growth factor receptor (EGFR) gene mutations [11].

Breast Cancer

A greater incidence of breast cancer was noticed among Latinas living in the Southwestern United States and South Florida [12]. However, in a cohort of breast cancer patients from Puerto Rico, the prominent subtypes were found to be Luminal

A (69%), followed by triple negative (15%), Luminal B (10%), and human epidermal growth factor receptor 2 positive (HER2+; 6%). The clinicopathological characterization of breast cancer in this cohort was incomplete because of study limitations (late-stage diagnosis, missing mammography records) and lack of insurance coverage, which presents a health disparity [13].

Liver Cancer (Hepatocellular Carcinoma; HCC)

Chronic liver disease, including cancer, ranked fourth in terms of deaths for Latino men between ages 55 and 64, and Latinos are 1.6 times more likely to die from liver disease compared to the US general population [14]. Consumption of contaminated diet and viral infections were the reported contributors to liver cancer in Latinos. A study conducted by Ramirez et al. [15] found that Latinos in Texas who had liver cancer had greater levels of aflatoxins (carcinogenic chemicals found in contaminated corn, nuts, seeds, and rice) than those without the disease. The Ramirez team also reported that Latinos in Texas had the highest incidence of liver cancer in the United States [16].

Hepatitis C virus (HCV) infection is another risk factor for liver cancer. HCV infection was found to be significantly higher in Latinos from South Texas compared to controls [16]. Aflatoxin exposures and Hepatitis B infections were reported to show an additive effect toward development of HCC [17]. A systematic review of HCC among Latinos in South Texas revealed that metabolic syndrome (diabetes and obesity), viral hepatitis (B and C), genetic predisposition, environmental exposures, diet (consumption of aflatoxin-contaminated diet), and lifestyle (smoking) were the most likely risk factors [18].

Colorectal Cancer (CRC)

CRC was the second most diagnosed cancer accounting for 13% of cancer deaths (in each sex) in Puerto Rico, and lack of knowledge about this disease was responsible for a low screening rate [19]. The incidence of CRC was reported to be high in Latinos living near the United States–Mexico border [20] and also in New Mexico [21]. Latinos were reported to develop distal colon tumors more frequently compared to the general population [22] and when detected they were at a late-stage CRC compared to their non-Latino counterparts [21]. The development of CRC has been attributed to environmental exposures, smoking, diet, and obesity [20].

Prostate Cancer

Even though prostate cancer incidence among Latino men is lower than other racial groups, it still ranks fourth in terms of mortalities [23], and first among the new cancer cases to be detected [8]. Prostate cancer shows heterogeneity among Latinos. A 20-year Surveillance Epidemiology and End Results Program (SEER) data analysis revealed that prostate cancer characteristics in Latinos living in the United States were specific to their country of origin. Mexicans, Cubans, and Puerto Ricans registered higher prostate-specific antigen scores and advanced stage cancer compared to Dominicans and South-Central Americans [24].

Thyroid Cancer

The SEER data revealed that the age-adjusted incidence of papillary thyroid carcinoma was high in Puerto Rican women compared to the mainland Latinos, non-Latino Whites and Blacks [25]. Thyroid cancer in Puerto Rican men showed a similar trend, with a lower incidence than women. The follicular histology, occurrence of large tumors, localization of disease, and single nucleotide polymorphisms are some characteristics of Latino thyroid cancer patients [26].

Uterine and Cervical Cancer

The SEER database review revealed that both endometrioid and non-endometrioid carcinoma rates are on the rise among Latinos [27]. Latinos had more advanced cervical cancer disease and higher mortalities compared to Caucasians, African Americans, Asians, and other racial groups [28, 29]. The incidence of HPV-related cancers was also high in Latinos, and the risk was higher among HIV-infected Latinos than in the general population [30].

Biomarkers of Cancer

Biomarkers from the Perspective of Exposure Biology

As mentioned, environmental and life-style factors play a major role in assessing the etiology of cancer. In this regard, biomarkers play a dominant role in delineating the exposome as they are measures of either healthy or carcinogenic processes. The three major categories of biomarkers that assist in cancer risk assessment are as follows.

Biomarkers of Susceptibility These are markers of increased vulnerability to the effects of suspected environmental carcinogens, which can be measured in a tumor sample or organ system. As most cancers arise from gene–environment interactions (individuals' genetic susceptibilities against their chemical exposure histories), these markers are used to identify individuals/populations that are at risk from carcinogenic exposures. The biomarkers that come under this category are variants in genes that encode biotransformation enzymes such as cytochrome P450 (CYP) isozymes CYP1A1, CYP2C9, CYP2E1; N-acetyltransferase 2 (NAT2); serum paraoxonase and arylesterase 1 (PON1); epoxide hydrolase 1 (EPHX1); aryl hydrocarbon receptor (AhR); glutathione S-transferase theta 1 (GSTT1) null phenotype; DNA repair and oxidative damage repair genes (risks for leukemia and non-Hodgkins Lymphoma) [31].

Biomarkers of Exposure These markers highlight the significance of various exposure pathways and cancer risk; they allow measurement of carcinogens of interest in the body from an accessible biological matrix such as blood, urine, normal, and tumor tissues. For individuals who are either occupationally or dietarily exposed to polycyclic aromatic hydrocarbons (PAHs) (risks for lung cancer [32]) or aflatoxin B (risks for liver cancer [15]) either individually or in mixtures, metabolites of these chemicals in serum or urine serve as markers of exposure.

Biomarkers of Effect These markers are responses elicited as a result of interaction of an organism with the exposome mentioned in the earlier sections. The responses are measured at the level of tissue, organ, and whole organism etiology. The widely measured biomarkers of cancer are F2 isoprostanes (risks for prostate cancer [33], C-reactive protein (CRP), interleukin (IL) 6 (risks for lung cancer [34]), expression of p53, estrogen receptor α and β, progesterone receptor, cytokeratin 5 and 6, cell proliferation marker Ki-67, cancer antigen 125 marker (risks for breast and ovarian cancers [13]), and micro RNAs (risks for CRC [35]).

Biomarkers from the Perspective of Systems Biology

Most of the cellular macromolecules such as proteins, DNA, RNA, and lipids are regulated in cancer through various pathways. Their altered profiles in blood and tissues provide clues on their role in tumor formation, progression, and metastasis. Some omics data are potential biomarkers of aggressiveness of dysplastic cells and underlying pathways (diagnostic markers), while in some instances the altered pathways may serve as markers of intermediate steps or likelihood of more changes downstream (prognostic markers). Gaining awareness of the dynamics of various systems in the body and how vulnerabilities in one system and the associated symptoms (tumor growth) could impact other systems brought into light the importance of the systems biology concept in cancer research [36]. The systems biology approach could be capitalized by employing "omics" approaches. These approaches will unravel new biomarkers, which when standardized and validated could provide information on mechanism of action for carcinogens and the key biochemical and molecular pathways involved. Mentioned below are some examples of different omics approaches used by researchers to study the cancer disparities in Latinos. Most of the studies reported herein are one-step omics studies (discovery only). Very few studies have conducted two-step studies (discovery and validation). In addition to lack of literature, the small sample size used in the published studies is another limitation.

Genomics Single nucleotide polymorphism (SNP) studies have revealed that polymorphisms associated with nicotine metabolism and DNA repair genes are responsible for higher lung cancer risk in Latinos. Additionally, the predominant driver oncogenes reported were EGFR, Kirsten Rat Sarcoma (KRAS), and c-raf murine sarcoma viral oncogene homolog B1 (BRAF) [37]. Genome-wide association studies (GWAS) conducted to find SNPs associated with colon cancer in Latinos discovered 17 genetic variants across four independent regions [38]. Another GWAS with Latino breast cancer patients revealed SNPs at 6q25 locus were associated with a low risk of estrogen receptor (ER) negative breast cancer risk in Latinas with indigenous American ancestry [39]. A significant association between thyroid cancer and five specific SNPs were detected in Latinos living in Columbia [26].

Epigenomics Changes in DNA methylation, a well-known epigenetic modification, are dynamic and influenced by both intrinsic (genetic) and extrinsic (environmental, lifestyle) factors [40]. Unlike DNA sequence mutations, DNA methylation can be changeable throughout a lifetime and can be altered by environmental exposure [41]. Associated with cancer, DNA methylation can alter the regulation of diverse cellular processes [42]. The global loss of methylation, often measured by Long Interspersed Element-1 (LINE-1), is associated with cancer incidence and mortality [43–46]. Additionally, genome-wide methylation studies have revealed numbers of cancer site-specific, hyper- and hypo-methylation across the genome as potential biomarkers for diagnosis, treatment, and prognosis [47–49]. Thus, many studies have focused on the relationship between DNA methylation and cancer, but notably in Caucasians [50, 51] and far more limited for Latinos. Based on individuals (*n* = 573) from diverse Hispanic origins, one study identified 916 methylation sites that differ between ethnic subgroups (Mexican, Puerto Rican, Mixed Latino, Other Latino) [52]. Among those sites, 66% were associated with intrinsic factors (ancestry) and 34% were associated with extrinsic factors (e.g., cultural, economic, environmental, and social exposures) [52]. Compared to non-Latino whites, Latinos have increased risk for hypermethylation of some lung cancer-related tumor suppressor genes, for example, transcription factors that bind to the DNA sequence GATA, sulfatase 2 (SULF2), and protocadherin 20 (PCDH20) in exfoliated lung cells [53]. In global DNA, significantly lower levels of LINE-1 were found in Latinos relative to non-Latino whites [54]. A family history of breast cancer (mother with breast cancer susceptibility protein 1 [BRCA1] or BRCA2 mutations) influences lower LINE-1 methylation (18.8%, 95% CI = −42.7%, 5.1%), indicating

DNA methylation as a marker of inherited breast cancer susceptibility among Latina women [55]. Thus, in Latinos, DNA methylation differs by a combination of factors, including genetic susceptibility, socioeconomic status, lifestyle factors, and the environment, suggesting an epigenetic biomarker for understanding cancer disparities.

Transcriptomics Latino patients have been reported to experience a greater incidence of gastric cancer compared to Asians and Whites, and they have a greater proportion of genomically stable subtype tumors. Transcriptomic studies (whole-exome and RNA sequencing) revealed that 16% of patients possess unique molecular signatures, including a high proportion of cadherin 1 (CDH1) germline variants, which could be responsible for the aggressive gastric cancer phenotypes [56]. Transcriptomic studies of kidney cancer patients showed differential expression of almost 300 genes between tumors with different stage, size, and stage of kidney tumors, while advanced stage tumors showed overexpression of glucose-6-phosphate dehydrogenase (G6PD), amyloid-like protein 1 (APLP1), glucosaminyl (N-acetyl) transferase 3, mucin type (GCNT3), and phospholipid phosphatase 2 (PLPP2) genes [57].

Proteomics A proteomics study of Puerto Rican CRC patients revealed lower frequency of microsatellite instability (MSI)-related proteins, which result from DNA mismatch repair genes (MMR). Higher prevalence of the mismatch repair gene MutL homolog 1, colon cancer, nonpolyposis type 2 (MLH1) was found in 6–9% of colon tumors [58].

Metabolomics In a study on plasma metabolic profiling of breast cancer patients, Zhao et al. [59] reported that 14 metabolites showed a significant difference between Latino and non-Latino African American women. The identified metabolites were associated with citrate cycle, arginine-, proline-, and linoleic acid metabolic pathways.

Lipidomics No studies have been done on altered lipid profiles in US-based Latino breast cancer patients. However, lipidomic and metabolomic fingerprints of Latina women from Columbia who had breast cancer revealed a specific pattern of metabolites that were associated with glycerolipid, glycerophospholipid, amino acid, and fatty acid metabolism. These profiles were similar but not identical to those from non-Latina women [60].

Knowledge Gaps and Future Directions

The trans-omics approach, also known as multi-omics, poly-omics, and pan-omics, embraces integration of multidimensional omics data to provide a comprehensive assessment of a cancer in question [61]. This is an interesting approach to adopt because the etiology of a disease such as cancer is complex owing to its multiple causative factors. Single-level omics approaches help in identifying specific cancer-related mutations, epigenetic changes, and molecular characterization of tumors to different subtypes on the basis of gene–protein expressions. However, multi-omics approaches offer several advantages as they can dissect cancer cells in multiple dimensions and probe deeper to bring into light the mechanisms (molecular and biochemical) that underlie different phenotypes of a particular cancer. Additionally, these strategies can not only examine the response to suspected causative agent (carcinogen) exposure but also to chemo- and/or immunotherapies. Another beneficial outcome of these trans-omics approaches is the discovery of new diagnostic/prognostic markers for various types of cancer [62].

One shortcoming in assessing cancer disparities in Latinos is viewing health outcomes as a whole instead of taking subgroup heterogeneity into consideration [63]. Given the fact that Latinos comprise European, Native American (Amerindian), and African ancestries [23], assessing health disparities among Latinos is a daunting task. In this context, employing the trans-omics approach is expected to yield robust information.

These advantages aside, the trans-omics approach has some challenges as well. Each omics cancer dataset by itself is complex for reasons such as the quality of output in analytical platform and heterogeneity of data [64]. Issues pertaining to processing these enormous data volumes could be resolved by the Big Data to Knowledge (BD2K) technologies mentioned in Paten et al. [65] and Juarez et al. [66].

Another research area worth considering from a trans-omics perspective is the microbiome. Microbiota of the gut has been implicated in cancer [67]. Microbes contribute to cancer both in direct and indirect ways. While some microbes such as the bacterium *Helicobacter pylori* contribute to gastric cancer and some viruses such as HPV and HIV contribute to cervical cancers, other microbes contribute to cancer through altered metabolism. However, the role of microbiome in cancer is not completely understood and may require additional investigations [68].

References

1. Wild CP. Complementing the genome with an "exposome": the outstanding challenge of environmental exposure measurement in molecular epidemiology. Cancer Epidemiol Biomark Prev. 2005;14(8):1847–50. https://doi.org/10.1158/1055-9965.Epi-05-0456.
2. Juarez PD. (2019). The public health exposome. In Unraveling the Exposome (pp. 23–61). Springer, Cham. https://doi.org/10.1007/978-3-319-89321-1_2
3. Juarez PD, Matthews-Juarez P, Hood DB, Im W, Levine RS, Kilbourne BJ, et al. The public health exposome: a population-based, exposure science approach to health disparities research. Int J Environ Res Public Health. 2014;11(12):12866–95. https://doi.org/10.3390/ijerph111212866.
4. Miller GW, Jones DP. The nature of nurture: refining the definition of the exposome. Toxicol Sci. 2014;137(1):1–2. https://doi.org/10.1093/toxsci/kft251.

5. Agache I, Miller R, Gern JE, Hellings PW, Jutel M, Muraro A, et al. Emerging concepts and challenges in implementing the exposome paradigm in allergic diseases and asthma: a Practall document. Allergy. 2019;74(3):449–63. https://doi.org/10.1111/all.13690.
6. Juarez PD, Matthews-Juarez P. Applying an exposome-wide (ExWAS) approach to cancer research. Front Oncol. 2018;8:313. https://doi.org/10.3389/fonc.2018.00313.
7. Juarez PD, Tabatabai M, Valdez RB, Hood DB, Im W, Mouton C, et al. The effects of social, personal, and behavioral risk factors and PM$^{2.5}$ on cardio-metabolic disparities in a cohort of community health center patient. Int J Environ Res Public Health. 2020;17:3561.
8. American Cancer Society. Cancer facts & figures for Hispanics/Latinos 2018–2020. Atlanta: American Cancer Society, Inc.; 2018.
9. Miller K, Goding Sauer A, Ortiz A, Fedewa S, Pinheiro P, Tortolero-Luna G, et al. Cancer statistics for Hispanics/Latinos, 2018. CA Cancer J Clin. 2018;68(9):425–45. https://doi.org/10.3322/caac.21494.
10. Pinheiro PS, Callahan KE, Koru-Sengul T, Ransdell J, Bouzoubaa L, Brown CP, et al. Risk of cancer death among white, black, and Hispanic populations in South Florida. Prev Chronic Dis. 2019;16:E83. https://doi.org/10.5888/pcd16.180529.
11. Steuer C, Behera M, Berry L, Kim S, Rossi M, Sica G, et al. Role of race in oncogenic driver prevalence and outcomes in lung adenocarcinoma: results from the Lung Cancer Mutation Consortium. Cancer. 2016;122(5):766–72. https://doi.org/10.1002/cncr.29812.
12. Moore JX, Royston KJ, Langston ME, Griffin R, Hidalgo B, Wang HE, et al. Mapping hot spots of breast cancer mortality in the United States: place matters for Blacks and Hispanics. Cancer Causes Control. 2018;29(8):737–50. https://doi.org/10.1007/s10552-018-1051-y.
13. Rodriguez-Velazquez A, Velez R, Lafontaine JC, Colon-Echevarria CB, Lamboy-Caraballo RD, Ramirez I, et al. Prevalence of breast and ovarian cancer subtypes in Hispanic populations from Puerto Rico. BMC Cancer. 2018;18(1):1177. https://doi.org/10.1186/s12885-018-5077-z.
14. Centers for Disease Control and Prevention. Web-based injury statistics query and reporting system (WISQARS) 2020. http://www.cdc.gov/injury/wisqars/fatal.html. Accessed 23 June 2020.
15. Ramirez AG, Muñoz E, Parma DL, Michalek JE, Holden AEC, Phillips TD, et al. Lifestyle and clinical correlates of hepatocellular carcinoma in South Texas: a matched case-control study. Clin Gastroenterol Hepatol. 2017;15(8):1311–2. https://doi.org/10.1016/j.cgh.2017.03.022.
16. Ramirez AG, Munoz E, Holden AEC, Adeigbe RT, Suarez L. Incidence of hepatocellular carcinoma in Texas Latinos, 1995–2010: an update. PLoS One. 2014;9(6):e99365.
17. Wu HC, Santella R. The role of aflatoxins in hepatocellular carcinoma. Hepat Mon. 2012;12(10HCC):e7238.
18. Ha J, Chaudhri A, Avirineni A, Pan JJ. Burden of hepatocellular carcinoma among Hispanics in South Texas: a systematic review. Biomark Res. 2017;5(15). https://doi.org/10.1186/s40364-017-0096-5.
19. Ramírez-Amill R, Soto-Salgado M, Vázquez-Santos C, Corzo-Pedrosa M, Cruz-Correa MR. Assessing colorectal cancer knowledge among Puerto Rican Hispanics: implications for cancer prevention and control. J Community Health. 2017;42(6):1141–7. https://doi.org/10.1007/s10900-017-0363-2.
20. Robles A, Bashashati M, Contreras A, Chávez LO, Cerro-Rondón AD, Cu C, et al. Colorectal cancer in Hispanics living near the U.S.-Mexico border. Rev Invest Clin. 2019;71(5):306–10. https://doi.org/10.24875/RIC.19003026.
21. Gonzales M, Qeadan F, Mishra SI, Rajput A, Hoffman RM. Racial-ethnic disparities in late-stage colorectal cancer among Hispanics and Non-Hispanic Whites of New Mexico. Hisp Health Care Int. 2017;15(4):180–8. https://doi.org/10.1177/1540415317746317.
22. Chattar-Cora D, Onime GD, Coppa GF, Valentine IS, Rivera L. Anatomic, age, and sex distribution of colorectal cancer in a New York City Hispanic population. J Natl Med Assoc. 1998;90(1):19–24.

23. Stern MC. Prostate cancer in US Latinos; what have we learned and where should we focus our attention. In: Ramirez AG, Trapido EJ, editors. Advancing the science of cancer in Latinos. Cham: Springer; 2020. p. 57–67.

24. Dobbs RW, Malhotra NR, Abern MR, Moreira DM. Prostate cancer disparities in Hispanics by country of origin: a nationwide population-based analysis. Prostate Cancer Prostatic Dis. 2019;22(1):159–67. https://doi.org/10.1038/s41391-018-0097-y.

25. Tortolero-Luna G, Torres-Cintrón CR, Alvarado-Ortiz M, Ortiz-Ortiz KJ, Zavala-Zegarra DE, Mora-Piñero E. Incidence of thyroid cancer in Puerto Rico and the US by racial/ethnic group, 2011–2015. BMC Cancer. 2019;19(1). https://doi.org/10.1186/s12885-019-5854-3.

26. Estrada-Florez AP, Bohórquez ME, Sahasrabudhe R, Prieto R, Lott P, Duque CS, et al. Clinical features of Hispanic thyroid cancer cases and the role of known genetic variants on disease risk. Medicine. 2016;95(32):e4148. https://doi.org/10.1097/MD.0000000000004148.

27. Clarke MA, Devesa SS, Harvey SV, Wentzensen N. Hysterectomy-corrected uterine corpus cancer incidence trends and differences in relative survival reveal racial disparities and rising rates of nonendometrioid cancers. J Clin Oncol. 2019;37(22):1895–908. https://doi.org/10.1200/JCO.19.00151.

28. Mann L, Foley KL, Tanner AE, Sun CJ, Rhodes SD. Increasing cervical cancer screening among US Hispanics/Latinas: a qualitative systematic review. J Cancer Educ. 2015;30(2):165–8.

29. Eng TY, Chen T, Vincent J, Patel AJ, Clyburn V, Ha CS. Persistent disparities in Hispanics with cervical cancer in a major city. J Racial Ethn Health Disparities. 2017;4(2):165–8.

30. Ortiz AP, Engels EA, Nogueras-González GM, Colón-López V, Soto–Salgado M, Vargas A, et al. Disparities in human papillomavirus-related cancer incidence and survival among human immunodeficiency virus-infected Hispanics living in the United States. Cancer. 2018;124(23):4520–8.

31. Kelly RS, Vineis P. Biomarkers of susceptibility to chemical carcinogens: the example of non-Hodgkin lymphomas. Br Med Bull. 2014;111(1):89–100. https://doi.org/10.1093/bmb/ldu015.

32. Grebenshchikov IS, Studennikov AE, Ivanov VI, Ivanova NV, Titov VA, Vergbickaya NE, et al. Idiotypic and anti-idiotypic antibodies against polycyclic aromatic hydrocarbon in human blood serum are new biomarkers of lung cancer. Oncotarget. 2019;10(49):5070–81.

33. Barocas DA, Motley S, Cookson MS, Chang SS, Penson DF, Dai Q, et al. Oxidative stress measured by urine F2-isoprostane level is associated with prostate cancer. J Urol. 2011;85(6):2102–7. https://doi.org/10.1016/j.juro.2011.02.020.

34. Zhou B, Liu J, Wang ZM, Xi T. C-reactive protein, interleukin 6 and lung cancer risk: a meta-analysis. PLoS One. 2012;7(8):e43075. https://doi.org/10.1371/journal.pone.0043075.

35. Yang Y, Meng WJ, Wang ZQ. MicroRNAs in colon and rectal cancer--novel biomarkers from diagnosis to therapy. Endocr Metab Immune Disord Drug Targets. 2020. Published online ahead of print, 2020 May 5. https://doi.org/10.2174/1871530320666200506075219.

36. Knox SS. From 'omics' to complex disease: a systems biology approach to gene-environment interactions in cancer. Cancer Cell Int. 2010;10(11). https://doi.org/10.1186/1475-2867-10-11.

37. Cress WD, Chiappori A, Santiago P, Muñoz-Antonia T. Lung cancer mutations and use of targeted agents in Hispanics. Rev Recent Clin Trials. 2014;9(4):225–32. https://doi.org/10.2174/1574887110666150127103555.

38. Schmit SL, Schumacher FR, Edlund CK, Conti DV, Ihenacho U, Wan P, et al. Genome-wide association study of colorectal cancer in Hispanics. Carcinogenesis. 2016;37(6):547–56. https://doi.org/10.1093/carcin/bgw046.

39. Hoffman J, Fejerman L, Hu D, Huntsman S, Li M, John EM, et al. Identification of novel common breast cancer risk variants at the 6q25 locus among Latinas. Breast Cancer Res Treat. 2019;21(1):3. https://doi.org/10.1186/s13058-018-1085-9.

40. Jaenisch R, Bird A. Epigenetic regulation of gene expression: how the genome integrates intrinsic and environmental signals. Nat Genet. 2003;33(Suppl):345–54.

41. Dor Y, Cedar H. Principles of DNA methylation and their implications for biology and medicine. Lancet. 2018;392(10149):777–86.

42. Luo C, Hajkova P, Ecker JR. Dynamic DNA methylation: in the right place at the right time. Science. 2018;361(6409):1336–40.
43. Ehrlich M. DNA hypomethylation in cancer cells. Epigenomics. 2009;1(2):239–59.
44. Joyce BT, Gao T, Zheng Y, Liu L, Zhang W, Dai Q, et al. Prospective changes in global DNA methylation and cancer incidence and mortality. Br J Cancer. 2016;115(4):465–72.
45. King WD, Ashbury JE, Taylor SA, Yat Tse M, Pang SC, Louw JA, et al. A cross-sectional study of global DNA methylation and risk of colorectal adenoma. BMC Cancer. 2014;14:488.
46. Saghafinia S, Mina M, Riggi N, Hanahan D, Ciriello G. Pan-cancer landscape of aberrant DNA methylation across human tumors. Cell Rep. 2018;25(4):1066–80.
47. Fan J, Li J, Guo S, Tao C, Zhang H, Wang W, et al. Genome-wide DNA methylation profiles of low- and high-grade adenoma reveals potential biomarkers for early detection of colorectal carcinoma. Clin Epigenetics. 2020;12(1):56.
48. Ding W, Chen G, Shi T. Integrative analysis identifies potential DNA methylation biomarkers for pan-cancer diagnosis and prognosis. Epigenetics. 2019;14(1):67–80.
49. Hao X, Luo H, Krawczyk M, Wei W, Wang W, Wang J, et al. DNA methylation markers for diagnosis and prognosis of common cancers. Proc Natl Acad Sci U S A. 2017;114(28):7414–9.
50. Yang Y, Wu L, Shu XO, Cai Q, Shu X, Li B, et al. Genetically predicted levels of DNA methylation biomarkers and breast cancer risk: data from 228 951 women of European descent. J Natl Cancer Inst Monogr. 2020;112(3):295–304.
51. Yang Y, Wu L, Shu X, Lu Y, Shu XO, Cai Q, et al. Genetic data from nearly 63,000 women of European descent predicts DNA methylation biomarkers and epithelial ovarian cancer risk. Cancer Res. 2019;79(3):505–17.
52. Galanter JM, Gignoux CR, Oh SS, Torgerson D, Pino-Yanes M, Thakur N, et al. Differential methylation between ethnic sub-groups reflects the effect of genetic ancestry and environmental exposures. Elife. 2017;6:e20532.
53. Leng S, Liu Y, Thomas CL, Gauderman WJ, Picchi MA, Bruse SE, et al. Native American ancestry affects the risk for gene methylation in the lungs of Hispanic smokers from New Mexico. Am J Respir Crit Care Med. 2013;188(9):1110–6.
54. Zhang FF, Cardarelli R, Carroll J, Fulda KG, Kaur M, Gonzalez K, et al. Significant differences in global genomic DNA methylation by gender and race/ethnicity in peripheral blood. Epigenetics. 2011;6(5):623–9.
55. Delgado-Cruzata L, Wu HC, Liao Y, Santella RM, Terry MB. Differences in DNA methylation by extent of breast cancer family history in unaffected women. Epigenetics. 2014;9(2):243–8.
56. Wang SC, Yeu Y, Hammer STG, Xiao S, Zhu M, Hong C, et al. Adenocarcinoma have distinct molecular profiles including a high rate of germline CDH1 variants. Cancer Res. 2020;80(11):2114–24. https://doi.org/10.1158/0008-5472.CAN-19-2918.
57. Batai K, Imler E, Pangilinan J, Bell R, Lwin A, Price E, et al. Whole-transcriptome sequencing identified gene expression signatures associated with aggressive clear cell renal cell carcinoma. Genes Cancer. 2018;9(5–6):247–56. https://doi.org/10.18632/genesandcancer.183.
58. Reverón D, López C, Gutiérrez S, Sayegh ZE, Antonia T, Dutil J, et al. Frequency of mismatch repair protein deficiency in a Puerto Rican population with colonic adenoma and adenocarcinoma. Cancer Genomics Proteomics. 2018;15(4). https://doi.org/10.21873/cgp.20084.
59. Zhao H, Shen J, Moore SC, Ye Y, Wu X, Esteva FJ, et al. Breast cancer risk in relation to plasma metabolites among Hispanic and African American women. Breast Cancer Res Treat. 2019;6(3). https://doi.org/10.1007/s10549-019-05165-4687-96.
60. Cala MP, Aldana J, Medina J, Sánchez J, Guio J, Wist J, et al. Multiplatform plasma metabolic and lipid fingerprinting of breast cancer: a pilot control-case study in Colombian Hispanic women. PLoS One. 2018;13(2):e0190958. https://doi.org/10.1371/journal.pone.0190958.
61. Srivastava A, Kulkarni C, Mallick P, Huang K, Machiraju R. Building trans-omics evidence: using imaging and 'omics' to characterize cancer profiles. Pac Symp Biocomput. 2018;26:377–87.

62. Chakraborty S, Hosen MI, Ahmed M, Shekhar HU. Onco-multi-OMICS approach: a new frontier in cancer research. Biomed Res Int. 2018:9836256(e-collection). https://doi.org/10.1155/2018/9836256.
63. Velasquez MC, Chinea FM, Kwon D, Prakash NS, Barboza MP, Gonzalgo ML, et al. The influence of ethnic heterogeneity on prostate cancer mortality after radical prostatectomy in Hispanic or Latino men: a population-based analysis. Urology. 2018;117:108–14. https://doi.org/10.1016/j.urology.2018.03.036.
64. Buescher JM, Driggers EM. Integration of omics: more than the sum of its parts. Cancer Metab. 2016;4(4). https://doi.org/10.1186/s40170-016-0143-y.
65. Paten B, Diekhans M, Druker BJ, Friend S, Guinney J, Gassner N, et al. The NIH BD2K center for big data in translational genomics. J Am Med Inform Assoc. 2015;22(6):1143–7. https://doi.org/10.1093/jamia/ocv047.
66. Juarez PD, Hood DB, Song MA, Ramesh A. Use of an exposome approach to understand the effects of exposures from the natural, built, and social environments on cardio-vascular disease onset, progression, and outcomes. Front Public Health. 2020;17(10):3661. https://doi.org/10.3390/ijerph17103561.
67. Schwabe RF, Jobin C. The microbiome and cancer. Nat Rev Cancer. 2013;13(11):800–12. https://doi.org/10.1038/nrc3610.
68. Xavier JB, Young VB, Skufca J, Ginty F, Testerman T, Pearson AT, et al. The cancer microbiome: distinguishing direct and indirect effects requires a systemic view. Trends Cancer. 2020;8(3):192–204. https://doi.org/10.1016/j.trecan.2020.01.004.

Open Access   This chapter is licensed under the terms of the Creative Commons Attribution 4.0 International License (http://creativecommons.org/licenses/by/4.0/), which permits use, sharing, adaptation, distribution and reproduction in any medium or format, as long as you give appropriate credit to the original author(s) and the source, provide a link to the Creative Commons license and indicate if changes were made.

The images or other third party material in this chapter are included in the chapter's Creative Commons license, unless indicated otherwise in a credit line to the material. If material is not included in the chapter's Creative Commons license and your intended use is not permitted by statutory regulation or exceeds the permitted use, you will need to obtain permission directly from the copyright holder.

Chapter 3
Population Health Challenges for Latinos in the United States

Alexander N. Ortega

Latino Health-Care Access and the Patient Protection and Affordable Care Act

The Patient Protection and Affordable Care Act (ACA) became law in 2010 and was nationally implemented in 2014 to make insurance more affordable and accessible. This comprehensive health insurance reform emphasizes community engagement and population health and has multiple provisions—insurance plans that are offered through marketplaces, Medicaid expansion, and incentives to improve cost and quality of care.

Racial and Ethnic Disparities in Health-Care Access and Utilization Under the ACA

Shortly after the roll out of the Affordable Care Act, our research team wanted to answer a simple question: What impact has the ACA had on health-care inequities, particularly for African Americans and Latinos? Using a pre-post study design, we analyzed combined data from the National Health Interview Survey (NHIS) and Medical Expenditure Panel Survey (MEPS) [1]. We found that all groups—non-Latino whites, African Americans, Latinos, and other race/ethnicity—experienced improvements in health-care access and utilization post-ACA, but that Latinos fared worse than all the other groups. For example, from 2011 to 2014, the probability of being uninsured dropped from 0.14 to 0.11 for non-Latino whites; from 0.24 to 0.17

A. N. Ortega (✉)
Department of Health Management and Policy, Center for Population Health and Community Impact, Drexel Dornsife School of Public Health, Drexel University, Philadelphia, PA, USA
e-mail: ano37@drexel.edu

© The Author(s) 2023
A. G. Ramirez, E. J. Trapido (eds.), *Advancing the Science of Cancer in Latinos*, https://doi.org/10.1007/978-3-031-14436-3_3

33

for African Americans; and from 0.39 to 0.32 for Latinos. The other race/ethnicity category dropped from 0.18 to 0.14. The probability of delaying any necessary care also improved for every group; African Americans fared worse than Latinos (probability dropped from 0.17 to 0.14 and 0.18 to 0.12, respectively). The probability of having any physician visit increased post-ACA in all groups, but Latinos were consistently lower for all four years.

ACA's Impact Among Latino Subgroups

Are these observed trends in health-care access and utilization consistent for all Latinos or for just some Latino subgroups? To answer this question, we performed a simple analysis of trends in Latinos by subgroups defined by heritage group (Puerto Rican, Mexican, Cuban, Central American, and other Latino), citizenship status, and interview language (Spanish or English) [2]. Measures of access to health care included health insurance status and forgoing necessary care because of cost; measures of utilization included any emergency department (ED) visit and any physician visit within the past 12 months. Our findings showed that the ACA, which was implemented in 2014, has reduced gaps in access and utilization of health care, and most reductions in disparities were experienced between Puerto Ricans and non-Latino whites; disparities remain for noncitizens [2].

Insurance Coverage Central American and Mexican Latinos showed the lowest percentage of being insured currently (72.26% and 68.47% after the ACA, respectively); Puerto Ricans, who are citizens at birth, fared better (88.57%).

Forgoing Care Results showed that Cubans and Mexicans were more likely to forgo necessary care in the past 12 months because of costs, and Puerto Ricans did better in forgoing care pre- and post-ACA.

Emergency Department Visit We observed that emergency department utilization improved for all groups. Interestingly, while Puerto Ricans were much more likely to be insured and less likely to forgo seeking care, they had significantly higher percentage of visiting the emergency department in the last 12 months. We observed that ED use among other Latinos followed second to Puerto Ricans and that ED use among non-Latino whites did not change from 2011 to 2015.

Physician Visit Trends were flat for any physician visits in the past 12 months; Mexican Latinos fared worse than the other heritage groups, followed by Cuban Latinos.

Citizenship and Language Use We were also interested in knowing whether or not these associations were moderated by citizenship status or language use. We found that noncitizens had lower odds than US-born citizens of being insured

(OR = 0.34; 95% CI, 0.31–0.37; P < .01), visiting an ED (OR = 0.78, 95% CI, 0.69–0.88; P < .01), and seeing a physician (OR = 0.74, 95% CI, 0.68–0.80; P < .01). Those whose interview language was Spanish had lower odds than those whose interview language was English of being insured (OR = 0.79; 95% CI, 0.71–0.87; P < .01), visiting an ED (OR = 0.62; 95% CI, 0.55–0.71; P < .01), and seeing a physician (OR = 0.80; 95% CI, 0.74–0.87; P < .01) [2].

ACA's Impact on Reducing Disparities in Hypertension Treatment Among Mexican-Heritage Latinos

The cardiovascular literature shows that Latinos, in general, have lower rates of cardiovascular disease than other groups [3, 4]. Mexican-heritage Latinos, in particular, have lower rates of hypertension than non-Latino whites, but they are more likely to be undiagnosed; they are also more likely to be diagnosed later in disease, are much more difficult to treat, and are less likely to be on hypertensive medication.

In light of these disparities, we asked the question: Has the ACA made a difference in the treatment of hypertension in Mexican-heritage Latinos? Using data from the 2009–2014 California Health Interview Survey [5], we predicted trends in access, utilization, and hypertension control under the ACA for Mexican-heritage Latinos and non-Latino whites with hypertension. We found a significant initial uptake in insurance coverage for Mexican-heritage Latinos in 2013 followed by a slight decline in 2014, and there was a clear disparity in predicted insurance when compared to non-Latino whites even after implementation of ACA provisions. (These data reflect the fact that California adopted several provisions of the ACA before 2014.) Notably, the odds of taking hypertension medication increased among Mexican-heritage Latinos; that is, they were significantly more likely to report taking the medication after the ACA.

Impact of the ACA on Latino Children

Disparities Among Latino Children: Pre-ACA

About one in four US children under the age of 18 are Hispanic/Latino, making up the largest minority group among US children [6]. We thus had an interest in documenting disparities in health care among Latino children that existed before the ACA was implemented. Because family-centered care has been demonstrated to reduce disparities and improve the quality of health care, we examined racial and ethnic disparities in the receipt of family-centered care among the general pediatric population in the United States [7]. Using a linked dataset of MEPS and the NHIS from 2003 to 2006 (pre-ACA), we measured family-centered care using four questions adopted by the NHIS: "How often did your child's doctors or other health providers (1) listen carefully to you, (2) explain things in a way you could understand, (3) show respect for what you had to say, and (4) spend enough time with you?" We found that compared to non-Latino whites, Latino youth experienced pediatric care with less of the four core processes of family-centered care—showing respect, sharing information, encouraging participation, and promoting collaboration. Their parents were less likely to say that their child's doctors listened to them, explained things carefully, or spent enough time with them.

What is the source of the health-care disparities between Latino youth and other children? To identify explanatory factors, we used the Blinder-Oaxaca decomposition method to analyze the 2006–2011 NHIS (pre-ACA) data on parent-reported health-care access and utilization for white, Latino, and African American children in the United States [8]. We found that Latino children were less likely than non-Latino white children to have a usual source of care, receive at least one preventive care visit, and visit a doctor; Latino children were also more likely to have delayed care. These disparities could largely be explained by differences in socioeconomic status and health policy factors, such as having health insurance and having access to care.

Insurance Coverage and Latino Youth: Post-ACA

Did the ACA change the level of insurance coverage and health-care utilization or improve health-care disparities among Latino youth? Did Latino children show the same pattern of insurance coverage as Latino adults before and after implementation of the ACA? We analyzed national data from the 2011–2015 NHIS child component, which included parent-reported health-care utilization and access for youth aged 0–17 years. Using a pre-post study design, we found that insurance coverage and well-child visits improved for all youth post-ACA, but like their adult counterparts, Latino youth lagged significantly behind non-Hispanic whites, non-Hispanic blacks, and other race/ethnicity [9]. Even though Latino youth showed the largest gain in insurance coverage, they made up the highest proportion of uninsured post-ACA, largely because they had a much higher uninsured rate pre-ACA (Fig. 3.1). Although differences for well-child visits were minimal, Latino youth were also less likely to have a well-child visit.

Since our original analysis of insurance coverage for youth and well-child visits post-ACA [9], there have been changes in the implementation of the ACA. In an effort to determine if insurance coverage and disparity levels are still improving, we reanalyzed our original data to include more recent 2018 NHIS data [10]. For the total of all youth, the prevalence of uninsured initially decreased from 6.6% in 2011–2013 (pre-ACA) to 4.8% in 2014–2015 (post-ACA); however, there was an uptick to 5.1% by 2016–2018. While these percentage differences may seem small, note that the denominator is in the millions—the 0.3% increase in uninsured from 2014–2015 to 2016–2018 is 196,000 uninsured children. The uninsured rate for

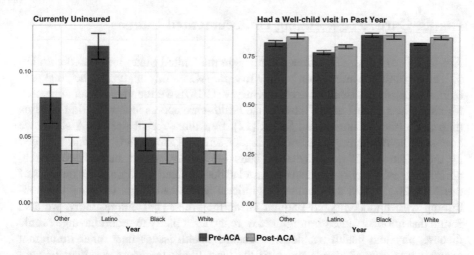

Fig. 3.1 Insurance coverage and well-child visits for youth (0–17 years) in the United States pre-ACA (2011–2013) and post-ACA (2014–2015). (Reprinted from Ortega et al. [9]. © 2018 with permission from Elsevier)

non-Latino white and non-Latino black youth showed a similar pattern of change as the total of all youth, but Latino youth continued to improve over the three time periods (11.4%, 2011–2013; 8.4%, 2014–2015; 7.6%, 2016–2018). Significant disparities remain, however, as the uninsured rate for Latino youth is still higher than non-Latino white and non-Latino black youth. All the three groups continued to improve on well-child visits over the three time periods. We hypothesize that this is largely attributable to the mandatory preventive visits that are provided by the ACA, so children are going in for immunizations and screening well-child visits, which are covered regardless of insurance coverage.

It has been established that the effect of the ACA on health-care disparities between Latinos and non-Latino whites varies among Latino-heritage groups [2], and the question is whether the same disparity patterns exist among Latino youth. Using data from the 2011–2016 NHIS, we compared insurance coverage and health-care utilization by subgroups of Latino youth (Puerto Rican, Mexican, Cuban, Central or South American, and other subgroups) [11]. We found that the uninsured rate dropped significantly post-ACA for most Latino subgroups and non-Latino whites; children of Mexican heritage and Central or South American heritage experienced the greatest decline in uninsured rate (13.1% pre-ACA to 9.9% post-ACA and 12.4% to 9.1%, respectively)—a similar pattern to their adult counterparts [11]. However, disparities remained as both subgroups still experienced greater uninsured rates post-ACA than the other subgroups and non-Latino whites. Similarly, the proportion for a well-child visit in the past 12 months increased for most groups post-ACA, but the proportion of Mexican children going to a well-child visit still lagged behind all other groups both pre-ACA and post-ACA [11]. Interestingly and contrary to popular belief, Mexican-heritage children were very low utilizers of the emergency department [11]. This was true for both citizens and noncitizens.

Health-Care Access Among Undocumented Latinos

Are health-care disparities among Latinos in the United States associated with US citizenship and documentation status? In a pre-ACA study analyzing the 2003 data from the California Health Interview Survey (CHIS), we found that undocumented Mexicans and other Latinos have worse health-care access and utilization patterns than those born in the United States [12]. In a more recent post-ACA study, we compared health-care access and utilization among Latinos in California stratified by the continuum of documentation status—US-born citizen, naturalized citizen, permanent resident with a green card, and undocumented immigrant. An analysis of the 2011–2015 CHIS data showed significant health-care disparity along this continuum with undocumented Latinos faring the worst [13]. Interestingly, we also found that undocumented immigrants were the least likely to report having chronic disease, physical health problems or mental health issues than other immigrant groups, even though they were also the least likely to report excellent or very good health.

The Affordable Care Act holds the promise of ameliorating some of the health disparities that the Latino population experiences in the United States, but coverage needs to be extended to undocumented immigrants to narrow disparities and improve utilization and access to health care [14]. For example, California offers Medicaid to eligible children who are undocumented and also provides health benefits to adult undocumented immigrants through Medicaid, which is covered by state funds.

Conclusion

The ACA has positively impacted health-care disparities in the United States for both adults and children. While there have been gains in insurance coverage and primary health-care access and utilization across all racial and ethnic groups, disparities remain, especially for Latinos in states that have not expanded Medicaid. Moreover, among Latinos, disparities are particularly striking for Mexican and Central American subgroups and for noncitizen and undocumented immigrants. Any revision in the implementation of the ACA must consider these unremitting disparities, especially as the Latino population continues to grow and expand across the country. Some states, like California, are leading the way in implementing policies that ensure health care is a right afforded to all its citizens, which includes noncitizens who have been in the country for less than five years and undocumented immigrants, and this should be a model for national health-care reform.

References

1. Chen J, Vargas-Bustamante A, Mortensen K, Ortega AN. Racial and ethnic disparities in health care access and utilization under the Affordable Care Act. Med Care. 2016;54(2):140–6. https://doi.org/10.1097/mlr.0000000000000467.
2. Alcalá HE, Chen J, Langellier BA, Roby DH, Ortega AN. Impact of the Affordable Care Act on health care access and utilization among Latinos. J Am Board Family Med. 2017;30(1):52–62. https://doi.org/10.3122/jabfm.2017.01.160208.
3. Keenan NL, Rosendorf KA. Centers for Disease Control and Prevention. Prevalence of hypertension and controlled hypertension-United States. 20052008. Morb Mortal Wkly Rep. 2011;60:94–7.
4. Sorlie PD, Allison MA, Avilés-Santa ML, Cai J, Daviglus ML, Howard AG, et al. Prevalence of hypertension, awareness, treatment, and control in the Hispanic Community Health Study/Study of Latinos. Am J Hypertens. 2014;27(6):793–800. https://doi.org/10.1093/ajh/hpu003.
5. McKenna R, Alcalá H, Lê-Scherban F, Roby D, Ortega A. The Affordable Care Act reduces hypertension treatment disparities for Mexican-heritage Latinos. Med Care. 2017;55:654–60. https://doi.org/10.1097/MLR.0000000000000726.
6. Kids Count Data Center. Child population by race in the United States. The Annie E Casey Foundation. 2016. https://datacenter.kidscount.org/data/line/103-child-population-by-race?loc=1&loct=1#1/any/false/870,35,11/asc/67,12,66/424. Accessed 17 April 2021.
7. Guerrero AD, Chen J, Inkelas M, Rodriguez HP, Ortega AN. Racial and ethnic disparities in pediatric experiences of family-centered care. Med Care. 2010;48(4):388–93. https://doi.org/10.1097/MLR.0b013e3181ca3ef7.
8. Langellier BA, Chen J, Vargas-Bustamante A, Inkelas M, Ortega AN. Understanding healthcare access and utilization disparities among Latino children in the United States. J Child Health Care. 2016;20(2):133–44. https://doi.org/10.1177/1367493514555587.
9. Ortega AN, McKenna RM, Chen J, Alcalá HE, Langellier BA, Roby DH. Insurance coverage and well-child visits improved for youth under the Affordable Care Act, but Latino youth still lag behind. Acad Pediatr. 2018;18(1):35–42. https://doi.org/10.1016/j.acap.2017.07.006.
10. Ortega AN, Pintor JK, Alberto CK, Roby DH. Inequities in insurance coverage and well-child visits improve, but insurance gains for white and black youth reverse. Acad Pediatr. 2020;20(1):14–5. https://doi.org/10.1016/j.acap.2019.08.005.
11. Kemmick Pintor J, Chen J, Alcalá HE, Langellier BA, McKenna RM, Roby DH, et al. Insurance coverage and utilization improve for Latino youth but disparities by heritage group persist following the ACA. Med Care. 2018;56(11):927–33. https://doi.org/10.1097/mlr.0000000000000992.
12. Ortega AN, Fang H, Perez VH, Rizzo JA, Carter-Pokras O, Wallace SP, et al. Health care access, use of services, and experiences among undocumented Mexicans and other Latinos. Arch Intern Med. 2007;167(21):2354–60. https://doi.org/10.1001/archinte.167.21.2354.
13. Ortega AN, McKenna RM, Kemmick Pintor J, Langellier BA, Roby DH, Pourat N, et al. Health care access and physical and behavioral health among undocumented Latinos in California. Med Care. 2018;56(11):919–26. https://doi.org/10.1097/mlr.0000000000000985.
14. Ortega AN, Rodriguez HP, Vargas BA. Policy dilemmas in Latino health care and implementation of the Affordable Care Act. Annu Rev Public Health. 2015;36:525–44. https://doi.org/10.1146/annurev-publhealth-031914-122421.

Open Access   This chapter is licensed under the terms of the Creative Commons Attribution 4.0 International License (http://creativecommons.org/licenses/by/4.0/), which permits use, sharing, adaptation, distribution and reproduction in any medium or format, as long as you give appropriate credit to the original author(s) and the source, provide a link to the Creative Commons license and indicate if changes were made.

The images or other third party material in this chapter are included in the chapter's Creative Commons license, unless indicated otherwise in a credit line to the material. If material is not included in the chapter's Creative Commons license and your intended use is not permitted by statutory regulation or exceeds the permitted use, you will need to obtain permission directly from the copyright holder.

Part III
Vulnerable Populations and Cancer Health Disparities

Chapter 4
Acute and Long-term Neurological Complications of Acute Lymphoblastic Leukemia (ALL) Therapy in Latino Children

Austin L. Brown, Kimberly P. Raghubar, Michael E. Scheurer, and Philip J. Lupo

Introduction

Acute lymphoblastic leukemia (ALL) is the most common malignancy diagnosed during childhood [1]. Once considered a terminal diagnosis, pediatric ALL is now curable in approximately 90% of cases with contemporary therapy [2]. Despite significant improvements in the treatment of pediatric ALL, racial and ethnic disparities still persist. In particular, compared to non-Latino White populations, Latinos have both a higher incidence of pediatric ALL and less favorable outcomes [3]. Disparities in pediatric ALL outcomes are likely due to a number of factors, including ethnic variability in somatic molecular profiles, comorbidities, treatment adherence, and response to chemotherapy. Notably, exposure to central nervous system (CNS)-directed chemotherapy during ALL treatment is associated with a risk of acute and long-term neurotoxicity [4, 5]. Emerging research from our group and others suggests Latino patients with ALL may be particularly vulnerable to the adverse neurologic side effects of CNS-directed therapy [6–8]. Therefore, we provide an overview of ethnic disparities in treatment-related neurotoxicity and recommendations for future research directions.

A. L. Brown · K. P. Raghubar · M. E. Scheurer · P. J. Lupo (✉)
Baylor College of Medicine, Houston, TX, USA

Texas Children's Hospital, Houston, TX, USA
e-mail: philip.lupo@bcm.edu

© The Author(s) 2023
A. G. Ramirez, E. J. Trapido (eds.), *Advancing the Science of Cancer in Latinos*, https://doi.org/10.1007/978-3-031-14436-3_4

Acute Neurotoxicity During ALL Therapy

The antifolate agent methotrexate is an important component of contemporary curative pediatric ALL protocols. Current ALL chemotherapy regimens typically include intravenous (IV), intrathecal (IT), and oral methotrexate. The antineoplastic effects of methotrexate are attributed to the competitive inhibition of the dihydrofolate reductase (DHFR) enzyme involved in tetrahydrofolate synthesis. The resulting tetrahydrofolate deficiency disrupts DNA and RNA synthesis, leading to cell cycle arrest. Methotrexate preferentially inhibits rapidly dividing cells, such as leukemic cells. However, because methotrexate is a folic acid analogue, prolonged use or exposure to high doses of methotrexate may deplete folate stores and result in adverse side effects. Specifically, approximately 10% of pediatric patients with ALL experience acute or subacute neurotoxicity, typically occurring within 14 days of receiving CNS-directed high-dose IV or IT methotrexate [4, 5]. Acute and subacute methotrexate-related neurotoxicity often manifests clinically as a combination of seizure, aphasia, altered mental status, stroke-like symptoms, and encephalopathy [6–8]. Although these symptoms are typically transient [9], the clinical management of methotrexate-related neurotoxicity often leads to delays or modification of cancer therapy, potentially limiting treatment efficacy. In fact, recent evidence from our group suggests that patients with suspected neurotoxic events during ALL therapy receive an average of two fewer doses of IT methotrexate [8]. Although follow-up was limited in this cohort, we also observed a statistically significant ($p < 0.05$) trend toward an increased risk of relapse in patients with a history of methotrexate-related neurotoxicity.

Despite neurotoxicity being a serious complication of methotrexate chemotherapy, information on the factors which modify the risk of methotrexate-related neurotoxicity is limited. Several independent studies have reported associations between older age at diagnosis and treatment intensity and the incidence of acute and subacute neurotoxicity [4, 5, 8, 10]. Recent case series further suggest that susceptibility to methotrexate-related neurotoxicity may vary across racial and ethnic groups. Giordano et al. [7] presented information on five ALL patients with acute or subacute neurotoxicity, all of whom were Latino, while Afshar et al. [6] described the presentation of clinical neurotoxicity in 18 pediatric oncology patients, including 12 Latino cases. Most recently, we conducted one of the largest evaluations of acute and subacute methotrexate-related neurotoxicity in a multisite study of patients treated on recent pediatric ALL protocols [8] and found significant differences in the incidence of neurotoxicity by ethnic group (Fig. 4.1). This analysis of 280 newly diagnosed (between 2012 and 2017) patients found that neurotoxicity occurred in 21.8% of Latino compared to 6.8% of non-Latino patients, corresponding to a nearly 2.5-fold increased risk of neurotoxicity after accounting for other clinical and demographic factors.

Growing evidence supports an association between genome-wide genetic ancestry and racial/ethnic disparities in pediatric ALL outcomes, including relapse [11], suggesting that genetic variants, which impact antileukemia therapy

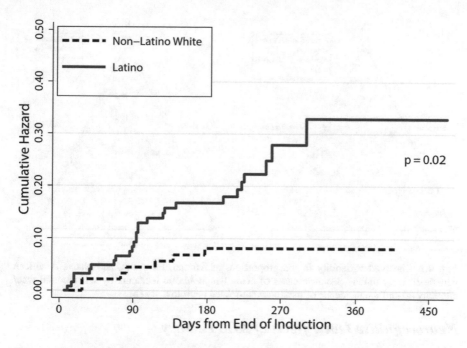

Fig. 4.1 Cumulative hazard of acute and subacute methotrexate-related neurotoxicity between Latino and non-Latino White patients with pediatric ALL

pharmacodynamics and pharmacokinetics, may co-segregate with areas of the genome associated with differing ancestral populations [12]. Because Latino ethnicity encompasses a genetically diverse population with various degrees of European, African, and Native American genetic admixture, we sought to evaluate the association between genetic ancestry and methotrexate-related neurotoxicity in a prospective cohort of pediatric patients with ALL. We estimated the proportions of European, African, East Asian, and Native American genetic ancestry using genome-wide genotype data available on 190 pediatric patients with ALL, including 35 individuals with a history of acute and subacute methotrexate-associated neurotoxicity, and publicly available reference populations [13, 14]. The proportion of genetic variation that co-segregates with Native American ancestry was overrepresented in individuals with methotrexate-related neurotoxicity (mean = 34.9%; Fig. 4.2) compared to individuals without a history of neurotoxicity (mean = 23.2%, $p = 0.025$). In multivariable proportional hazards regression models accounting for sex, age at diagnosis, and treatment risk group, every 10% increase in the proportion of Native American genetic ancestry was associated with a 16% increase in neurotoxicity incidence (HR = 1.16; 95% CI: 1.02–1.32). These findings highlight that ethnic-specific differences in inherited genetic variation likely contribute to disparities in the incidence of treatment-related toxicity.

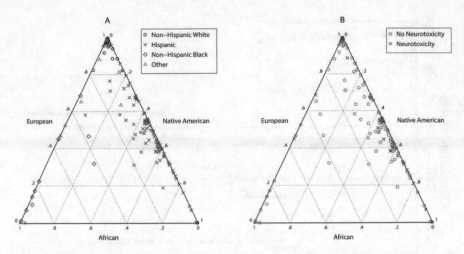

Fig. 4.2 Observed variability in the proportions of African, European, and Native American genetic ancestry among pediatric cases of acute lymphoblastic leukemia by self-reported race/ethnicity (**a**) and the incidence of methotrexate-related neurotoxicity (**b**)

Neurocognitive Late Effects of ALL Therapy

Contemporary treatment protocols for childhood ALL have largely eliminated the use of prophylactic cranial radiation in favor of CNS-directed chemotherapy [4, 15, 16]. Efforts to reduce exposure to cranial radiation have also reduced many adverse effects of ALL therapy, including neurocognitive deficits. Although cognitive functioning in survivors treated with contemporary chemotherapy is better preserved than in those treated with cranial radiation, survivors treated with chemotherapy alone continue to demonstrate deficits relative to their unaffected peers [17–21]. In fact, neurocognitive difficulties are estimated to be one of the most prevalent late effects of childhood ALL chemotherapy, affecting nearly 50% of survivors [22]. Neurocognitive difficulties are commonly detected in the domains of attention, executive functioning, working memory, and processing speed among long-term survivors of childhood ALL [17, 23, 24]. Neurocognitive changes in this population appear to be related to the effects of methotrexate, which have been associated with demyelinating white matter injury and vascular damage in the developing brain. Specifically, survivors treated with chemotherapy only have been found to have total white matter volume loss [25], notably in the frontal [26] and subcortical regions [27], and abnormal or reduced white matter connectivity [27–29], with children diagnosed at younger ages being particularly vulnerable to these adverse effects of treatment [27]. Children and adolescents experiencing clinical findings of acute or subacute methotrexate neurotoxicity during treatment may be at particularly increased risk for long-term neurocognitive deficits [30]. For example, children who experienced seizures during treatment for ALL demonstrated reduced attention, working memory, and processing speed relative to children who did not develop seizures and had normative scores at the end of treatment; additionally, these difficulties persisted over a two-year follow-up period [30]. However, other therapeutic exposures, including anesthesia, have been associated with persistent neurocognitive issues among survivor [31]. These cognitive deficits not only impede learning and academic achievement but also have long-term educational and economic consequences [32–34].

Despite increased incidence of ALL and neurotoxic events during therapy among Latino patients coupled with increased neurocognitive risk among Latinos more broadly, there is an extreme lack of population diversity in neurocognitive outcomes research for pediatric ALL to date. According to recent meta-analyses summarizing sociodemographic factors and neurocognitive outcomes in ALL, only one-third of studies reported the ethnic/racial composition of their sample, and when race/ethnicity was reported, the overwhelming majority (almost 80%) self-identified as White or Caucasian [21, 35]. Two studies have been conducted among Latino cohorts, and they indicate that survivors are at risk for neurocognitive late effects and school-based learning difficulties [36, 37]. Specifically, Latino survivors of pediatric ALL demonstrated reduced performance relative to the normative mean in neurocognitive domains typically affected in non-Latino patients including working memory, processing speed, visual reasoning, executive functioning, and visual learning [37]. In addition, Latino survivors demonstrated reduced verbal reasoning and reading comprehension skills, which are not typically implicated in late effects research of predominantly non-Latino populations. Despite a focus on Latino survivors, models did not account for socioeconomic status (SES), though proxies for the general socioeconomic standing of the sample were described.

Emerging Research Needs

Most models of neurotoxicity in pediatric patients with ALL have focused on clinical predictors, often excluding sociodemographic and molecular factors known to influence neurologic development and outcomes in unaffected populations. For example, neurocognitive abilities of children in the general population are adversely impacted by many factors, including SES and native language [38, 39], which disproportionately affect racial and ethnic minorities. Despite the fact that ethnic disparities in ALL outcomes and toxicity are well documented [3, 11, 40–43], few studies have evaluated neurotoxicity in multiethnic populations, much less evaluated the role of SES and acculturation [24, 36, 37, 44]. Moreover, the considerable inter-patient variability in susceptibility to neurotoxicity might be partly explained by underlying molecular variation. However, the role of these factors in treatment-related neurotoxicity has received limited attention. Additional research on the roles of socioeconomic, cultural, and biologic factors in ethnically diverse populations is needed to advance our understanding of neurological outcomes in vulnerable populations.

Incorporating Information on SES and Acculturation

Survivors of childhood ALL who are from racial/ethnic minority groups and lower SES are at increased risk for cognitive deficits. SES refers to a combination of income, education, and occupation [45]. Therefore, generally speaking, the relationship between ethnicity and neurocognitive outcome is complex, given that ethnicity and SES can be highly related, particularly among Latino families [46]. In particular, Latinos who immigrate to the United States have, on average, a lower SES [47], though there is considerable variability depending on country of origin. For example, Cuban-Americans graduate from college at three times the rate of Mexican-Americans [48]. Among healthy children, associations are documented between SES and cognitive abilities. The domains most affected by SES disparities include language abilities, executive functioning, attention, and memory [38, 39]. Overall, few studies have considered SES in relation to neurocognitive outcome among survivors of childhood leukemia; however, when these factors are considered the observed associations are typically consistent with individuals of lower SES having an increased risk of impairment [49].

Among Latino families, acculturation may simultaneously impact cognitive and academic skill development along with socioeconomic factors, though acculturation is not necessarily related to such factors. Language is an important aspect of determining an individual's level of acculturation. Parent language acculturation in Latino families, namely English proficiency and primary language in the home, is important for children's academic readiness and academic success in higher grades [50, 51]. Furthermore, Latino children whose native language is Spanish perform significantly worse than non-Latino children on the Wechsler Intelligence Scales, the most commonly used measure of intelligence in childhood, with specific adverse effects exhibited on verbal subtests [52]. While there are a number of proxies for acculturation, such as generational status and number of years of US residency, none of them are adequate for providing insight into the influence on the acculturative experience on neurocognitive development and performance.

Molecular Predictors of Neurotoxicity

In addition to variability in patient characteristics and therapeutic exposures, a number of factors likely contribute to disparities in pediatric ALL toxicity and outcomes, including underlying genetic variation. To date, few studies have evaluated inherited single nucleotide variants; however, associations have been reported between clinical neurotoxicity and candidate variants in *SHMT1*, *MTHFR*, and *GSTP1* [53, 54]. In particular, the missense C677T polymorphism in *MTHFR* (rs1801133) has been associated with adverse responses to methotrexate therapy in pediatric and adult patients treated for rheumatoid arthritis and various malignancies [55–57]. Several publications have speculated that inherited variation in *MTHFR* may also contribute to the risk of methotrexate-related neurotoxicity in children with ALL [54, 58], but direct evidence that *MTHFR* genetic variation affects neurotoxicity susceptibility is limited. Compared to individuals who are homozygous for the reference allele (CC), carriers of the alternate allele (CT/TT) exhibit decreased *MTHFR* enzymatic activity and increased plasma homocysteine levels [59]. Homocysteine concentrations are transiently elevated following methotrexate therapy, and cerebrospinal fluid levels of homocysteine have been linked to neurotoxicity in children undergoing treatment of ALL [60, 61]. Notably, the frequency of the C677T missense variant appears to vary across ancestral populations. Based on the 1000 Genomes data [62], the C677T alternate allele frequency is approximately 9.0% in individuals of African ancestry, 36.5% in individuals of European ancestry, and 47.0% in admixed American populations comprised individuals of Latino ethnicity. Additional research is needed to better characterize the genetic contribution to methotrexate-related neurotoxicity and disparities in susceptibility. However, genome-wide association studies have not yet successfully identified and replicated susceptibility loci due to challenges in assembling large cohorts to sufficiently power these studies [4]. Alternative approaches that examine the association between local Native American genetic ancestry and neurotoxicity risk using methods such as admixture mapping may prove more powerful at identifying novel susceptibility loci responsible for the ethnic disparities observed in neurotoxicity risk.

Conclusion

Current treatment strategies for pediatric ALL are associated with acute and long-term neurotoxicity. The incidence of acute and subacute neurotoxicity during pediatric ALL therapy potentially jeopardizes treatment efficacy, while long-term neurocognitive impairment profoundly affects quality of life in survivors of ALL. Emerging evidence indicates that Latino patients may be particularly susceptible to these adverse side effects of therapy. In fact, we recently reported that Latino patients with ALL experience acute and subacute neurotoxic events at a rate far exceeding their non-Latino counterparts [8]. Some evidence suggests that acute toxicity predisposes affected individuals to long-term neurocognitive and behavior complications as survivors [30]; therefore, Latino survivors may be particularly vulnerable. Unfortunately, studies of neurotoxicity during pediatric ALL therapy have largely neglected Latino populations. Future well-designed studies are needed to characterize neurotoxicity outcomes in Latino patients, while considering factors associated with disparities in cognitive performance in the general population, including SES and acculturation. Ultimately, a better understanding of the various factors likely responsible for disparities in neurotoxicity, including inherited genetic variation, clinical characteristics, and sociocultural differences, is needed to improve outcomes for Latino populations.

References

1. Linabery AM, Ross JA. Trends in childhood cancer incidence in the U.S. (1992–2004). Cancer. 2008;112(2):416–32. https://doi.org/10.1002/cncr.23169.
2. Hunger SP, Mullighan CG. Acute lymphoblastic leukemia in children. N Engl J Med. 2015;373(16):1541–52. https://doi.org/10.1056/NEJMra1400972.
3. Kadan-Lottick NS, Ness KK, Bhatia S, Gurney JG. Survival variability by race and ethnicity in childhood acute lymphoblastic leukemia. JAMA. 2003;290(15):2008–14. https://doi.org/10.1001/jama.290.15.2008.
4. Bhojwani D, Sabin ND, Pei D, Yang JJ, Khan RB, Panetta JC, et al. Methotrexate-induced neurotoxicity and leukoencephalopathy in childhood acute lymphoblastic leukemia. J Clin Oncol. 2014;32(9):949–59. https://doi.org/10.1200/jco.2013.53.0808.
5. Mahoney DH Jr, Shuster JJ, Nitschke R, Lauer SJ, Steuber CP, Winick N, et al. Acute neurotoxicity in children with B-precursor acute lymphoid leukemia: an association with intermediate-dose intravenous methotrexate and intrathecal triple therapy--a Pediatric Oncology Group study. J Clin Oncol. 1998;16(5):1712–22. https://doi.org/10.1200/jco.1998.16.5.1712.
6. Afshar M, Birnbaum D, Golden C. Review of dextromethorphan administration in 18 patients with subacute methotrexate central nervous system toxicity. Pediatr Neurol. 2014;50(6):625–9. https://doi.org/10.1016/j.pediatrneurol.2014.01.048.
7. Giordano L, Akinyede O, Bhatt N, Dighe D, Iqbal A. Methotrexate-induced neurotoxicity in Hispanic adolescents with high-risk acute leukemia-A case series. J Adolesc Young Adult Oncol. 2017;6(3):494–8. https://doi.org/10.1089/jayao.2016.0094.
8. Taylor OA, Brown AL, Brackett J, Dreyer ZE, Moore IK, Mitby P, et al. Disparities in neurotoxicity risk and outcomes among pediatric acute lymphoblastic leukemia patients. Clin Cancer Res. 2018;24(20):5012–7. https://doi.org/10.1158/1078-0432.Ccr-18-0939.
9. Magge RS, DeAngelis LM. The double-edged sword: neurotoxicity of chemotherapy. Blood Rev. 2015;29(2):93–100. https://doi.org/10.1016/j.blre.2014.09.012.
10. Dufourg MN, Landman-Parker J, Auclerc MF, Schmitt C, Perel Y, Michel G, et al. Age and high-dose methotrexate are associated to clinical acute encephalopathy in FRALLE 93 trial for acute lymphoblastic leukemia in children. Leukemia. 2007;21(2):238–47. https://doi.org/10.1038/sj.leu.2404495.
11. Yang JJ, Cheng C, Devidas M, Cao X, Fan Y, Campana D, et al. Ancestry and pharmacogenomics of relapse in acute lymphoblastic leukemia. Nat Genet. 2011;43(3):237–41. https://doi.org/10.1038/ng.763.
12. Karol SE, Larsen E, Cheng C, Cao X, Yang W, Ramsey LB, et al. Genetics of ancestry-specific risk for relapse in acute lymphoblastic leukemia. Leukemia. 2017;31(6):1325–32. https://doi.org/10.1038/leu.2017.24.
13. Altshuler DM, Gibbs RA, Peltonen L, Altshuler DM, Gibbs RA, Peltonen L, et al. Integrating common and rare genetic variation in diverse human populations. Nature. 2010;467(7311):52–8. https://doi.org/10.1038/nature09298.
14. Mao X, Bigham AW, Mei R, Gutierrez G, Weiss KM, Brutsaert TD, et al. A genomewide admixture mapping panel for Hispanic/Latino populations. Am J Hum Genet. 2007;80(6):1171–8. https://doi.org/10.1086/518564.
15. Duffner PK, Armstrong FD, Chen L, Helton KJ, Brecher ML, Bell B, et al. Neurocognitive and neuroradiologic central nervous system late effects in children treated on Pediatric Oncology Group (POG) P9605 (standard risk) and P9201 (lesser risk) acute lymphoblastic leukemia protocols (ACCL0131): a methotrexate consequence? A report from the Children's Oncology Group. J Pediatr Hematol Oncol. 2014;36(1):8–15. https://doi.org/10.1097/mph.0000000000000000.
16. Cole PD, Kamen BA. Delayed neurotoxicity associated with therapy for children with acute lymphoblastic leukemia. Ment Retard Dev Disabil Res Rev. 2006;12(3):174–83. https://doi.org/10.1002/mrdd.20113.

17. Conklin HM, Krull KR, Reddick WE, Pei D, Cheng C, Pui CH. Cognitive outcomes following contemporary treatment without cranial irradiation for childhood acute lymphoblastic leukemia. J Natl Cancer Inst. 2012;104(18):1386–95. https://doi.org/10.1093/jnci/djs344.

18. Pui CH, Campana D, Pei D, Bowman WP, Sandlund JT, Kaste SC, et al. Treating childhood acute lymphoblastic leukemia without cranial irradiation. N Engl J Med. 2009;360(26):2730–41. https://doi.org/10.1056/NEJMoa0900386.

19. Peterson CC, Johnson CE, Ramirez LY, Huestis S, Pai AL, Demaree HA, et al. A meta-analysis of the neuropsychological sequelae of chemotherapy-only treatment for pediatric acute lymphoblastic leukemia. Pediatr Blood Cancer. 2008;51(1):99–104. https://doi.org/10.1002/pbc.21544.

20. von der Weid N, Mosimann I, Hirt A, Wacker P, Nenadov Beck M, Imbach P, et al. Intellectual outcome in children and adolescents with acute lymphoblastic leukaemia treated with chemotherapy alone: age- and sex-related differences. Eur J Cancer. 2003;39(3):359–65.

21. Campbell LK, Scaduto M, Sharp W, Dufton L, Van Slyke D, Whitlock JA, et al. A meta-analysis of the neurocognitive sequelae of treatment for childhood acute lymphocytic leukemia. Pediatr Blood Cancer. 2007;49(1):65–73. https://doi.org/10.1002/pbc.20860.

22. Krull KR, Okcu MF, Potter B, Jain N, Dreyer Z, Kamdar K, et al. Screening for neurocognitive impairment in pediatric cancer long-term survivors. J Clin Oncol. 2008;26(25):4138–43. https://doi.org/10.1200/jco.2008.16.8864.

23. Cheung YT, Krull KR. Neurocognitive outcomes in long-term survivors of childhood acute lymphoblastic leukemia treated on contemporary treatment protocols: a systematic review. Neurosci Biobehav Rev. 2015;53:108–20. https://doi.org/10.1016/j.neubiorev.2015.03.016.

24. Jacola LM, Krull KR, Pui CH, Pei D, Cheng C, Reddick WE, et al. Longitudinal assessment of neurocognitive outcomes in survivors of childhood acute lymphoblastic leukemia treated on a contemporary chemotherapy protocol. J Clin Oncol. 2016;34(11):1239–47. https://doi.org/10.1200/jco.2015.64.3205.

25. Reddick WE, Taghipour DJ, Glass JO, Ashford J, Xiong X, Wu S, et al. Prognostic factors that increase the risk for reduced white matter volumes and deficits in attention and learning for survivors of childhood cancers. Pediatr Blood Cancer. 2014;61(6):1074–9. https://doi.org/10.1002/pbc.24947.

26. Carey ME, Haut MW, Reminger SL, Hutter JJ, Theilmann R, Kaemingk KL. Reduced frontal white matter volume in long-term childhood leukemia survivors: a voxel-based morphometry study. AJNR Am J Neuroradiol. 2008;29(4):792–7. https://doi.org/10.3174/ajnr.A0904.

27. Kesler SR, Tanaka H, Koovakkattu D. Cognitive reserve and brain volumes in pediatric acute lymphoblastic leukemia. Brain Imaging Behav. 2010;4(3–4):256–69. https://doi.org/10.1007/s11682-010-9104-1.

28. Aukema EJ, Caan MW, Oudhuis N, Majoie CB, Vos FM, Reneman L, et al. White matter fractional anisotropy correlates with speed of processing and motor speed in young childhood cancer survivors. Int J Radiat Oncol Biol Phys. 2009;74(3):837–43. https://doi.org/10.1016/j.ijrobp.2008.08.060.

29. Khong PL, Leung LH, Fung AS, Fong DY, Qiu D, Kwong DL, et al. White matter anisotropy in post-treatment childhood cancer survivors: preliminary evidence of association with neurocognitive function. J Clin Oncol. 2006;24(6):884–90. https://doi.org/10.1200/jco.2005.02.4505.

30. Nassar SL, Conklin HM, Zhou Y, Ashford JM, Reddick WE, Glass JO, et al. Neurocognitive outcomes among children who experienced seizures during treatment for acute lymphoblastic leukemia. Pediatr Blood Cancer. 2017;64(8). https://doi.org/10.1002/pbc.26436.

31. Banerjee P, Rossi MG, Anghelescu DL, Liu W, Breazeale AM, Reddick WE, et al. Association between anesthesia exposure and neurocognitive and neuroimaging outcomes in long-term survivors of childhood acute lymphoblastic leukemia. JAMA Oncol. 2019;5(10). https://doi.org/10.1001/jamaoncol.2019.1094.

32. Jacola LM, Edelstein K, Liu W, Pui CH, Hayashi R, Kadan-Lottick NS, et al. Cognitive, behaviour, and academic functioning in adolescent and young adult survivors of childhood acute lymphoblastic leukaemia: a report from the Childhood Cancer Survivor Study. Lancet Psychiatry. 2016;3(10):965–72. https://doi.org/10.1016/s2215-0366(16)30283-8.

33. Kanellopoulos A, Andersson S, Zeller B, Tamnes CK, Fjell AM, Walhovd KB, et al. Neurocognitive outcome in very long-term survivors of childhood acute lymphoblastic leukemia after treatment with chemotherapy only. Pediatr Blood Cancer. 2016;63(1):133–8. https://doi.org/10.1002/pbc.25690.

34. Holmqvist AS, Wiebe T, Hjorth L, Lindgren A, Øra I, Moëll C. Young age at diagnosis is a risk factor for negative late socio-economic effects after acute lymphoblastic leukemia in childhood. Pediatr Blood Cancer. 2010;55(4):698–707. https://doi.org/10.1002/pbc.22670.

35. Pierson C, Waite E, Pyykkonen B. A meta-analysis of the neuropsychological effects of chemotherapy in the treatment of childhood cancer. Pediatr Blood Cancer. 2016;63(11):1998–2003. https://doi.org/10.1002/pbc.26117.

36. Patel SK, Lo TT, Dennis JM, Bhatia S. Neurocognitive and behavioral outcomes in Latino childhood cancer survivors. Pediatr Blood Cancer. 2013;60(10):1696–702. https://doi.org/10.1002/pbc.24608.

37. Bava L, Johns A, Kayser K, Freyer DR. Cognitive outcomes among Latino survivors of childhood acute lymphoblastic leukemia and lymphoma: a cross-sectional cohort study using culturally competent, performance-based assessment. Pediatr Blood Cancer. 2018;65(2). https://doi.org/10.1002/pbc.26844.

38. Hackman DA, Farah MJ. Socioeconomic status and the developing brain. Trends Cogn Sci. 2009;13(2):65–73. https://doi.org/10.1016/j.tics.2008.11.003.

39. Lawson GM, Farah MJ. Executive function as a mediator between SES and academic achievement throughout childhood. Int J Behav Dev. 2017;41(1):94–104. https://doi.org/10.1177/0165025415603489.

40. Dores GM, Devesa SS, Curtis RE, Linet MS, Morton LM. Acute leukemia incidence and patient survival among children and adults in the United States, 2001–2007. Blood. 2012;119(1):34–43. https://doi.org/10.1182/blood-2011-04-347872.

41. Bhatia S, Sather HN, Heerema NA, Trigg ME, Gaynon PS, Robison LL. Racial and ethnic differences in survival of children with acute lymphoblastic leukemia. Blood. 2002;100(6):1957–64. https://doi.org/10.1182/blood-2002-02-0395.

42. Lim JY, Bhatia S, Robison LL, Yang JJ. Genomics of racial and ethnic disparities in childhood acute lymphoblastic leukemia. Cancer. 2014;120(7):955–62. https://doi.org/10.1002/cncr.28531.

43. Yang JJ, Landier W, Yang W, Liu C, Hageman L, Cheng C, et al. Inherited NUDT15 variant is a genetic determinant of mercaptopurine intolerance in children with acute lymphoblastic leukemia. J Clin Oncol. 2015;33(11):1235–42. https://doi.org/10.1200/jco.2014.59.4671.

44. Moore IM, Lupo PJ, Insel K, Harris LL, Pasvogel A, Koerner KM, et al. Neurocognitive predictors of academic outcomes among childhood leukemia survivors. Cancer Nurs. 2016;39(4):255–62. https://doi.org/10.1097/ncc.0000000000000293.

45. Adler NE, Stewart J. Preface to the biology of disadvantage: socioeconomic status and health. Ann N Y Acad Sci. 2010;1186:1–4. https://doi.org/10.1111/j.1749-6632.2009.05385.x.

46. Llorente AM. Principles of neuropsychological assessment with Hispanics: theoretical foundations and clinical practice. New York: Springer Science & Business Media; 2007.

47. Advisers CoE. Changing America: indicators of social and economic well-being by race and Hispanic origin. Washington, DC: US Government Printing Office; 1998.

48. Williams DR, Mohammed SA, Leavell J, Collins C. Race, socioeconomic status, and health: complexities, ongoing challenges, and research opportunities. Ann N Y Acad Sci. 2010;1186:69–101. https://doi.org/10.1111/j.1749-6632.2009.05339.x.

49. Hardy KK, Embry L, Kairalla JA, Helian S, Devidas M, Armstrong D, et al. Neurocognitive functioning of children treated for high-risk B-acute lymphoblastic leukemia randomly assigned to different methotrexate and corticosteroid treatment strategies: a report from the Children's Oncology Group. J Clin Oncol. 2017;35(23):2700–7. https://doi.org/10.1200/jco.2016.71.7587.

50. Baker CE. Mexican mothers' English proficiency and children's school readiness: mediation through home literacy involvement. Early Educ Dev. 2014;25(3):338–55.

51. Quiroz BG, Snow CE, Jing Z. Vocabulary skills of Spanish—English bilinguals: impact of mother–child language interactions and home language and literacy support. Int J Biling. 2010;14:379–99.

52. Harris JG, Llorente AM. Cultural considerations in the use of the Wechsler Intelligence Scale for Children—fourth edition (WISC-IV). In: WISC-IV clinical use and interpretation. San Diego: Elsevier; 2005. p. 381–413.
53. Kishi S, Cheng C, French D, Pei D, Das S, Cook EH, et al. Ancestry and pharmacogenetics of antileukemic drug toxicity. Blood. 2007;109(10):4151–7. https://doi.org/10.1182/blood-2006-10-054528.
54. Vagace JM, Caceres-Marzal C, Jimenez M, Casado MS, de Murillo SG, Gervasini G. Methotrexate-induced subacute neurotoxicity in a child with acute lymphoblastic leukemia carrying genetic polymorphisms related to folate homeostasis. Am J Hematol. 2011;86(1):98–101. https://doi.org/10.1002/ajh.21897.
55. Xiao H, Xu J, Zhou X, Stankovich J, Pan F, Zhang Z, et al. Associations between the genetic polymorphisms of MTHFR and outcomes of methotrexate treatment in rheumatoid arthritis. Clin Exp Rheumatol. 2010;28(5):728–33.
56. Yousef AM, Farhad R, Alshamaseen D, Alsheikh A, Zawiah M, Kadi T. Folate pathway genetic polymorphisms modulate methotrexate-induced toxicity in childhood acute lymphoblastic leukemia. Cancer Chemother Pharmacol. 2019;83(4):755–62. https://doi.org/10.1007/s00280-019-03776-8.
57. Zhao M, Liang L, Ji L, Chen D, Zhang Y, Zhu Y, et al. MTHFR gene polymorphisms and methotrexate toxicity in adult patients with hematological malignancies: a meta-analysis. Pharmacogenomics. 2016;17(9):1005–17. https://doi.org/10.2217/pgs-2016-0004.
58. Muller J, Kralovanszky J, Adleff V, Pap E, Nemeth K, Komlosi V, et al. Toxic encephalopathy and delayed MTX clearance after high-dose methotrexate therapy in a child homozygous for the MTHFR C677T polymorphism. Anticancer Res. 2008;28(5b):3051–4.
59. Frosst P, Blom HJ, Milos R, Goyette P, Sheppard CA, Matthews RG, et al. A candidate genetic risk factor for vascular disease: a common mutation in methylenetetrahydrofolate reductase. Nat Genet. 1995;10(1):111–3. https://doi.org/10.1038/ng0595-111.
60. Kishi S, Griener J, Cheng C, Das S, Cook EH, Pei D, et al. Homocysteine, pharmacogenetics, and neurotoxicity in children with leukemia. J Clin Oncol. 2003;21(16):3084–91. https://doi.org/10.1200/jco.2003.07.056.
61. Quinn CT, Griener JC, Bottiglieri T, Hyland K, Farrow A, Kamen BA. Elevation of homocysteine and excitatory amino acid neurotransmitters in the CSF of children who receive methotrexate for the treatment of cancer. J Clin Oncol. 1997;15(8):2800–6. https://doi.org/10.1200/jco.1997.15.8.2800.
62. Auton A, Brooks LD, Durbin RM, Garrison EP, Kang HM, Korbel JO, et al. A global reference for human genetic variation. Nature. 2015;526(7571):68–74. https://doi.org/10.1038/nature15393.

Open Access This chapter is licensed under the terms of the Creative Commons Attribution 4.0 International License (http://creativecommons.org/licenses/by/4.0/), which permits use, sharing, adaptation, distribution and reproduction in any medium or format, as long as you give appropriate credit to the original author(s) and the source, provide a link to the Creative Commons license and indicate if changes were made.

The images or other third party material in this chapter are included in the chapter's Creative Commons license, unless indicated otherwise in a credit line to the material. If material is not included in the chapter's Creative Commons license and your intended use is not permitted by statutory regulation or exceeds the permitted use, you will need to obtain permission directly from the copyright holder.

Part IV
Cancer Outcomes and Survivorship in Latinos

Part IV
Cancer Outcomes and Survivorship
in Latinos

Chapter 5
Supportive Care Needs and Coping Strategies Used by Latino Men Cancer Survivors

Dinorah Martinez Tyson and Erik L. Ruiz

Introduction

Over 1.8 million Americans will be diagnosed and over 600,000 are estimated to die from cancer by the end of 2020, making it the second leading cause of death in the United States [1]. Modern developments in cancer treatment have facilitated increased survival, and there is a growing population of cancer survivors that is expected to reach 18 million within the next decade [2, 3]. Cancer survivors may experience long-term physical and psychosocial effects which extend beyond the treatment phase and which require additional supportive care to cope with these effects and enhance quality of life [1, 4–7].

In this chapter we will provide a brief overview of the epidemiology of cancer within the US Hispanic population with a specific focus on health disparities experienced by Hispanic men cancer survivors (HMCS). Next, we explore the emerging themes derived from research of the cultural, social, and environmental supportive care needs of HMCS and the coping mechanisms they use. Finally, we propose implications for research and practice for those working with HMCS. In this chapter we will use the terms Hispanic/Latino and Latinx interchangeably. While we recognize the term Latinx has recently emerged, many of the communities we work with still prefer and use the terms Hispanic/Latino.

D. Martinez Tyson (✉) · E. L. Ruiz
College of Public Health, University of South Florida, Tampa, FL, USA
e-mail: dmtyson@usf.edu; elruiz@usf.edu

© The Author(s) 2023
A. G. Ramirez, E. J. Trapido (eds.), *Advancing the Science of Cancer in Latinos*, https://doi.org/10.1007/978-3-031-14436-3_5

57

Epidemiology of Cancer Within the Latinx Population

Overall, Hispanics in the United States experience lower incidence and mortality rates of most cancers compared to other racial and ethnic groups within the nation; however, they experience a significantly higher rate of infection-associated cancers including cervical, liver, and gastrointestinal [1]. It should be noted that the Hispanic population is not homogeneous; cancer incidence, morbidity, mortality rates, and quality of life can vary by a Hispanic person's country of origin, generational status, and time spent in the United States. For example, US Hispanic men are 85% more likely to die from stomach cancer than non-Hispanic Whites [8]. Additionally, when compared to US non-Hispanic White men, Cuban born men experience higher incidence and mortality rates of prostate cancer, and the incidence of colorectal cancers has been observed to be lower for Hispanics with low socioeconomic status (SES) compared to those with high SES [8–10]. Finally, whereas the population of Hispanic cancer survivors is growing, the psychosocial distress experienced by these survivors also varies according to sociocultural factors; more acculturated US Hispanics have reported a lower quality of life than less acculturated Hispanics due in part to a lack of supportive care [10–12].

Disparities in Diagnosis and Survivorship

Although US Hispanics experience lower incidence rates of most cancer types, they do suffer from disproportionately high barriers to care access and have lower cancer survival rates when compared to non-Hispanic Whites [11, 13–16]. For example, 18% of US Hispanics are likely to be uninsured compared to only 5% of non-Hispanic Whites, which can make US Hispanics vulnerable to delayed cancer diagnosis, resulting in more involved, costlier, and potentially less successful treatments [1]. Similarly, Hispanic men and women experience lower rates of cancer-related mortality compared to their non-Hispanic counterparts. However, Hispanic men of all country-of-origin subgroups experience higher incidence rates of all cancer types, except gallbladder cancer, and higher rates of cancer-related mortality compared to Hispanic women [13, 17]. Special attention to the supportive care needs of Hispanic men is required as they are a part of the largest ethnic minority group in the United States and their number of cancer survivors continues to grow [15, 18]. The remainder of this chapter focuses on understanding the supportive care needs of Hispanic men cancer survivors and describes how they cope with cancer. At the end of the chapter, we describe strategies to address these identified needs.

Supportive Care Needs of Hispanic Men Cancer Survivors

Hispanic men report worse cancer-related morbidities including reduced sexual and physical functioning, increased bowel-related issues, decreased quality of life, and worse mental health outcomes compared to their non-White male counterparts [19–22]. These poor conditions are further complicated by disparities in and access to culturally competent care, health information exchange, and disease management education [4, 19]. Additionally, compared to Hispanic women, Hispanic men who have been diagnosed with cancer may have more psychosocial needs and tend to engage less with supportive care services [23, 24]. Finally, there is a dearth of data and research pertaining to the supportive care needs of HMCS, so the full extent of their needs both during and after cancer treatment is not yet fully understood.

An emerging body of research has sought to capture the unique needs of Hispanic men diagnosed with cancer [10, 14, 15, 25]. We draw on findings from recent research that has sought to explore and understand the needs of HMCS. A detailed description of the mixed methods used is described elsewhere [26–29]. The overarching themes expressed by HMCS include the needs: for better communication with providers and for culturally competent care; for comprehensive survivorship care and more cancer treatment-related information; to still provide for their family and also navigate changing gender role expectations; and to connect with other cancer survivors.

Need for Better Communication with Providers and for Culturally Competent Care

HMCS discussed the need for culturally competent care; they specifically identified language barriers which inhibit communication relating to care, barriers associated with the use of interpreters, and a lack of *confianza* (confidence in the personal relationship with the care provider) [28]. HMCS who mentioned language barriers cited a need for bilingual communication of cancer-specific treatment information due in part to a lack of confidence in their English-speaking abilities which inhibited them from asking clarifying questions. Furthermore, even with the use of a bilingual interpreter, some HMCS had reservations about their care as they expressed a lack of confidence that the interpreter was accurately describing their sentiments and concerns. An additional element that surfaced was the importance of having *confianza* (trust) and *personalismo* (friendly and personal relationships) with providers, which allows men to build rapport and be able to talk more openly with providers. This affects disclosure of potentially important information about treatment side effect management [28].

Need for Comprehensive Survivorship Care and More Cancer Treatment-Related Information

In addition to cancer recurrence, the major concerns and sources of stress discussed by participants were related to not having enough information about the availability of other treatment options and/or alternative/complimentary medicine, the treatment they received, and the long-term side effects (e.g., impotency, incontinence, and fatigue) [28]. Additionally, many HMCS participants indicated that they lacked understanding of posttreatment care and follow-up, including additional cancer screenings that may need to be done. Many HMCS felt as if the care they received for their cancer should have been more comprehensive and holistic with goals which extended beyond treatment and that were more focused on maintaining overall health and well-being.

Need to Provide for Family While Navigating Changing Gender Role Expectations

HMCS identified impairment of both physical and social aspects of their masculine identities [28]. Common physical complaints centered around impotence and incontinence (potential side effects of prostate cancer treatments), whereas common social complaints identified were the financial and emotional burden placed on female family members due to employment changes or the physical demands of cancer treatments. Both physical and social concerns troubled HMCS because they brought into question their traditional masculine roles in their families, and many HMCS did not feel they were equipped to navigate those expectations.

Need to Connect with Other Cancer Survivors

Finally, HMCS expressed a need to socialize with other HMCS in order to connect and *distraerse* (to distract themselves) through the discussion of shared experiences in the final emergent needs-based theme [28]. Some HMCS indicated that the only time they had discussed their cancer process with other HMCS was during the interview or focus groups for this study. We observed that participants openly shared their experiences and concerns without inhibition. They expressed a desire to connect with others who had gone through similar experiences.

Data from the S-CaSUN survey (Table 5.1) show that the most highly endorsed items included needs related to comprehensive care/provider communication (46% said yes to their worries about their health being adequately addressed and 45% need to feel their opinion is important to their doctors), information needs and emotional support (42% said they need more information about follow-up care that is

Table 5.1 Key supportive care needs of Hispanic men cancer survivors taken from the 37 question S-CaSUN survey [26]

Selected supportive care needs of Hispanic men cancer survivors (N = 84)				
During the last month I have needed:	No (%)	Yes, a little (%)	Yes, somewhat (%)	Yes, a lot (%)
That my worries about my health are adequately addressed	53.6	9.5	13.1	23.8
To feel that my opinion is important to my doctor	54.8	9.5	16.7	19.0
More information about the follow-up care that I need and how often I should see the doctor	58.3	7.1	19.0	15.5
Help with my concerns about the cancer coming back	65.1	6.0	15.7	13.3
Help to deal with the impact that cancer has had on my relationship with my partner	65.5	10.7	9.5	14.3

needed), and existential survivorship (35% said they need help with their concerns about cancer coming back and knowledge about what to do to stay healthy) [26]. With regards to interpersonal/partner-related issues, 35% said they needed help to deal with the impact that cancer has had on the relationship with their partner.

Coping Mechanisms for Hispanic Men Cancer Survivors

Next, we will describe the coping mechanisms of HMCS in response to their cancer diagnosis, which include maintaining a positive attitude, optimism, humor, faith, incorporation of home remedies into the broader care plan, and lifestyle changes [29]. Having a positive outlook and utilizing optimism and humor were identified as important factors in navigating through a successful care plan after the initial shock of cancer diagnosis. In this way, HMCS felt that the overall attitude was a significant factor in succumbing to or overcoming the disease process. Having faith in God was also observed to be a significant coping mechanism as HMCS perceived their faith to facilitate positive cancer treatment outcomes. Finally, incorporating home remedies and engaging in lifestyle changes, including diet and exercise, were important coping mechanisms for HMCS, as they provided a sense of agency and self-efficacy over their cancer diagnosis and treatment processes. HMCS identified relying on their social support systems, both proximate and distal family members, as an important mechanism to alleviate the feeling of isolation associated with their cancer diagnosis and also as a way to facilitate the physical and logistical demands of attending appointments, receiving treatment, and managing treatment side effects. Similarly, maintaining a positive and supportive relationship between the HMCS and their care provider was identified as an essential coping mechanism because the care provider's attitude throughout the cancer treatment process carried a significant weight on the HMCS' positive outlook as it reduced their perceived stress.

Implications for Research and Practice

Innovative public health research and practice is essential for addressing the disparities in supportive care needs experienced by HMCS. This work will require the focused efforts of public health researchers, practitioners, HMCS, Latinx community stakeholders, and care providers in order to identify and implement culturally relevant interventions, which may reduce the illness burden of HMCS. Efforts should center on provision of culturally competent care delivery, transcreation of existing evidence-based interventions to engage and meet the psychosocial needs of HMCS, and the dissemination of research findings to Latinx community members to address the health information needs of HMCS and their families. We also need to develop programs that build on the strengths of the Latino community and facilitate opportunities for HMCS to connect with one another and build their support networks to relieve the burden of isolation frequently experienced by HMCS [30–32].

Our findings illustrate the importance of health-care provider communication through listening and building a relationship built on trust with both the HMCS and their families. We also need to address the survivorship care planning needs of HMCS and provide ample health information and psychosocial resources to ease the transition from cancer treatment to survivorship and to enhance quality of life. Finally, public health practitioners in clinical settings should evaluate the role of interpreters in HMCS care as they are pivotal to successful patient-provider communication for both monolingual and bilingual Spanish-speaking patients. We need to ensure that the physical, psychosocial, and supportive care needs of HMCS are adequately addressed.

Conclusion

Although US Hispanics experience lower incidence of most cancer types, cancer remains a leading health burden for the population, particularly for Hispanic men. Additionally, disparities in access to care and delayed diagnoses pose continuing threats to the health of Hispanics in the United States. Furthermore, advances in cancer treatment have facilitated the growth of the HMCS population, which experiences unique supportive care needs and coping styles, many of which remain unaccounted for and unaddressed. We need to build on and recognize community strengths and acknowledge personal agency and coping strategies that will enable HMCS to not only survive but thrive after a cancer diagnosis and treatment.

Acknowledgments A special thanks to the members of our community advisory board, LUNA Inc., Hispanic Health Initiatives, *Creando Conciencia por Reina*, Dr. Pow-Sang, Mr. Jim West, Dr. Cathy Meade, Dr. Paul Jacobsen, and the Tampa Bay Community Cancer Network. This work was supported by the NCI under Grant R03CA168403. The content is solely the responsibility of the authors and does not necessarily represent the official views of the National Institutes of Health.

References

1. American Cancer Society. Cancer facts and figures 2020. Atlanta: American Cancer Society; 2020.
2. Fitzmaurice C, Dicker D, Pain A, Hamavid H, Moradi-Lakeh M, MacIntyre MF, et al. The global burden of cancer 2013. JAMA Oncol. 2015;1(4):505–27. https://doi.org/10.1001/jamaoncol.2015.0735.
3. Hodgkinson K, Butow P, Hunt GE, Pendlebury S, Hobbs KM, Lo SK, et al. The development and evaluation of a measure to assess cancer survivors' unmet supportive care needs: the CaSUN (Cancer Survivors' Unmet Needs measure). Psychooncology. 2007;16(9):796–804. https://doi.org/10.1002/pon.1137.
4. Adler NE, Page AEK. Cancer care for the whole patient meeting psychosocial health needs. Washington: The National Academies Press; 2008.
5. de Moor JS, Mariotto AB, Parry C, Alfano CM, Padgett L, Kent EE, et al. Cancer survivors in the United States: prevalence across the survivorship trajectory and implications for care. Cancer Epidemiol Biomark Prev. 2013;22(4):561–70. https://doi.org/10.1158/1055-9965.EPI-12-1356.
6. Hui D, De La Cruz M, Mori M, Parsons HA, Kwon JH, Torres-Vigil I, et al. Concepts and definitions for "supportive care," "best supportive care," "palliative care," and "hospice care" in the published literature, dictionaries, and textbooks. Support Care Cancer. 2013;21(3):659–85. https://doi.org/10.1007/s00520-012-1564-y.
7. Martinez Tyson D. The social context of stress and social support among immigrant Latinas diagnosed with breast cancer. Tampa. University of South Florida; 2008.
8. Pinheiro PS, Callahan KE, Siegel RL, Jin H, Morris CR, Trapido EJ, et al. Cancer mortality in Hispanic ethnic groups. Cancer Epidemiol Biomark Prev. 2017;26(3):376–82. https://doi.org/10.1158/1055-9965.EPI-16-0684.
9. Baquero B, Parra-Medina DM. Chronic disease and the Latinx population: threats, challenges, and opportunities. In: Martinez AD, Rhodes SD, editors. New and emerging issues in Latinx health. Cham: Springer Nature AG; 2020. p. 19–45.
10. Yanez B, McGinty HL, Buitrago D, Ramirez AG, Penedo FJ. Cancer outcomes in Hispanics/Latinos in the United States: an integrative review and conceptual model of determinants of health. J Lat Psychol. 2016;4(2):114–29. https://doi.org/10.1037/lat0000055.
11. Alcalá HE. Differential mental health impact of cancer across racial/ethnic groups: findings from a population-based study in California. BMC Public Health. 2014;14:930. https://doi.org/10.1186/1471-2458-14-930.
12. Stephens C, Stein K, Landrine H. The role of acculturation in life satisfaction among Hispanic cancer survivors: results of the American Cancer Society's study of cancer survivors. Psychooncology. 2010;19(4):376–83. https://doi.org/10.1002/pon.1566.
13. Martinez Tyson D, Medina-Ramirez P, Flores AM, Siegel R, Aguado LC. Unpacking Hispanic ethnicity-cancer mortality differentials among Hispanic subgroups in the United States, 2004–2014. Front Public Health. 2018;6:219.
14. Moreno PI, Ramirez AG, San Miguel-Majors SL, Fox RS, Castillo L, Gallion KJ, et al. Satisfaction with cancer care, self-efficacy, and health-related quality of life in Latino cancer survivors. Cancer. 2018;124(8):1770–9. https://doi.org/10.1002/cncr.31263.
15. Penedo FJ, Yanez B, Wortman K, Castaneda SF, Gonzalez P, Gallo L, et al. Self-reported cancer prevalence among Hispanics in the US: results from the Hispanic community health study/study of Latinos. PLoS One. 2016;11(1):e0146268.
16. Siegel R, Naishadham D, Jemal A. Cancer statistics, 2013. CA Cancer J Clin. 2013;63(1):11–30. https://doi.org/10.3322/caac.21166.
17. Miller KD, Goding Sauer A, Ortiz AP, Fedewa SA, Pinheiro PS, Tortolero-Luna G, et al. Cancer statistics for Hispanics/Latinos, 2018. CA Cancer J Clin. 2018;68(6):425–45. https://doi.org/10.3322/caac.21494.

18. Siegel RL, Fedewa SA, Miller KD, Goding-Sauer A, Pinheiro PS, Martinez-Tyson D, et al. Cancer statistics for Hispanics/Latinos, 2015. CA Cancer J Clin. 2015;65(6):457–80. https://doi.org/10.3322/caac.21314.
19. Gore JL, Krupski T, Kwan L, Fink A, Litwin MS. Mental health of low income uninsured men with prostate cancer. J Urol. 2005;173(4):1323–6. https://doi.org/10.1097/01.ju.0000152312.28002.ad.
20. Krupski TL, Sonn G, Kwan L, Maliski S, Fink A, Litwin MS. Ethnic variation in health-related quality of life among low-income men with prostate cancer. Ethn Dis. 2005;15(3):461–8.
21. Ramsey SD, Zeliadt SB, Hall IJ, Ekwueme DU, Penson DF. On the importance of race, socio-economic status and comorbidity when evaluating quality of life in men with prostate cancer. J Urol. 2007;177(6):1992–9.
22. Traeger L, Penedo FJ, Gonzalez JS, Dahn JR, Lechner SC, Schneiderman N, et al. Illness perceptions and emotional well-being in men treated for localized prostate cancer. J Psychosom Res. 2009;67(5):389–97. https://doi.org/10.1016/j.jpsychores.2009.03.013.
23. Im EO, Chee W, Guevara E, Lim HJ, Liu Y, Shin H. Gender and ethnic differences in cancer patients' needs for help: an internet survey. Int J Nurs Stud. 2008;45(8):1192–204. https://doi.org/10.1016/j.ijnurstu.2007.09.006.
24. Lintz K, Moynihan C, Steginga S, Norman A, Eeles R, Huddart R, et al. Prostate cancer patients' support and psychological care needs: survey from a non-surgical oncology clinic. Psychooncology. 2003;12(8):769–83. https://doi.org/10.1002/pon.702.
25. Valdovinos C, Penedo FJ, Isasi CR, Jung M, Kaplan RC, Giacinto RE, et al. Perceived discrimination and cancer screening behaviors in US Hispanics: the Hispanic Community Health Study/Study of Latinos Sociocultural Ancillary Study. Cancer Causes Control. 2016;27(1):27–37. https://doi.org/10.1007/s10552-015-0679-0.
26. Martinez Tyson D, Medina-Ramirez P, Vazquez-Otero C, Gwede CK, Babilonia MB, McMillan SC. Initial evaluation of the validity and reliability of the culturally adapted Spanish CaSUN (S-CaSUN). J Cancer Surviv. 2018;12(4):509–18. https://doi.org/10.1007/s11764-018-0689-5.
27. Martinez Tyson D, Medina-Ramirez P, Vazquez-Otero C, Gwede CK, Bobonis M, McMillan SC. Cultural adaptation of a supportive care needs measure for Hispanic men cancer survivors. J Psychosoc Oncol. 2018;36(1):113–31. https://doi.org/10.1080/07347332.2017.1370763.
28. Martinez Tyson DD, Vazquez-Otero C, Medina-Ramirez P, Arriola NB, McMillan SC, Gwede CK. Understanding the supportive care needs of Hispanic men cancer survivors. Ethn Health. 2017;22(1):1–16. https://doi.org/10.1080/13557858.2016.1196649.
29. Sommariva S, Vázquez-Otero C, Medina-Ramirez P, Aguado Loi C, Fross M, Dias E, et al. Hispanic male cancer survivors' coping strategies. Hisp J Behav Sci. 2019;41(2):267–84. https://doi.org/10.1177/0739986319840658.
30. Napoles AM, Stewart AL. Transcreation: an implementation science framework for community-engaged behavioral interventions to reduce health disparities. BMC Health Serv Res. 2018;18(1):710. https://doi.org/10.1186/s12913-018-3521-z.
31. Nápoles AM. A vision for improving quality of life among Spanish-speaking Latina breast cancer survivors. In: Ramirez AG, Trapido EJ, editors. Advancing the science of cancer in Latinos. Cham: Springer International Publishing; 2020. p. 157–65.
32. Pineiro B, Diaz DR, Monsalve LM, Martinez U, Meade CD, Meltzer LR, et al. Systematic transcreation of self-help smoking cessation materials for Hispanic/Latino smokers: improving cultural relevance and acceptability. J Health Commun. 2018;23(4):350–9. https://doi.org/10.1080/10810730.2018.1448487.

Open Access   This chapter is licensed under the terms of the Creative Commons Attribution 4.0 International License (http://creativecommons.org/licenses/by/4.0/), which permits use, sharing, adaptation, distribution and reproduction in any medium or format, as long as you give appropriate credit to the original author(s) and the source, provide a link to the Creative Commons license and indicate if changes were made.

The images or other third party material in this chapter are included in the chapter's Creative Commons license, unless indicated otherwise in a credit line to the material. If material is not included in the chapter's Creative Commons license and your intended use is not permitted by statutory regulation or exceeds the permitted use, you will need to obtain permission directly from the copyright holder.

Chapter 6
Cancer Care Delivery Among Breast Cancer Patients: Is it the Same for All?

Catalina Malinowski and Mariana Chavez Mac Gregor

Introduction

Breast cancer is the most common cancer among women worldwide [1]. In the United States, it also represents the most common cancer in women – in 2019, it is estimated that 268,600 women were diagnosed with invasive breast cancer and 41,760 died of the disease. Among Hispanic women, breast cancer is the most common cancer accounting for close to 30% of the total cancer cases. It is estimated that in 2018 alone, 24,000 Hispanics were diagnosed with invasive breast cancer [2]. Of significant importance is that breast cancer is the leading cause of cancer death (16%) among Hispanic women, with over 3000 patients dying in 2018 secondary to this disease [2].

Despite the decrease in breast cancer mortality rates seen in recent years, the magnitude of that decrease among Hispanics is lower compared to the decrease seen among non-Hispanic White women [3]. Potential contributing factors associated with this phenomenon include the fact that Hispanics are more likely to be diagnosed with more advanced stages and to have tumors with aggressive biology. In addition, sociodemographic factors and difficulty accessing medical care are likely to play an important role. It has been described that Hispanic women are less likely than non-Hispanic Whites to receive appropriate and timely breast cancer treatment [4]. Unfortunately, cancer care delivery is not the same for all and this can seriously hinder the cancer outcomes of those affected. In this chapter, we will discuss the complexities associated with breast cancer treatment and some of the challenges in

C. Malinowski
Health Services Research Department, The University of Texas MD Anderson Cancer Center, Houston, TX, USA

M. Chavez Mac Gregor (✉)
Health Services Research Department, Breast Medical Oncology Department, The University of Texas MD Anderson Cancer Center, Houston, TX, USA
e-mail: Mchavez1@mdanderson.org

© The Author(s) 2023
A. G. Ramirez, E. J. Trapido (eds.), *Advancing the Science of Cancer in Latinos*, https://doi.org/10.1007/978-3-031-14436-3_6

cancer care delivery that Hispanics experience. In addition, we will expand on data describing the detrimental impact that treatment delays can have among minorities and some of the unique challenges that Hispanics experience.

Understanding the Magnitude of the Problem: Breast Cancer

Breast cancer is the deadliest cancer among women worldwide, with a total of over half a million deaths annually impacting both developed and developing countries [1]. There are an estimated 912,930 new cancer cases expected to occur in the United States in 2020 – breast cancer alone is projected to account for 30% of these cases despite numbers accounting solely for cases among women. With an esti-mated 276,480 breast cancer cases projected to occur in women, it is estimated that 42,170 women will die in 2020 due to this devastating disease [5].

Currently, one in eight women in the United States are likely to develop breast cancer in their lifetime [5]. While a decrease in breast cancer incidence is being seen overall due to continued screening efforts and therapeutic improvements, this trend is disparate across race and ethnicity. Hispanics make up the largest minority group in the United States with a population that is expected to double over the next four decades [2]. Although Hispanic women experience lower breast cancer incidence compared to Blacks and non-Hispanic Whites (93.9, 126.7, and 130.8 per 100,000, respectively) [5], the projected population growth coupled with increasing lifestyle risk factors through acculturation could contribute to a higher breast cancer inci-dence and mortality overall.

Breast Cancer Outcomes in Minorities: Why the Difference?

Despite minority groups having lower rates of breast cancer incidence among women, Black and Hispanic women are more likely to: (1) be diagnosed with more aggressive forms of breast cancer [4], (2) experience higher rates of delays in breast cancer treatment, and (3) have worse survival outcomes compared to their non-Hispanic White counterparts [4, 6]. In order to better explain the differences in breast cancer outcomes among minorities, we must analyze this phenomenon through the complex interaction of social, cultural, and structural factors between minorities and the health-care system.

One of the cornerstones of breast cancer control is early detection of abnormali-ties to improve outcomes and survival – yet there are significant differences in adherence to screening guidelines among Hispanic, Black, and non-Hispanic White women, with foreign-born women being less likely to have ever had a mammogram [7, 8]. According to the last mammography utilization rates reported by the Center for Disease Control in 2015, Black and non-Hispanic White women both have higher breast cancer screening rates (69.7% and 65.8%, respectively) than Hispanics (60.9%), reported as the percent of women having had a mammogram in the last 2 years [9]. The disparity in screening among foreign-born women compared to US-born women is even greater (88.3% compared to 94.1%), with even lower rates of screening among recently immigrated women (76.4%) [8].

Hispanics in particular are more likely to not adhere to screening guidelines, be diagnosed with advanced stages of disease, have longer time to definitive diagnosis and treatment initiation, and experience poorer quality of life relative to non-Hispanic Whites [3]. Inequities in cancer and quality of life outcomes are impacted by intermediate and modifiable targets that act as barriers to accessing breast cancer treatment, including but not limited to psychosocial, health care, cancer-specific, medical factors, and cultural factors [10].

It has been reported that foreign-born minorities experience a unique process of acculturation in regard to American culture and lifestyle [10, 11]. Acculturation is a multidimensional process of culture change among Hispanics through integration of cultural values and habits of their surrounding social environment relative to their native culture. Interestingly, studies have revealed that acculturation carries both positive and negative impacts on health outcomes.

Benefits of acculturation can encompass an increase in English literacy and the ability to communicate with health-care providers as well as a shift in cultural perspectives of susceptibility to disease, all of which can increase breast cancer screening among Hispanic women. However, acculturation can also have detrimental impacts on breast cancer outcomes among Hispanics by assumption of lifestyle behaviors similar to those of American women which has been studied as a possible factor in the stagnancy of decreasing incidence rates among Hispanic women beyond nonadherence to screening [6, 10].

Foreign-born Hispanics experience a unique protective benefit from a combination of their native values and lifestyle factors, a phenomenon referred to as the Hispanic paradox [10, 12]. The Hispanic paradox emerged from observations showing that middle-aged to elderly Hispanics had similar or improved mortality compared to their non-Hispanic White counterparts [13]. This immigrant paradox highlights the negative impacts of acculturation on foreign-born Hispanic's health outcomes. The Hispanic paradox suggests significant correlations between varying levels of American acculturation, socioeconomic factors, and native cultural factors influencing health statuses [12]. Recent research suggests that the benefits from the Hispanic paradox may also carry over to cancer outcomes [10].

Is Breast Cancer Care Delivery Equal for All?

Breast Cancer Treatment, Biology, and Social Factors

Today, a large proportion of patients with early-stage breast cancer are cured due to the high effectiveness of breast cancer treatment. Breast cancer treatment by nature is multidisciplinary and most patients receive multi-modality treatment, usually including surgery, radiation therapy, and systemic therapy (chemotherapy, targeted therapy, and endocrine therapy) [3]. The complex, and in many cases long, treatments that are needed to achieve the desired outcomes force patients to face issues associated with navigating the health-care system, timely treatment, and adherence.

It is well known that breast cancer is a biologically heterogenous disease. While it is possible that some biological features are different among Hispanic populations, many cancer-specific biological factors are not well studied in Hispanic populations [10]. Evaluating biological or molecular characteristics of cancer in Hispanics is inherently challenging, given the great heterogeneity and diversity that defines Hispanics and Latinx populations. Despite this, our group and many others have tried to determine whether the differences in outcomes seen among Hispanics can be explained based on biological factors alone.

In a study evaluating 2074 breast cancer patients treated with similar preoperative (neoadjuvant) chemotherapy regimens, we determined that after adjusting for breast cancer subtype, the rates of complete pathological response were not different among Hispanics, suggesting that treatment effect is not associated with race or ethnicity [14]. Similarly, using transcriptional profiling in a cohort of 376 breast cancer patients, unsupervised hierarchical clustering of protein expression data showed no distinct clusters by race. An analysis of patients registered to participate in phase II/III clinical trials showed that when Hispanic breast cancer patients receive uniform treatment and follow-up in a highly controlled setting, no differences in survival are observed when compared to non-Hispanics [15]. This study emphasizes that when Hispanic cancer patients receive state-of-the-art treatment, disparate outcomes among race and ethnicity groups are reduced. The evidence described above suggests that differential outcomes are not derived from differences in biology or differential treatment, but rather that social determinants of health are at the root of the problem.

Social determinants of health encompass a complex interplay of factors. The place where an individual lives, learns, and works influences a wide range of health decisions, risks, and both quality-of-life and health outcomes [16]. Among some Hispanics, issues like lower rates of economic stability, language differences, low health literacy, and lack of access to regular medical services and/or health insurance determine poor health outcomes [17]. For Hispanic women, some of these social determinants and their interconnections are shown in Fig. 6.1, which graphically depicts how all these factors can have a critical impact on breast cancer outcomes.

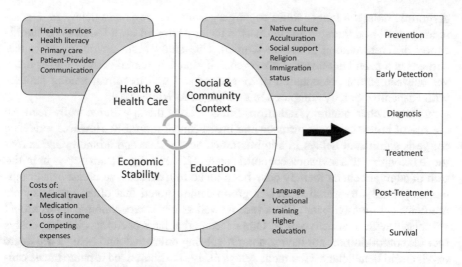

Fig. 6.1 Schematic representation of sociodemographic factors that impact Hispanic women through the breast cancer care continuum

Ideally, the first steps in cancer care include prevention and early detection. Breast cancer screening programs are aimed at evaluating healthy women prior to the presentation of symptoms to detect abnormalities at an early stage. Hispanic women tend to have low screening rates, a phenomenon has been connected to cultural factors, financial factors, and limited access to health care [10, 18]. Given the low participation rates in screening programs, many Hispanic women begin their breast cancer journey after symptoms have presented, most commonly the detection of a palpable mass [6]. The difference between screening and diagnosis based on symptoms can have a significant impact on cancer outcomes, as presentation of symptoms can indicate breast cancer that has progressed to a more advanced stage. Advanced presentation of cancer is not confined to older Hispanic women, as younger Hispanic women tend to experience diagnostic delays due to providers' lack of suspicion of cancer at first presentation [19]. Suboptimal cancer care disproportionately impacts Hispanic patients throughout the continuum of breast cancer treatments [20].

The Impact of Treatment Delays

Treatment delays have been known to have significant detrimental impacts on survival outcomes among vulnerable populations [10, 21–23]. Shortened times to surgery along with timely initiation and administration of treatment can be a turning point for survival outcomes [24] – yet treatment delays persist. Hispanic women's disparate experience with cancer care does not stop at screening nonadherence or diagnostic delays – longer times to surgery from diagnosis and delays in chemo-therapy, radiation therapy, and endocrine therapy have all been found to be signifi-cantly different among Hispanic women. One study focusing on breast cancer patients in a safety net hospital observed 3.38 times increased odds of longer inter-val between initial presentation of symptoms and first treatment among patients with Hispanic ethnicity compared to non-Hispanic Whites [20].

Adjuvant chemotherapy, radiation, and endocrine therapy dramatically decrease the risk of breast cancer recurrence and breast cancer mortality. However, evidence suggests significant delays in administration across race and ethnicity and across those belonging to a low socioeconomic status [25–27]. Significant delays in initia-tion of adjuvant chemotherapy have been found to have adverse breast cancer out-comes [21–23]. Research from our group demonstrated that older age, Hispanic ethnicity, and non-Hispanic Black race as well as low socioeconomic status are all associated with treatment delays. Other factors that have been associated to delays include comorbidities, not having a partner, being uninsured, and being a Medicare or Medicaid beneficiary. Treatment delays likely contributed to Hispanic breast can-cer patients having 1.53 higher risk of experiencing worse overall survival and 1.27 higher risk of worse breast-cancer specific survival compared to Whites [21–23].

Since patients that experience delays in the administration of chemotherapy are at an increased risk of death, every effort should be made to understand and remove barriers associated with treatment delays. However, in order to fully understand this complex phenomenon, it is imperative to evaluate factors at the operational, medi-cal, and personal/social level. Our group is currently recruiting participants to proj-ect START (NCT04087057), a qualitative study in which we aim to comprehensively assess and identify determinants of delays in chemotherapy initiation among breast cancer patients. In addition to deeply evaluating operational and personal factors, we are evaluating social support, health literacy, and trust in medical professionals using validated instruments. We believe that understanding the complexities of the problem at hand is critical in the design and implementation of highly effective strategies for decreasing treatment delays.

Impact of COVID-19

In 2020, the global health-care system was overwhelmed by the Coronavirus Disease 2019 (COVID-19), which was declared a global pandemic by the World Health Organization. As of September 2020, the global health crisis had seen over three million cases of COVID-19 caused by infection with severe acute respiratory syndrome coronavirus 2 (SARS-CoV-2), with almost one million fatalities [28].

Since the first case of COVID-19 was diagnosed in the United States, screening tests for early detection of cervical, breast, and colon cancer plummeted by over 85% [29]. It is estimated that 79% of cancer patients actively undergoing treatment experienced some type of a delay in care due to COVID-19, with 17% specifically experiencing a delay in cancer therapy (chemotherapy, radiation, endocrine therapy) [30]. Communities of color and minorities have disproportionately shouldered the COVID-19 burden, with Hispanics accounting for 34% of cases despite only representing 18% of the US population [31] – this unequal burden exacerbates the poor survival outcomes among Hispanic women with cancer as they are at higher risk for mortality if infected with SARS-CoV-2 than non-cancer patients [29]. The disproportionate impact of COVID-19 among cancer patients and minorities is yet to be determined; however, the National Cancer Institute estimates an additional 10,000 associated deaths from breast cancer and colorectal cancers over the next decade due to the global pandemic's impact on screening and treatment [32].

How to Improve Cancer Care Delivery for All?

Success in improving cancer care delivery for all hinges on a holistic approach to reducing disparities across race, ethnicity, and the socioeconomic strata. Increasing adherence to screening guidelines for early detection is critical for overall improvement in survival outcomes, but we cannot ignore the complex dynamics of factors that infringe on cancer care access among minorities. Expansion of culturally effective health education programs and social assistance alongside research of biological differences in Hispanic tumor characteristics are crucial in improving cancer care delivery and long-term breast cancer outcomes.

Patient navigation programs are known to play a role in reducing cancer disparities by empowering patients to take an active role in their health-care experience – this is accomplished by the use of patient navigators, people who work with patients to eliminate barriers to accessing care once they are admitted into the health-care system [3]. Traditional patient navigation only comes into play when an individual has been admitted into the health-care system with the intention to decrease delays in treatment initiation and delivery with little to no impact on adherence to timely screening. Community patient navigation can bridge the gap between the community and clinical setting by expanding the traditional patient navigation program beyond the existing internal system within the health care. The implementation of community-based navigation programs among Hispanics, such as *Naveguemos con Salud* in Philadelphia, extends social assistance to target individuals from prescreening outreach to posttreatment follow-up [18] in order to improve quality of life and outcomes among Hispanics [10]. This form of community planning highlights the need for culturally sensitive health education programming and implementation, which can successfully address cultural factors contributing to screening nonadherence by targeting not just Hispanic women but also their family units and supporting communities.

Increasing access and availability of financial assistance programs for minorities along with expanding eligibility criteria is key in reducing financial toxicity derived from breast cancer treatment and care. Financial assistance programs provide additional support to mitigate treatment costs, yet limited assistance programs exist to cover family expenses, cost of living, or indirect medical costs, such as housing and travel [26]. There are a number of theoretical models showing that Hispanic breast cancer patients tend to emphasize survival at any cost over financial concerns; however, resulting financial stress from limited pretreatment knowledge and delays in financial planning have long-lasting impact even beyond post-cancer treatment [26].

Further investigation of the differences among Hispanic subgroups in regard to cultural differences and their impact on health decision-making and education is necessary to develop increasingly culturally effective health education interventions to reduce breast cancer disparities. Quantitative research provides insight into the treatment delays among women with breast cancer by identifying key factors that elucidate the complex interaction of social determinants of health. Future research should focus on expanding breast cancer patient narratives to enrich qualitative understanding of treatment delays among racial and ethnic populations to develop a culturally effective framework for reducing health disparities and improving breast cancer outcomes for all.

Acknowledgments MCM is funded by Susan G. Komen, CIPRIT, Conquer Cancer and BCRF. CM is funded by Susan G. Komen.

References

1. World Health Organization. WHO | Breast cancer. WHO; 2018.
2. American Cancer Society. Cancer facts & figures for Hispanics/Latinos 2018–2020. Atlanta; 2018.
3. American Cancer Society. Breast cancer facts & figures 2019–2020. Am Cancer Soc. 2019.
4. Farias AJ, Wu WH, Du XL. Racial differences in long-term adjuvant endocrine therapy adherence and mortality among Medicaid-insured breast cancer patients in Texas: findings from TCR-Medicaid linked data. BMC Cancer [Internet]. 2018 Dec 4 [cited 2020 Sep 20];18(1). Available from: /pmc/articles/PMC6280479/?report=abstract.
5. Siegel RL, Miller KD, Jemal A. Cancer statistics, 2020. CA Cancer J Clin [Internet]. 2020 Jan 1 [cited 2020 Sep 20];70(1):7–30. Available from: https://acsjournals.onlinelibrary.wiley.com/doi/full/10.3322/caac.21590.
6. Miller BC, Bowers JM, Payne JB, Moyer A. Barriers to mammography screening among racial and ethnic minority women. Soc Sci Med. Elsevier Ltd. 2019;239:112494.
7. Bolton CD, Sunil TS, Hurd T, Guerra H. Hispanic men and women's knowledge, beliefs, perceived susceptibility, and barriers to clinical breast examination and mammography practices in South Texas Colonias. J Community Health [Internet]. 2019 Dec 1 [cited 2020 Sep 20];44(6):1069–75. Available from: https://pubmed.ncbi.nlm.nih.gov/31161398/
8. Clarke TC, Duran D, Saraiya M. Breast cancer screening among women by nativity, birthplace, and length of time in the United States [Internet]. Vol. 129. National Health Statistics Reports Number; 2019 [cited 2020 Sep 20]. Available from: https://www.cdc.gov/nchs/products/index.htm.
9. Center for Health Statistics N. Health, United States 2018 Chartbook [Internet]. Health. 2018 [cited 2020 Sep 20]. Available from: https://www.cdc.gov/nchs/hus/hus_infographic.htm.
10. Yanez B, McGinty HL, Buitrago D, Ramirez AG, Penedo FJ. Cancer outcomes in Hispanics/Latinos in the United States: an integrative review and conceptual model of determinants of health. J Lat Psychol [Internet]. 2016 May [cited 2020 Sep 20];4(2):114–29. Available from: /pmc/articles/PMC4943845/?report=abstract.

11. John EM, Phipps AI, Davis A, Koo J. Migration history, acculturation, and breast cancer risk in Hispanic women. Cancer Epidemiol Biomarkers Prev [Internet]. 2005 Dec 1 [cited 2020 Sep 20];14(12):2905–13. Available from: https://cebp.aacrjournals.org/content/14/12/2905.

12. Teruya SA, Bazargan-Hejazi S. The immigrant and Hispanic paradoxes: a systematic review of their predictions and effects. Hisp J Behav Sci [Internet]. 2013 Nov 5 [cited 2020 Sep 19];35(4):486–509. Available from: http://journals.sagepub.com/doi/10.1177/0739986313499004.

13. Turra CM, Goldman N. Socioeconomic differences in mortality among U.S. adults: insights into the Hispanic paradox. J Gerontol B Psychol Sci Soc Sci [Internet]. 2007 May 1 [cited 2020 Sep 19];62(3):S184–92. Available from: https://academic.oup.com/psychsocgerontology/article/62/3/S184/600844.

14. Chavez-MacGregor M, Litton J, Chen H, Giordano SH, Hudis CA, Wolff AC, et al. Pathologic complete response in breast cancer patients receiving anthracycline- and taxane-based neoadjuvant chemotherapy: evaluating the effect of race/ethnicity. Cancer [Internet]. 2010 Sep 1 [cited 2020 Sep 23];116(17):4168–77. Available from: https://pubmed.ncbi.nlm.nih.gov/20564153/.

15. Chavez-MacGregor M, Unger JM, Moseley A, Ramsey SD, Hershman DL. Survival by Hispanic ethnicity among patients with cancer participating in SWOG clinical trials. Cancer. 2018;124(8):1760–9.

16. Social Determinants of Health | Healthy People 2020 [Internet]. [cited 2020 Sep 20]. Available from: https://www.healthypeople.gov/2020/topics-objectives/topic/social-determinants-of-health.

17. Karimi SE, Rafiey H, Sajjadi H, Nejad FN. Identifying the social determinants of breast health behavior: a qualitative content analysis. Asian Pacific J Cancer Prev [Internet]. 2018 Jul 1 [cited 2020 Sep 20];19(7):1867–77. Available from: /pmc/articles/PMC6165651/?report=abstract.

18. Keith JD, Kang NE, Bodden MR, Miller C, Karamanian V, Banks T. Supporting Latina breast health with community-based navigation. J Cancer Educ [Internet]. 2019 Aug 15 [cited 2020 Sep 20];34(4):654–7. Available from: https://pubmed.ncbi.nlm.nih.gov/29574540/.

19. Unger-Saldaña K, Fitch-Picos K, Villarreal-Garza C. Breast cancer diagnostic delays among young Mexican women are associated with a lack of suspicion by health care providers at first presentation. J Glob Oncol. 2019;5:1–12.

20. Jaiswal K, Hull M, Furniss AL, Doyle R, Gayou N, Bayliss E. Delays in diagnosis and treatment of breast cancer: a safety-net population profile. JNCCN J Natl Compr Cancer Netw [Internet]. 2018 Dec 1 [cited 2020 Sep 20];16(12):1451–7. Available from: https://jnccn.org/view/journals/jnccn/16/12/article-p1451.xml.

21. Chavez-MacGregor M, Clarke CA, Lichtensztajn DY, Giordano SH. Delayed initiation of adjuvant chemotherapy among patients with breast cancer. JAMA Oncol. 2016;2(3):322–9.

22. Smith-Graziani D, Lei X, Giordano SH, Zhao H, Karuturi M, Chavez-MacGregor M. Delayed initiation of adjuvant chemotherapy in older women with breast cancer. Cancer Med. 2020;9(19):6961–71.

23. De Melo Gagliato D, Gonzalez-Angulo AM, Lei X, Theriault RL, Giordano SH, Valero V, et al. Clinical impact of delaying initiation of adjuvant chemotherapy in patients with breast cancer. J Clin Oncol. 2014;32(8):735–44.

24. Bleicher RJ, Ruth K, Sigurdson ER, Beck JR, Ross E, Wong YN, et al. Time to surgery and breast cancer survival in the United States. JAMA Oncol [Internet]. 2016 Mar 1 [cited 2020 Sep 20];2(3):330–9. Available from: https://pubmed.ncbi.nlm.nih.gov/26659430/.

25. Rossi L, Stevens D, Pierga J-Y, Lerebours F, Reyal F, Robain M, et al. Impact of adjuvant chemotherapy on breast cancer survival: a real-world population. Bathen TF, editor. PLoS One [Internet]. 2015 Jul 27 [cited 2020 Sep 20];10(7):e0132853. Available from: https://dx.plos.org/10.1371/journal.pone.0132853.

26. Chebli P, Lemus J, Avila C, Peña K, Mariscal B, Merlos S, et al. Multilevel determinants of financial toxicity in breast cancer care: perspectives of healthcare professionals and Latina

survivors. Support Care Cancer [Internet]. 2020 Jul 1 [cited 2020 Sep 20];28(7):3179–88. Available from: https://pubmed.ncbi.nlm.nih.gov/31712953/.

27. Wöckel A, Wolters R, Wiegel T, Novopashenny I, Janni W, Kreienberg R, et al. The impact of adjuvant radiotherapy on the survival of primary breast cancer patients: a retrospective multicenter cohort study of 8935 subjects. Ann Oncol [Internet]. 2014 Mar 1 [cited 2020 Sep 20];25(3):628–32. Available from: http://www.annalsofoncology.org/article/S0923753419342760/fulltext.

28. WHO Coronavirus Disease (COVID-19) Dashboard I WHO Coronavirus Disease (COVID-19) Dashboard [Internet]. [cited 2020 Sep 20]. Available from: https://covid19.who.int/.

29. AACR cancer disparities progress report 2020 I Cancer Progress Report [Internet]. [cited 2020 Sep 19]. Available from: https://cancerprogressreport.aacr.org/disparities/.

30. COVID-19 pandemic ongoing impact on cancer patients and survivors survey findings summary [Internet]. [cited 2020 Sep 20]. Available from: https://www.kff.org/other/state-indicator/total-population/.

31. COVID-19 data from the National Center for Health Statistics [Internet]. [cited 2020 Sep 20]. Available from: https://www.cdc.gov/nchs/covid19/index.htm.

32. Sharpless NE. COVID-19 and cancer [Internet]. Vol. 368. Science. American Association for the Advancement of Science; 2020 [cited 2020 Sep 20]. p. 1290. Available from: www.cancer.gov.

Open Access This chapter is licensed under the terms of the Creative Commons Attribution 4.0 International License (http://creativecommons.org/licenses/by/4.0/), which permits use, sharing, adaptation, distribution and reproduction in any medium or format, as long as you give appropriate credit to the original author(s) and the source, provide a link to the Creative Commons license and indicate if changes were made.

The images or other third party material in this chapter are included in the chapter's Creative Commons license, unless indicated otherwise in a credit line to the material. If material is not included in the chapter's Creative Commons license and your intended use is not permitted by statutory regulation or exceeds the permitted use, you will need to obtain permission directly from the copyright holder.

Chapter 7
Genetic Ancestry and Breast Cancer Subtypes in Hispanic/Latina Women

Lizeth I. Tamayo, Elam Day-Friedland, Valentina A. Zavala, Katie M. Marker, and Laura Fejerman

Introduction

The terms Hispanic and Latino are used in the United States to refer to Americans who trace their heritage to Latin America or Spain. The US Census takes a self-identification approach to categorizing race/ethnicity, including those who identify themselves as Hispanic or Latino [1]. Beyond any debate of who is or is not Hispanic/Latino, in this review we use the categories of Hispanic/Latino (Latina for women) to refer to the heterogeneous group of individuals who self-identify as such, and who are assumed to have been born or have ancestors who were born in a Latin American country. Genetic studies of the distribution of continental ancestry proportions in US Hispanics/Latinos and Latin Americans show that individuals in this group are genetically diverse, with varying proportions of European, Indigenous American, African, and to a lesser extent, Asian continental ancestry [2–7]. This

L. I. Tamayo
Department of Public Health Sciences, The University of Chicago, Chicago, IL, USA

E. Day-Friedland
Albany High School, Albany, CA, USA

V. A. Zavala
Department of Public Health Sciences, Division of Epidemiology, University of California, Davis, CA, USA

K. M. Marker
Human Medical Genetics and Genomics Program, School of Medicine, University of Colorado Anschutz Medical Campus, Aurora, CO, USA

L. Fejerman (✉)
Department of Public Health Sciences, Division of Epidemiology, University of California, Davis, CA, USA

UC Davis Comprehensive Cancer Center, University of California, Davis, CA, USA
e-mail: lfejerman@ucdavis.edu

© The Author(s) 2023
A. G. Ramirez, E. J. Trapido (eds.), *Advancing the Science of Cancer in Latinos*, https://doi.org/10.1007/978-3-031-14436-3_7

heterogeneous group has often been treated as a monolithic unit in cancer epidemiology, partly out of necessity because of small sample sizes and the concomitant limitations in statistical power. The number of datasets with extensive information about Latino subgroups is limited, despite the fact that individuals who self-identify as Hispanics/Latinos make up the second-largest group within the US racial/ethnic categories [8].

Breast cancer is the most common cancer among US Hispanics/Latinas [9]; however, Hispanic/Latina women in the United States have historically shown a relatively low breast cancer incidence compared to non-Hispanic White (NHW) or African American/Black (AA/B) women [10]. In addition to the differences among racial/ethnic groups, variation within different Hispanic/Latina populations in the distribution of breast cancer subtypes by ancestry has been reported [11–13].

Breast cancer is a heterogeneous disease with intrinsic biological subtypes associated with different prognosis [14, 15]. Tumor profiling based on transcriptional profiles, such as PAM50, are considered the "gold standard" for intrinsic subtyping [14]. As routinely used in clinical practice, breast cancer intrinsic subtypes can be approximated by immunohistochemical markers, the most typically being estrogen receptor (ER), progesterone receptor (PR), and human epidermal growth factor receptor 2 (HER2) [16, 17]. Both population-based and hospital-based studies have shown that Hispanics/Latinas have about a 20–40% higher risk of developing ER−/ PR− HER2+ and triple negative breast cancer (TNBC, a tumor subtype that is ER−/ PR− HER2−) compared to NHW women [18–20]. ER/PR− tumors have fewer treatment options and poorer prognosis than other subtypes [21–28].

Ancestry-specific genetic variants have been shown to be associated with breast cancer risk in Hispanics/Latinas, and the strength of their association is tumor subtype-specific [29, 30]. Sample size in available data for breast cancer genetic studies in Hispanic/Latina populations has been limited, which represents a significant barrier for the further exploration of the possibility of additional germline variants that could predispose US Hispanics/Latinas or Latin American women to develop ER/PR− and HER2+ tumors [31–34]. Studies reporting associations between genetic ancestry and tumor subtype provide suggestive evidence that can be informative in the design of follow-up studies aimed at identifying factors that explain the observed association. These factors can be genetic, behavioral, environmental, and structural [29, 35, 36] . Additionally, observed associations could be the result of systematic sample bias [37].

This chapter summarizes results from studies that include breast cancer subtype and genetic ancestry information from women of Latin American origin, discusses possible explanations for observed associations, and proposes future studies that could contribute to a better understanding of tumor subtype-specific risk in US Hispanics/Latinas and Latin American women.

Indigenous American/European Genetic Ancestry and Breast Cancer Subtype in Hispanics/Latinas

The risk of developing breast cancer among Hispanics/Latinas varies by genetic ancestry [25, 38]. Women with higher proportion of Indigenous American ancestry (or lower European ancestry) have a lower risk of developing breast cancer [25]. An analysis based on data from the San Francisco Bay Area Breast Cancer Study (SFBCS) was the first to report on this association [25]. This study had a sample size of 440 cases and 597 controls and included 294 ER+ and 83 ER− patients, but had no information regarding HER2 status [25]. Genetic ancestry was estimated using a panel of ~100 ancestry informative markers. The investigators did not find a statistically significant difference in Indigenous American or European genetic ancestry proportion by ER status. However, higher European ancestry was found to be associated with increased breast cancer risk even after adjustment for known risk factors (OR = 1.39; 95% CI, 1.06–2.11; $P = 0.013$). A study of breast cancer survival and genetic ancestry conducted with additional cases from the SFBCS (476 ER+ and 169 ER− patients) with ancestry estimations based on genome-wide genotype data reported similar findings [39]. A subsequent study including cases from the Kaiser Permanente Pathways Cohort (408 ER+ and 94 ER−) also reported no association between ER/PR or HER2 status and Indigenous American or European ancestry proportions [36].

The Peruvian Genetics and Genomics of Breast Cancer (PEGEN-BC) is an ongoing case series study, including patients from the *Instituto Nacional de Enfermedades Neoplasicas* in Lima, Peru, diagnosed with invasive breast cancer since 2010 [40]. Results of an analysis including 1312 PEGEN-BC study patients showed a statistically significant association between proportion of Indigenous American ancestry and tumor subtype [40]. The average Indigenous American ancestry among participants with ER/PR− HER2+ tumors was 80%, compared with 75% among participants with the ER/PR+ HER2− subtype. Genetic ancestry was estimated from genome-wide genotype data and the program ADMIXTURE [41]. A multinomial logistic regression analysis was performed, which showed that the odds of ER/PR− HER2+ breast cancer increased by a factor of 1.22 per every 10% increase in Indigenous American ancestry when using ER/PR+ HER2− as the reference group (95% CI, 1.07–1.35; $P = 0.001$). This study included independent replication in a combined sample of Mexican and Colombian breast cancer patients from the COLUMBUS Consortium [40].

A study that analyzed breast tumor tissue samples from 232 Colombian women provided information on average Indigenous American ancestry proportions for luminal, HER2-enriched, and TNBC tumors [13]. Subtypes were inferred using immunohistochemical surrogates from the 2013 St. Gallen International Expert Consensus, and genetic ancestry was estimated using ~100 ancestry informative markers genotyped using DNA extracted from the tumor tissue [13]. Patients with luminal tumors had an average of 39% Indigenous American ancestry: those with HER2-enriched tumors had 35% and those with TNBC 37%. These differences in ancestry between subtypes, however, were not statistically significant. Another analysis in a subset of these Colombian study samples reported a suggestive correlation between expression of the ERBB2 gene, which is the gene that codes for the HER2 receptor, and Indigenous American ancestry. In this study, ERBB2 expression was higher among women above the median of Indigenous American ancestry compared to women below the median [42].

The Breast Cancer Health Disparities Consortium includes samples from the SFBCS, the Four Corners Study, and a case/control breast cancer study from Mexico [43]. A study using data from this consortium and including 1854 NHW women and 2326 Hispanics/Latinas analyzed the influence of risk factors and genetic ancestry on breast cancer risk in postmenopausal women. ER status information was available for a subset of the Hispanic/Latina patients, with 348 cases being ER+ and 106 ER−. They did not compare genetic ancestry proportions by subtype, and instead conducted analyses testing the association between quartiles of Indigenous American ancestry and overall breast cancer, ER+ breast cancer, and ER− breast cancer [43]. All analyses showed the same trend toward higher odds of developing breast cancer in the lower quartiles compared to the highest quartile of Indigenous American ancestry, which is consistent with results from previously published studies [25, 38].

African Genetic Ancestry and Tumor Subtype in Hispanic/ Latina Breast Cancer Patients

Average African genetic ancestry in Hispanics/Latinas tends to vary greatly between countries and regions, from 5% or less in samples from Chile, Argentina, and Mexico to 10% or higher in Brazil, Cuba, or Puerto Rico [3, 44–48]. Assessing the association between African ancestry and tumor subtype requires large sample sizes in areas where this is a relatively minor ancestral component.

The previously mentioned study of tumor tissue samples from Colombia [13] reported an association between African ancestry and ER status, with average African ancestry being higher in ER− compared to ER+ cases ($P = 0.02$) [13]. Women with HER2-enriched tumors had a higher proportion of African ancestry (14%), followed by those with triple negative (12%) and luminal tumors (7%). The SFBCS study did not report a statistically significant association between African ancestry proportion and ER status, which was to be expected in a relatively small set of samples with limited African ancestry representation [25]. Average African ancestry proportion in the PEGEN-BC study samples was reported at 4% and differences between tumor subtypes for this component were not statistically significant, ranging between 3 and 5% [40].

Possible Reasons Behind Genetic Ancestry and Tumor Subtype Association Results

Studies that include US Hispanics/Latinas or Latin American women are heterogeneous. Not only because of the diversity within the Hispanic/Latino category discussed in the introduction but also because of various research designs that have been used in these studies. Most studies are based on a convenience sampling strategy within hospitals, while population-based studies with information on tumor characteristics are harder to find. In the United States, studies using cancer registry data to recruit cases can approximate a population-based design. As a result of both the intrinsic heterogeneity of the Hispanic/Latino population and the biases brought by convenience sampling, studies reporting associative findings or lack of association have to be taken with caution and should be followed up with additional research that allows for further evaluation of potential causal relationships between cancer phenotypes and etiological factors.

Differences in sample size could likely explain inconsistencies in reported associations between genetic ancestry and tumor subtype. For example, studies including a few hundred cases might not detect differences of 2 or 3% in average genetic ancestry between groups, as was the case in the Kaiser Permanente Pathways study [36], which only included a small sample of HER2+ patients. The PEGEN-BC study, with a sample of 1312 cases, had more power and identified a ~22% increase in the odds of having HER2+ tumors per 10% increase in Indigenous American ancestry [40], but was not informative about African ancestry, given that this component is minor, on average, among the study patients.

Genetic heterogeneity across Latin American countries can contribute to differences in ancestry and tumor subtype associations. Disaggregating Latin American populations based on the main genetic ancestry components will allow the association between some less represented genetic components to be tested, such as African ancestry, with specific breast cancer subtypes. For example, a study including women from Cuba or Puerto Rico will have more power than a study in Peru, with only 4% average African ancestry among patients [40]. For this purpose, additional efforts to run larger studies including participants from diverse ancestry backgrounds from Latin American countries are still needed.

Observed associations might also be explained by sampling bias. For example, within the Peruvian or Colombian studies [13, 40], there might be over-representation of patients with aggressive tumors from remote regions (such as the coastal region in Colombia or the Amazonian region in Peru). If ancestry proportion were correlated with region of origin within these countries, then by analyzing patients recruited in the cancer center might lead to an association between ancestry proportion and tumor subtype if region of origin is not accounted for in the analysis [40].

Correlation between behavioral, environmental, or socioeconomic factors and genetic ancestry could partly explain observed associations between genetic ancestry and tumor subtype. For example, socioeconomic status (SES) has been shown to be correlated with genetic ancestry [20, 49]. A study exploring the association between SES and tumor subtype among Hispanics/Latinas in data from the California Cancer Registry, including women diagnosed with invasive breast cancer from 2005 to 2010, reported that women in lower SES neighborhoods had greater risk of TNBC and ER/PR− HER2+ subtypes relative to ER/PR+ HER2− ($P < 0.05$) [20]. Additionally, Hispanic/Latina women who resided in low SES neighborhoods had significantly increased the risk of developing and dying from hormone receptor negative tumors than hormone receptor positive tumors [20]. This information leads to plausible explanations for the association between ancestry and subtype being related to SES and behavioral or environmental exposures associated with it.

Lifestyle may also play a part in the association between ancestry and breast cancer subtype. A study, including 2023 Hispanic/Latinas from the previously mentioned Breast Cancer Health Disparities Consortium, found that among women not using menopausal hormone therapy, weight gain was associated with increased risk of ER/PR+ breast cancer, but only among those with a low young-adult BMI [50]. The association with weight gain, for those who had information on genetic ancestry, was limited to women with lower Indigenous American genetic ancestry within this group [50] and interactions were not tested. It is possible that given the association between BMI and genetic ancestry among Hispanics/Latinas, associations between BMI and tumor subtype might lead to the observed link between ancestry and subtype.

Finally, underlying population-specific genetic variation could predispose specific populations to particular subtypes, thereby explaining observed ancestry and subtype associations. In a breast cancer genome-wide association study in Hispanics/Latinas, researchers identified two variants (rs140068132 and rs7157845) within the region 6q25, upstream of the estrogen receptor 1 gene (ESR1), and breast cancer risk [29]. The minor allele is protective (associated with decreased risk) against ER− breast cancer (OR = 0.60; 95% CI, 0.53–0.67) [29]. Other genetic variants such as these could explain the differences in breast cancer subtype by ancestry [30, 51].

Next Steps and Conclusions

In this chapter, we summarized the studies that have described associations (or lack of) between breast cancer subtypes and genetic ancestry among Hispanics/Latinas. Yet, more and larger studies are needed to increase the statistical power and better representation of the ancestral, cultural, and environmental diversity of Latin America. Ongoing collaborative efforts are aiming to do so by improving the design and collection of epidemiological and genetic data from breast cancer patients and the healthy population [30].

Future research is needed to understand the potential molecular mechanisms of population-specific variants as drivers of specific subtypes during breast cancer etiology and progression. This could explain, for example, the association between African ancestry and ER− tumors or Indigenous American ancestry and HER2+

disease. Additionally, building diverse cohorts with measures that reflect exposures associated with the individual (behavioral and biological), neighborhood, and structural level variables will provide the necessary information to disentangle the different components that contribute to observed associations between genetic ancestry and overall as well as subtype-specific breast cancer risk [30].

Currently, there are insufficient studies on tumor subtype etiology and outcome predictors among Hispanics/Latinas and African Americans that include estimations of genetic ancestry [30]. Additional support toward the enhancement of existing studies or the creation of news ones will be fundamental to improve our understanding of subtype-specific breast cancer risk, treatment efficacy, and outcome prognosis in admixed minority populations.

References

1. Lopez MH, Krogstad JM, Passel JS. Who is Hispanic? PEW Res Cent 2019. https://www.pewresearch.org/fact-tank/2019/11/11/who-is-hispanic/. Accessed 3 Aug 2020.
2. Parolin ML, Toscanini UF, Velázquez IF, Llull C, Berardi GL, Holley A, et al. Genetic admixture patterns in Argentinian Patagonia. PLoS One. 2019;14:e0214830. https://doi.org/10.1371/journal.pone.0214830
3. Pena SDJ, Di Pietro G, Fuchshuber-Moraes M, Genro JP, Hutz MH, de Kehdy FSG, et al. The genomic ancestry of individuals from different geographical regions of Brazil is more uniform than expected. PLoS One. 2011;6:e17063. https://doi.org/10.1371/journal.pone.0017063.
4. Harris DN, Song W, Shetty AC, Levano KS, Cáceres O, Padilla C, et al. Evolutionary genomic dynamics of Peruvians before, during, and after the Inca Empire. Proc Natl Acad Sci U S A. 2018;115:E6526–35. https://doi.org/10.1073/pnas.1720798115.
5. Ossa H, Aquino J, Pereira R, Ibarra A, Ossa RH, Pérez LA, et al. Outlining the ancestry landscape of Colombian admixed populations. PLoS One. 2016;11 https://doi.org/10.1371/journal.pone.0164414.
6. Wang S, Ray N, Rojas W, Parra MV, Bedoya G, Gallo C, et al. Geographic patterns of genome admixture in Latin American mestizos. PLoS Genet. 2008;4 https://doi.org/10.1371/journal.pgen.1000037.
7. Avena S, Via M, Ziv E, Pérez-Stable EJ, Gignoux CR, Dejean C, et al. Heterogeneity in genetic admixture across different regions of Argentina. PLoS One. 2012;7:e34695. https://doi.org/10.1371/journal.pone.0034695.
8. Colby SL, Ortman JM. Projections of the size and composition of the U.S. population: 2014 to 2060. Current Population Reports, U.S. Census Bureau, Washington, DC; 2014. pp. 25–1143.
9. Howlader N, Noone AM, Krapcho M, Miller D, Brest A, Yu M, et al. (eds). SEER cancer statistics review, 1975–2017, National Cancer Institute. Bethesda, MD, https://seer.cancer.gov/csr/1975_2017/, based on November 2019 SEER data submission, posted to the SEER web site, April 2020. Accessed 1 Jul 2020.
10. Miller KD, Goding Sauer A, Ortiz AP, Fedewa SA, Pinheiro PS, Tortolero-Luna G, et al. Cancer statistics for Hispanics/Latinos, 2018. CA Cancer J Clin. 2018;68:425–45. https://doi.org/10.3322/caac.21494.
11. Serrano-Gómez SJ, Fejerman L, Zabaleta J. Breast cancer in Latinas: a focus on intrinsic subtypes distribution. Cancer Epidemiol Biomark Prev. 2017:cebp.0420.2017. https://doi.org/10.1158/1055-9965.EPI-17-0420.

12. Rey-Vargas L, Sanabria-Salas MC, Fejerman L, Serrano-Gomez SJ. Risk factors for triple-negative breast cancer among Latina women. 2019; https://doi.org/10.1158/1055-9965. EPI-19-0035.

13. Serrano-Gomez SJ, Sanabria-Salas MC, Hernández-Suarez G, García O, Silva C, Romero A, et al. High prevalence of luminal B breast cancer intrinsic subtype in Colombian women. Carcinogenesis. 2016;37:669–76. https://doi.org/10.1093/carcin/bgw043.

14. Bernard PS, Parker JS, Mullins M, Cheung MCU, Leung S, Voduc D, et al. Supervised risk predictor of breast cancer based on intrinsic subtypes. J Clin Oncol. 2009;27:1160–7. https://doi.org/10.1200/JCO.2008.18.1370.

15. Cejalvo JM, De Dueñas EM, Galván P, García-Recio S, Gasión OB, Paré L, et al. Intrinsic subtypes and gene expression profiles in primary and metastatic breast cancer. Cancer Res. 2017;77:2213–21. https://doi.org/10.1158/0008-5472.CAN-16-2717.

16. Perou CM, Sørile T, Eisen MB, Van De Rijn M, Jeffrey SS, Ress CA, et al. Molecular portraits of human breast tumours. Nature. 2000;406:747–52. https://doi.org/10.1038/35021093.

17. Blows FM, Driver KE, Schmidt MK, Broeks A, van Leeuwen FE, Wesseling J, et al. Subtyping of breast cancer by immunohistochemistry to investigate a relationship between subtype and short and long term survival: a collaborative analysis of data for 10,159 cases from 12 studies. PLoS Med. 2010;7 https://doi.org/10.1371/journal.pmed.1000279.

18. Ooi SL, Martinez ME, Li CI. Disparities in breast cancer characteristics and outcomes by race/ethnicity. Breast Cancer Res Treat. 2011;127:729–38. https://doi.org/10.1007/s10549-010-1191-6.

19. Parise CA, Bauer KR, Brown MM, Caggiano V. Breast cancer subtypes as defined by the estrogen receptor (ER), progesterone receptor (PR), and the human epidermal growth factor receptor 2 (HER2) among women with invasive breast cancer in California, 1999-2004. Breast J. 2009;15:593–602. https://doi.org/10.1111/j.1524-4741.2009.00822.x.

20. Banegas MP, Tao L, Altekruse S, Anderson WF, John EM, Clarke CA, et al. Heterogeneity of breast cancer subtypes and survival among Hispanic women with invasive breast cancer in California. Breast Cancer Res Treat. 2014;144:625–34. https://doi.org/10.1007/s10549-014-2882-1.

21. Newman LA, Griffith KA, Jatoi I, Simon MS, Crowe JP, Colditz GA. Meta-analysis of survival in African American and White American patients with breast cancer: ethnicity compared with socioeconomic status. J Clin Oncol. 2006;24(9):1342–9. https://doi.org/10.1200/jco.2005.03.3472.

22. de Macêdo Andrade AC, Ferreira Júnior CA, Dantes Guimarães B, Waleska Pessoa Barros A, Sarmento de Almeida G, Weller M. Molecular breast cancer subtypes and therapies in a public hospital of Northeastern Brazil. BMC Womens Health. 2014;14:110. https://doi.org/10.118 6/1472-6874-14-110.

23. Sans M. Admixture studies in Latin America: from the 20th to the 21st century. Hum Biol. 2000;72:155–77.

24. Gonzalez-Angulo AM, Timms KM, Liu S, Chen H, Litton JK, Potter J, et al. Incidence and outcome of BRCA mutations in unselected patients with triple receptor-negative breast cancer. Clin Cancer Res. 2011;17:1082–9. https://doi.org/10.1158/1078-0432.CCR-10-2560.

25. Fejerman L, John EM, Huntsman S, Beckman K, Choudhry S, Perez-Stable E, et al. Genetic ancestry and risk of breast cancer among U.S. Latinas Cancer Res. 2008;68:9723–8. https://doi.org/10.1158/0008-5472.CAN-08-2039.

26. John EM, Phipps AI, Davis A, Koo J. Migration history, acculturation, and breast cancer risk in Hispanic women. Cancer Epidemiol Biomark Prev. 2005;14:2905–13. https://doi.org/10.1158/1055-9965.EPI-05-0483.

27. Goldstein J, Jacoby E, Del Aguila R, Lopez A. Poverty is a predictor of non-communicable disease among adults in Peruvian cities. Prev Med (Baltim). 2005;41:800–6. https://doi.org/10.1016/j.ypmed.2005.06.001.

28. Srur-Rivero N, Cartin-Brenes M. Breast cancer characteristics and survival in a Hispanic population of Costa Rica. Breast Cancer (Auckl). 2014;8:103–8. https://doi.org/10.4137/BCBCR.S15854.
29. Fejerman L, Ahmadiyeh N, Hu D, Huntsman S, Beckman KB, Caswell JL, et al. Genome-wide association study of breast cancer in Latinas identifies novel protective variants on 6q25. Nat Commun. 2014;5:1–8. https://doi.org/10.1038/ncomms6260.
30. Zavala VA, Serrano-Gomez SJ, Dutil J, Fejerman L. Genetic epidemiology of breast cancer in Latin America. Genes (Basel). 2019;10:153. https://doi.org/10.3390/genes10020153.
31. Park SL, Cheng I, Haiman CA. Genome-wide association studies of cancer in diverse populations. Cancer Epidemiol Biomark Prev. 2018;27:405–17. https://doi.org/10.1158/1055-9965.EPI-17-0169.
32. Sirugo G, Williams SM, Tishkoff SA. The missing diversity in human genetic studies. Cell. 2019;177:26–31. https://doi.org/10.1016/j.cell.2019.02.048.
33. Popejoy AB, Fullerton SM. Genomics is failing on diversity. Nature. 2016;538:161–4. https://doi.org/10.1038/538161a.
34. Peterson RE, Kuchenbaecker K, Walters RK, Chen CY, Popejoy AB, Periyasamy S, et al. Genome-wide association studies in ancestrally diverse populations: opportunities, methods, pitfalls, and recommendations. Cell. 2019;179:589–603. https://doi.org/10.1016/j.cell.2019.08.051.
35. Ziv E, John EM, Choudhry S, Kho J, Lorizio W, Perez-Stable EJ, et al. Genetic ancestry and risk factors for breast cancer among Latinas in the San Francisco Bay area. Cancer Epidemiol Biomark Prev. 2006;15:1878–85. https://doi.org/10.1158/1055-9965.EPI-06-0092.
36. Engmann NJ, Ergas IJ, Yao S, Kwan ML, Roh JM, Ambrosone CB, et al. Genetic ancestry is not associated with breast cancer recurrence or survival in U.S. Latina women enrolled in the Kaiser Permanente pathways study. Cancer Epidemiol Biomark Prev. 2017;26:1466–9. https://doi.org/10.1158/1055-9965.EPI-17-0148.
37. Munafò MR, Tilling K, Taylor AE, Evans DM, Smith GD. Collider scope: when selection bias can substantially influence observed associations. Int J Epidemiol. 2018;226–35 https://doi.org/10.1093/ije/dyx206.
38. Fejerman L, Romieu I, John EM, Lazcano-Ponce E, Huntsman S, Beckman KB, et al. European ancestry is positively associated with breast cancer risk in Mexican women. Cancer Epidemiol Biomark Prev. 2010;19:1074–82. https://doi.org/10.1158/1055-9965.EPI-09-1193.
39. Fejerman L, Hu D, Huntsman S, John EM, Stern MC, Haiman CA, et al. Genetic ancestry and risk of mortality among U.S. Latinas with breast cancer. Cancer Res. 2013;73:7243–53. https://doi.org/10.1158/0008-5472.CAN-13-2014.
40. Marker KM, Zavala VA, Vidaurre T, Lott PC, Vásquez JN, Casavilca-Zambrano S, et al. Human epidermal growth factor receptor 2–positive breast cancer is associated with indigenous American ancestry in Latin American women. Cancer Res. 2020;80:1893–901. https://doi.org/10.1158/0008-5472.can-19-3659.
41. Alexander DH, Novembre J, Lange K. Fast model-based estimation of ancestry in unrelated individuals. Genome Res. 2009;19:1655–64. https://doi.org/10.1101/gr.094052.109.
42. Serrano-Gómez SJ, Sanabria-Salas MC, Garay J, Baddoo MC, Hernández-Suarez G, Mejía JC, et al. Ancestry as a potential modifier of gene expression in breast tumors from Colombian women. PLoS One. 2017;12 https://doi.org/10.1371/journal.pone.0183179.
43. Hines LM, Sedjo RL, Byers T, John EM, Fejerman L, Stern MC, et al. The interaction between genetic ancestry and breast cancer risk factors among Hispanic women: the breast cancer health disparities study. Cancer Epidemiol Biomark Prev. 2017;26:692–701. https://doi.org/10.1158/1055-9965.EPI-16-0721.
44. González Burchard E, Borrell LN, Choudhry S, Naqvi M, Tsai HJ, Rodriguez-Santana JR, et al. Latino populations: a unique opportunity for the study of race, genetics, and social environment in epidemiological research. Am J Public Health. 2005;95:2161–8. https://doi.org/10.2105/AJPH.2005.068668.

45. Fejerman L, Carnese FR, Goicoechea AS, Avena SA, Dejean CB, Ward RH. African ancestry of the population of Buenos Aires. Am J Phys Anthropol. 2005;128:164–70. https://doi.org/10.1002/ajpa.20083.
46. Fuentes M, Pulgar I, Gallo C, Bortolini M-C, Canizales-Quinteros S, Bedoya G, et al. Geografía génica de Chile: distribución regional de los aportes genéticos americanos, europeos y africanos. Rev Med Chil. 2014;142:281–9. https://doi.org/10.4067/S0034-98872014000300001.
47. Marcheco-Teruel B, Parra EJ, Fuentes-Smith E, Salas A, Buttenschøn HN, Demontis D, et al. Cuba: exploring the history of admixture and the genetic basis of pigmentation using autosomal and uniparental markers. PLoS Genet. 2014;10:e1004488. https://doi.org/10.1371/journal.pgen.1004488.
48. Fortes-Lima C, Bybjerg-Grauholm J, Marin-Padrón LC, Gomez-Cabezas EJ, Bækvad-Hansen M, Hansen CS, et al. Exploring Cuba's population structure and demographic history using genome-wide data. Sci Rep. 2018;8:11422. https://doi.org/10.1038/s41598-018-29851-3.
49. Via M, Gignoux CR, Roth LA, Fejerman L, Galanter J, Choudhry S, et al. History shaped the geographic distribution of genomic admixture on the island of Puerto Rico. PLoS One. 2011;6:e16513. https://doi.org/10.1371/journal.pone.0016513.
50. John EM, Sangaramoorthy M, Hines LM, Stern MC, Baumgartner KB, Giuliano AR, et al. Body size throughout adult life influences postmenopausal breast cancer risk among Hispanic women: the breast cancer health disparities study. Cancer Epidemiol Biomark Prev. 2015;24:128–37. https://doi.org/10.1158/1055-9965.EPI-14-0560.
51. Al-Alem U, Rauscher G, Shah E, Batai K, Mahmoud A, Beisner E, et al. Association of genetic ancestry with breast cancer in ethnically diverse women from Chicago. PLoS One. 2014;9:e112916. https://doi.org/10.1371/journal.pone.0112916.

Open Access This chapter is licensed under the terms of the Creative Commons Attribution 4.0 International License (http://creativecommons.org/licenses/by/4.0/), which permits use, sharing, adaptation, distribution and reproduction in any medium or format, as long as you give appropriate credit to the original author(s) and the source, provide a link to the Creative Commons license and indicate if changes were made.

The images or other third party material in this chapter are included in the chapter's Creative Commons license, unless indicated otherwise in a credit line to the material. If material is not included in the chapter's Creative Commons license and your intended use is not permitted by statutory regulation or exceeds the permitted use, you will need to obtain permission directly from the copyright holder.

Chapter 8
Precision Medicine Approaches for Stratification and Development of Novel Therapies of Latin(x) Patients at Risk of Lung Malignancy

Kenneth S. Ramos, Stefano Guerra, and Randa El-Zein

Unmet Needs in Lung Cancer Diagnosis and Treatment

Lung cancer remains the leading cause of cancer-related mortality worldwide [1], with deaths likely to remain elevated, in part, due to continued use of tobacco products among young adults [2], increasing recreational use of inhaled toxic substances [3], and worsening levels of environmental pollution in some parts of the world [4]. Every year, 1.8 million people are diagnosed with lung cancer, with 5-year survival rates ranging from 4% to 17%, depending on stage and regional differences [5]. Lung cancer deaths account for more lives lost every year than colon, breast, prostate, and pancreatic cancers combined [1, 6]. Non-small-cell lung cancer (NSCLC) accounts for ~85% of all lung cancer cases, with the majority of cases linked to tobacco smoke [7]. NSCLC disproportionately affects African Americans (AAs) compared to Caucasian Americans (CAs), even after adjusting for tobacco use [8]. Despite the introduction of low-dose computerized tomography screening, lung cancers in all racial and ethnic groups are often diagnosed late when curative surgical interventions are no longer an option [9]. Several targeted therapies are now available including: epidermal growth factor receptor inhibitors (such as the tyrosine kinase inhibitors erlotinib and gefitinib and the monoclonal antibody cetuximab); vascular endothelial growth factor inhibitors (such as bevacizumab); EML4-ALK inhibitors (such as crizotinib, with benefits mostly in relatively young,

K. S. Ramos (✉)
Texas A & M Health Science Center, Houston, TX, USA
e-mail: kramos@tamu.edu

S. Guerra
University of Arizona, Tucson, AZ, USA
e-mail: stefano@email.arizona.edu

R. El-Zein
Houston Methodist Hospital, Houston, TX, USA
e-mail: rel-zein2@houstonmethodist.org

© The Author(s) 2023
A. G. Ramirez, E. J. Trapido (eds.), *Advancing the Science of Cancer in Latinos*, https://doi.org/10.1007/978-3-031-14436-3_8

never, or light smokers with adenocarcinoma); and programmed cell death protein 1 (PD-1)/programmed cell death ligand 1 (PD-L1) checkpoint inhibitors (pembroli-zumab, with antitumor activity against immune-positive cancers) [10]. Targeted therapies are considerably more effective against specific NSCLC variants, thus leaving a large number of patients with limited options for treatment. These knowl-edge gaps emphasize the need for more precise stratification of racial and ethnic groups; development of noninvasive, early biomarkers of lung cancer; and addi-tional research to uncover molecular pathways of malignant conversion that can be targeted for therapeutic intervention.

COPD is a highly prevalent chronic disease, characterized by persistent airflow limitation, debilitating morbidity, and staggering mortality [11]. The public health burden of COPD has increased substantially throughout the world, with chronic respiratory diseases now ranked as the third leading cause of death worldwide [12]. There is only limited understanding of the genetic factors that predispose to disease and, other than smoking cessation, no therapies to specifically modify trajectory of disease. A focus on COPD within the context of lung cancer is critical given that 50–80% of lung cancer patients have COPD compared with a 15–20% prevalence of COPD in the general smoking population [13, 14], and growing evidence that smokers with COPD are at significantly increased risk of lung cancer development [15–21]. In fact, in some patients, COPD may be an intermediate phenotype between smoking and lung cancer, although the exact mechanisms driving this relationship remain uncertain.

Racial and Ethnic Differences in COPD and Lung Cancer

COPD and lung cancer are related diseases associated with substantial morbidity and mortality [22]. Both of these conditions present more severely in individuals with African ancestry compared to CAs [23, 24], although the root causes of these differences have not been studied in detail. A recent study of genomic samples from Colombia, Mexico, Peru, and Puerto Rico identified several ancestry-enriched sin-gle nucleotide polymorphisms (SNPs) in genes coding for cytokine receptors, T cell receptor signaling, and antigen presentation [25]. The study also described SNPs with excess African or European ancestry that were linked to ancestry-specific expression patterns of genes involved in both the innate and adaptive immune sys-tems, indicating their possible effects on health- and disease-related phenotypes in Latin(x) populations. In this regard, differential gene expression has been found in the lung tumors of AAs compared to CAs, along with significant differences in M1 and M2 macrophage infiltration into the tumor [26]. Other studies point to racial differences in genes involved in inflammation and oxidative stress in both lung can-cer and COPD [27]. Such differences may eventually help explain the lower 5-year survival rate for lung cancer in AAs (16%) relative to CAs (19%). Survival is lower in AAs at every stage of diagnosis, which has been attributed to differences in timely, high-quality medical care [28, 29]. However, racial disparities may persist even after accounting for socioeconomic factors and access to care [30–32]. Interestingly, AAs develop COPD with less cumulative smoking and at younger ages [33–35], suggesting greater susceptibility to tobacco smoke carcinogens. The racial differences in lung cancer outcomes found in AAs are relevant to Latin(x) populations because this ethnic group is characterized by pervasive admixture among European settlers, Native Americans, and Africans. The large degree of admixture among Latin(x) suggests that their relative susceptibility is highly variable, and that subgroups with large African ancestry may share the enhanced susceptibility of AAs. The same argument may be raised for many AAs, where considerable genetic admixture exists across the United States. Interestingly, despite lower socioeconomic status, Latin(x) have been found to be at lower risk of COPD and lung cancer compared to AAs or CAs, even after accounting for differences in smoking status and intensity [36–38]. While the debate continues to determine whether such differences are accounted for by social, behavioral, environmental, and economic factors, growing evidence supports that "protection" of Latin(x) may be partly accounted for by Native American ancestry [39, 40]. In sharp contrast, the proportion of African ancestry has been associated with increased risk [41], suggesting that ancestral heterogeneity generates a broad spectrum of susceptibility among Latin(x) depending on the balance of protection and susceptibility afforded by the Native American and African ancestry components. This scenario is consistent with the inverse relation of African ancestry to lung function among AAs [42, 43].

ORF1p in COPD and Lung Cancer

The search for circulating biomarkers has become a research priority in the study of complex diseases. Blood is readily accessible and provides a relatively noninvasive means to detect illness-related alterations and track disease trajectory over time, allowing for amplification of the signal of interest for association with other clinical measures. One of our focuses over the past 10 years has been the study of LINE-1 retroelements and their role in the regulation of lung epithelial cell phenotypes and genetic instability. We have also been interested in examining the utility of measurements of LINE-1-encoded proteins in tissue and the general circulation as biomarkers of lung cancer. Human LINE-1 is ~6 kb and consists of an internal promoter, two open reading frames encoding two proteins (ORF1p and ORF2p), and a poly (A) tail [44] (Fig. 8.1). LINE-1 propagates its own DNA and other DNAs through a copy-and-paste mechanism that uses an RNA intermediate, a process known as retrotransposition. This process can lead to full-length or truncated insertions of LINE-1 sequences or other sequences throughout the genome [45]. Approximately 100 full-length, retrotransposition-competent copies of LINE-1 remain in the human genome [46]. In healthy somatic cells, LINE-1 is epigenetically silenced through DNA methylation, histone covalent modifications, and nucleosome positioning (Fig. 8.2). Hypomethylation of selected CpG sites by DNA damage,

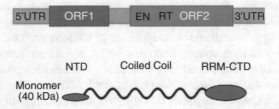

Fig. 8.1 Schematic representation of LINE-1. Full length LINE-1 is approximately 6 kb in length and consists of 5′ and 3′ untranslated regions (UTRs) and two proteins, ORF1 (orange) and ORF2 (blue). ORF1 is a nucleic acid binding protein consisting of an alpha helix in between the N- and C-terminal domains (NTD and CTD), with an RNA recognition motif (RRM) near the CTD. Coiled-coil interactions facilitate the formation of higher order multimers and polymers of ORF1p. ORF2p is approximately 150 kDa and contains both endonuclease (EN) and reverse transcriptase (RT) domains

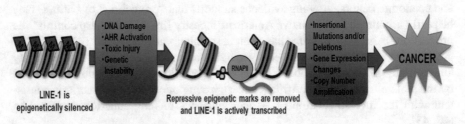

Fig. 8.2 Epigenetic regulation of LINE-1. LINE-1 is silenced by DNA methylation and repressive chromatin modifications in somatic tissues. Under stressful conditions, LINE-1 can be reactivated to cause genetic and epigenetic alterations associated with cancer development

activation of the aryl hydrocarbon receptor by lung carcinogens present in tobacco smoke, or various other forms of toxic injury mediate transcriptional activation of LINE-1 and result in cellular buildup of ORF1p. This protein in turn modulates oncogenic signaling and participates in retrotransposition [47, 48]. To date, we have extensively characterized the molecular effectors responsible for epigenetic silencing of LINE-1 [49], and more recently have begun to exploit this knowledge to develop prevention strategies and targeted therapeutics against lung cancer.

The genome of NSCLCs is strongly affected by LINE-1 insertions [50, 51]. Several studies by our group and others have shown that ORF1p accumulates in lung cancer cells [52, 53]. This buildup is consistent with increased LINE-1 hypomethylation in lung cancer [54, 55]. Because COPD may be viewed as a preneoplastic state, at least in a subset of NSCLC patients, we hypothesized that measurements of circulating ORF1p may inform the clinical evaluation of patients with COPD. To test this hypothesis, the association of ORF1p with lung function and airflow limitation (the hallmark of COPD) was examined in a population-based cohort of adults [56]. Stratification by smoking status showed consistent associations of ORF1p with FEV1, FVC, and airflow limitation in former smokers, after adjustment for the above covariates and active asthma. The observed increases in ORF1p after smoking cessation suggest that sustained alterations in genetic control of LINE-1 coupled with genetic instability occur in at least a subgroup of former smokers. Indeed, previous reports have shown that airway and systemic inflammation may persist in a proportion of smokers after smoking cessation, posing increased risk of inception and progression of COPD years after quitting [57]. Given that the cohort examined was mostly CAs, and that our sample size was only 427 subjects, additional studies are required to evaluate the generalizability of our findings and their relevance to different racial and ethnic groups. These limitations notwithstanding our findings suggest that ORF1p is associated with lower lung function and increased airflow limitation in former smokers. A preliminary study comparing self-identified Latin(x) and African Americans has suggested that ostensibly healthy AAs have higher levels of circulating ORF1p than Latin(x), and that females exhibit higher protein levels than males (Ramos et al., unpublished). These data are consistent with our working hypothesis and raise important questions about the impact of genetic admixture and sex on ORF1p levels in the general circulation.

ORF1p is a basic protein with conserved C- and N-terminal coiled-coil domains responsible for multimerization [58]. Coiled-coil proteins are involved in tethering of transport vesicles and regulation of cargo binding [59], functions consistent with the accumulation of ORF1p in circulating human exosomes [60]. ORF1p functions as a single-stranded RNA and DNA-binding protein with chaperone activity and is known to participate in retrotransposition [61–63]. As such, measurements of ORF1p reflect the LINE-1 status and serve as a tool for development of sensitive biomarkers of genetic instability in lung cancer. ORF1p interacts with a number of cellular proteins [64], including nucleolin (NCL). NCL is an RNA-binding protein with multiple roles in ribosome biogenesis, transcription, RNA turnover, translation, DNA repair, and apoptosis [65–67]. This protein accumulates in the cytoplasm and the cell surface in several cancer types, including lung cancer [68, 69]. We have recently shown that NCL regulates ORF1p expression and that this interaction can be targeted by NCL antagonists [70]. We also showed that pharmacological inhibition of NCL arrests NSCLC growth in a nude mouse xenograft model of lung cancer. These findings open the door to novel therapies for lung cancer treatment focused on inhibition of LINE-1 activity in cancer cells.

Concluding Remarks

Given the molecular heterogeneity that characterizes lung cancer, precision approaches that risk stratify individuals and populations, coupled with targeted therapies, are needed. Population stratification is particularly relevant for precise identification of individuals at risk of lung malignancy. While the increased susceptibility to lung cancer in individuals of African ancestry has been recognized for years, little is known about the genetic, environmental, and lifestyle determinants of this increased susceptibility. For Latin(x) groups, this gap in knowledge is significant given their large degree of genetic admixture, which may either afford protection or increased susceptibility depending on the relative degree of genetic admixture. Such differences in susceptibility also become relevant for future development of targeted therapies. Currently available therapies only benefit a small subset of NSCLC patients, mostly those who are either relatively young or never/light smokers. Thus, novel strategies are needed to increase the numbers of lung cancer patients who may benefit from precision therapies. Precision approaches will help to better define the root causes of lung cancer heterogeneity in different populations and address some of the shortcomings of low-dose computerized tomography screening. Together, the evidence reviewed here can be contextualized to develop novel risk stratification strategies and targeted therapies for lung cancer that take into account genetic admixture and health disparities among Latin(x) populations.

Acknowledgments The creative contributions of Dr. Emma Bowers in the design of figures and the editorial assistance of Ms. Kim Nguyen are gratefully acknowledged.

References

1. Dela Cruz CS, Tanoue LT, Matthay RA. Lung cancer: epidemiology, etiology and prevention. Clin Chest Med. 2011;32(4):605–44. https://doi.org/10.1016/j.ccm.2011.09.001.
2. Centers for Disease Control and Prevention. Tobacco use by youth is rising. https://www.cdc.gov/vitalsigns/youth-tobacco-use/index.html. Accessed 2 Sept 2020.
3. Centers for Disease Control and Prevention. Outbreak of lung injury associated with the use of e-cigarette, or vaping, products. https://www.cdc.gov/tobacco/basic_information/e-cigarettes/severe-lung-disease.html. Accessed 1 Sept 2020.
4. Song Q, Christiani DC, Wang X, Ren J. The global contribution of outdoor air pollution to the incidence, prevalence, mortality and hospital admission for chronic obstructive pulmonary disease: a systematic review and meta-analysis. Int J Environ Res Public Health. 2014;11(11):11822–32. https://doi.org/10.3390/ijerph111111822.
5. Travis WD. Pathology of lung cancer. Clin Chest Med. 2011;32(4):669–92. https://doi.org/10.1016/j.ccm.2011.08.005.
6. Alberg AJ, Brock MV, Ford JG, Samet JM, Spivack SD. Epidemiology of lung cancer: diagnosis and management of lung cancer, 3rd ed: American College of Chest Physicians evidence-based clinical practice guidelines. Chest. 2013;143(5 Suppl):e1S–e29S. https://doi.org/10.1378/chest.12-2345.
7. Molina JR, Yang P, Cassivi SD, Schild SE, Adjei AA. Non–small cell lung cancer: epidemiology, risk factors, treatment, and survivorship. Mayo Clin Proc. 2009;83(5):584–94. https://doi.org/10.4065/83.5.584.
8. Ryan BM. Lung cancer health disparities. Carcinogenesis. 2018;39(6):741–51. https://doi.org/10.1093/carcin/bgy047.
9. Schabath MB, Cress WD, Munoz-Antonia T. Racial and ethnic differences in the epidemiology of lung cancer and the lung cancer genome. Cancer Control. 2016;23(4):338–46. https://doi.org/10.1177/107327481602300405.
10. Halliday PR, Blakely CM, Bivona TG. Emerging targeted therapies for the treatment of non-small cell lung cancer. Curr Oncol Rep. 2019;21(3):21. https://doi.org/10.1007/s11912-019-0770-x.
11. Segal LN, Martinez FJ. Chronic obstructive pulmonary disease subpopulations and phenotyping. J Allergy Clin Immunol. 2018;141:1961–71. https://doi.org/10.1016/j.jaci.2018.02.035.
12. GBD Chronic Respiratory Disease Collaborators. Prevalence and attributable health burden of chronic respiratory diseases, 1990-2017: a systematic analysis for the Global Burden of

Disease Study 2017. Lancet Respir Med. 2020;8:585–96. Available from: https://www.thelancet.com/journals/lanres/article/PIIS2213-2600(20)30105-3/fulltext. Accessed 4 Sept 2020.

13. El-zein, RA, Young RP, Hopkins RJ, Etzel CJ. Genetic predisposition to chronic obstructive pulmonary disease and/or lung cancer: important considerations when evaluating risk. Cancer Prev Res. 2012;5(4):522–7. Available from: https://doi.org/10.1158/1940-6207.CAPR-12-0042.

14. Young RP, Hopkins RJ. How the genetics of lung cancer overlap with COPD. Respirology. 2011;16(7):1047–55. https://doi.org/10.1111/j.1440-1843.2011.02019.x.

15. Husebo GR, Nielsen R, Hardie J, Bakke PS, Lerner L, D'Alessandro-Gabazz C, Gyuris J, Gabazza E, Aukrust P, Eagan T. Risk factors for lung cancer in COPD – results from the Bergen COPD cohort study. Respir Med. 2019;152:81–8. https://doi.org/10.1016/j.rmed.2019.04.019.

16. Mannino DM, Aguayo SM, Petty TL, Redd SC. Low lung function and incident lung cancer in the United States: data from the first National Health and Nutrition Examination Survey follow-up. Arch Intern Med. 2003;163:1475–80.

17. Gagnat AA, Gulsvik A, Bakke P, Gjerdevik M. Comparison of two lung cancer screening scores among patients with chronic obstructive pulmonary disease: a community study. Clin Respir J. 2019;13(2):114–9. https://doi.org/10.1111/crj.12988.

18. Tockman MS, Anthonisen NR, Wright EC, Donithan MG. Airways obstruction and the risk for lung cancer. Ann Inter Med. 1987;106:512–8.

19. Lowry KP, Gazelle GS, Gilmore ME, Johanson C, Munshi V, Choi SE, et al. Personalizing annual lung cancer screening for patients with chronic obstructive pulmonary disease: a decision analysis. Cancer. 2015;121:1556–62. https://doi.org/10.1002/cncr.29225.

20. Wang J, Spitz MR, Amos CI, Wu X, Wetter DW, Cinciripini PM, et al. Method for evaluating multiple mediators: mediating effects of smoking and COPD on the association between the CHRNA5-A3 variant and lung cancer risk. PLoS One. 2012;7(10):e47705.

21. Yang IA, Relan V, Wright CM, Davidson MR, Sriram KB, Savarimuthu SM, et al. Common pathogenic mechanisms and pathways in the development of COPD and lung cancer. Expert Opin Ther Targets. 2011;15(4):439–56. https://doi.org/10.1517/14728222.2011.555400.

22. Young RP, Hopkins RJ, Gamble GD, Etzel C, El-Zein R, Crapo JD. Genetic evidence linking lung cancer and COPD: a new perspective. Appl Clin Genet. 2011;4:99–111. https://doi.org/10.2147/TACG.S20083.

23. Mina N, Soubani AO, Cote ML, Suwan T, Wenzlaff AS, Jhajhria S, et al. The relationship between COPD and lung cancer in African American patients. Clin Lung Cancer. 2012;13(2):149–56. https://doi.org/10.1016/j.cllc.2011.09.006.

24. Dransfield MT, Davis JJ, Gerald LB, Bailey WC, et al. Racial and gender differences in susceptibility to tobacco smoke among patients with chronic obstructive pulmonary disease. Respir Med. 2006;100(6):1110–6.

25. Bryc K, Durand EY, Macpherson JM, Reich D, Mountain JL. The genetic ancestry of African Americans, Latinos and European Americans across the United States. Am J Hum Genet. 2015;96(1):37–53. https://doi.org/10.1016/j.ajhg.2014.11.010.

26. Jacklute J, Zermaitis M, Pranys D, Sitkauskiene B, Miliauskas S, Vaitkiene S, et al. Distribution of M1 and M2 macrophages in tumor islets and stroma in relation to prognosis of non-small cell lung cancer. BMC Immunol. 2018;19:3. https://doi.org/10.1186/s12865-018-0241-4.

27. Barnes PJ. Molecular genetics of chronic obstructive pulmonary disease. Thorax. 1999;54:245–52. https://doi.org/10.1136/thx.54.3.245.

28. Bach PB, Schrag D, Brawley OW, Galaznik A, Yakren S, Begg CB. Survival of blacks and whites after a cancer diagnosis. JAMA. 2002;287(16):2106–13. https://doi.org/10.1001/jama.287.16.2106.

29. Schwartz AG, Prysak GM, Bock CH, Cote ML. The molecular epidemiology of lung cancer. Carcinogenesis. 2006;28(3):507–18. https://doi.org/10.1093/carcin/bgl253.

30. William DR, Priest N, Anderson N. Understanding associations between race, socioeconomic status and health: patterns and prospects. Health Psychol. 2016;35(4):407–11. https://doi.org/10.1037/hea0000242.

31. Centers for Disease Control and Prevention (CDC). Racial/ethnic disparities and geographic differences in lung cancer incidence – 38 States and the District of Columbia, 1998–2006. Morb Mortal Wkly Rep. 2010;59(44):1434–8.
32. American Cancer Society. Cancer facts & figures for African Americans 2019–2021. Atlanta: American Cancer Society; 2019. https://www.cancer.org/content/dam/cancer-org/research/cancer-facts-and-statistics/cancer-facts-and-figures-for-african-americans/cancer-facts-and-figures-for-african-americans-2019-2021.pdf. Accessed 1 Sept 2020.
33. Chatila WM, Wynkoop WA, Vance G, Criner CJ. Smoking patterns in African Americans and whites with advanced COPD. Chest. 2004;125(1):15–21. https://doi.org/10.1378/chest.125.1.15.
34. Putcha N, Han MK, Martinez CH, Foreman MG, Anzueto AR, Casaburi R, et al. Comorbidities of COPD have a major impact on clinical outcomes, particularly in African Americans. Chronic Obstr Pulm Dis. 2014;1(1):105–14. https://doi.org/10.15326/jcopdf.1.1.2014.0112.
35. Roberts ME, Colby SM, Lu B, Ferketich AK. Understanding tobacco use onset among African Americans. Nicotine Tob Res. 2016;18(S1):S49–56.
36. Diaz AA, Celli B, Celedon JC. Chronic obstructive pulmonary disease in Hispanics. A 9-year update. Am J Resp Crit Care Med. 2018;197:15–21. https://doi.org/10.1164/rccm.201708-1615PP.
37. Bruse S, Sood A, Petersen H, Liu Y, Leng S, Celedon JC, et al. New Mexican Hispanic smokers have lower odds of chronic obstructive pulmonary disease and less decline in lung function than non-Hispanic whites. Am J Respir Crit Care Med. 2011;184(11):1254–60. https://www.atsjournals.org/doi/full/10.1164/rccm.201103-0568OC. Accessed 3 Sept 2020.
38. Young RP, Hopkins RJ. A review of the Hispanic paradox: time to spill the beans? Eur Respir Rev. 2014;23(134):439–49. https://doi.org/10.1183/09059180.00000814.
39. Leng S, Liu Y, Thomas CL, Gauderman WJ, Picchi MA, Bruse SE, et al. Native American ancestry affects the risk for gene methylation in the lungs of Hispanic smokers from New Mexico. Am J Respir Crit Care Med. 2013;188(9):1110–6. https://www.atsjournals.org/doi/full/10.1164/rccm.201305-0925OC. Accessed 1 Sept 2020.
40. Stern MC, Fejerman L, Das R, Setiawan VW, Cruz-Correa MR, Perez-Stable EJ, et al. Variability in cancer risk and outcomes within US Latinos by national origin and genetic ancestry. Curr Epidemiol Rep. 2016;3:181–90. https://link.springer.com/article/10.1007/s40471-016-0083-7. Accessed 1 Sept 2020.
41. Haiman CA, Stram DO, Wilens LR, Pike MC, Kolonel LN, Henderson BE, et al. Ethnic and racial differences in the smoking-related risk of lung cancer. N Engl J Med. 2006;354:333–42. https://www.nejm.org/doi/full/10.1056/NEJMoa033250.
42. Kumar R, Seibold MA, Aldrich MC, Williams LK, Reiner AP, Colangelo L, et al. Genetic ancestry in lung-function predictions. N Engl J Med. 2010;363(4):321–30. https://doi.org/10.1056/NEJMoa0907897.
43. Aldrich MC, Kumar R, Colangelo LA, Williams LK, Sen S, Kritchevsky SB, et al. Genetic ancestry-smoking interactions and lung function in African Americans: a cohort study. PLoS One. 2012;7(6):e39541. https://doi.org/10.1371/journal.pone.0039541.
44. Khalid M, Bojang P, Hassanin AAI, Bowers EC, Ramos IN, Ramos KS. LINE-1: implications in the etiology of cancer, clinical applications and pharmacological targets. Mut Res Rev. 2018;778:51–60. https://doi.org/10.1016/j.mrrev.2018.09.003.
45. Bojang P, Roberts R, Anderton M, Ramos KS. De novo LINE-1 retrotransposition in HepG2 cells preferentially targets gene poor regions of chromosome 13. Genomics. 2014;104(2):96–104. https://doi.org/10.1016/j.ygeno.2014.07.001.
46. Beck CR, Collier P, Macfarlane C, Malig M, Kidd JM, Eichler EE, et al. LINE-1 retrotransposition activity in human genomes. Cell. 2010;141:1159–70. https://doi.org/10.1016/j.cell.2010.05.021.
47. Reyes-Reyes EN, Ramos I, Tavera-Garcia MA, Ramos KS. The aryl hydrocarbon receptor agonist benzo(a)pyrene reactivates LINE-1 in HepG2 cells through canonical TGF-β1 signaling:

implications in hepatocellular carcinogenesis. Am J Cancer Res. 2016:1066–77. https://www.ncbi.nlm.nih.gov/pmc/articles/PMC4889720/. Accessed 1 Sept 2020.

48. Reyes-Reyes EM, Aispuro I, Tavera-Garcia MA, Field M, Moore S, Ramos IN, et al. LINE-1 couples EMT programming with acquisition of oncogenic phenotypes in human bronchial epithelial cells. Oncotarget. 2017:103828–42. https://doi.org/10.18632/oncotarget.21953.

49. Bojang P, Ramos KS. Epigenetic reactivation of LINE-1 disrupts NuRD co-repressor functions and induces oncogenic transformation of human bronchial epithelial cells. Mol Oncol. 2018;12:1342–57. https://febs.onlinelibrary.wiley.com/doi/full/10.1002/1878-0261.12329. Accessed 1 Sept 2020.

50. Iskow RC, McCabe MT, Mills RE, Torene S, Pittard WS, Neuwald AF, et al. Natural mutagenesis of human genomes by endogenous retrotransposons. Cell. 2010;141:1253–61. https://doi.org/10.1016/j.cell.2010.05.020.

51. Rodic N, Sharma R, Sharma R, Zampella J, Dai L, Taylor MS, et al. Long interspersed element-1 protein expression is a hallmark of many human cancers. Am J Pathol. 2014;184:1280–6. https://doi.org/10.1016/j.ajpath.2014.01.007.

52. Asch HL, Eliacin E, Fanning TG, Connolly JL, Bratthauer G, Asch BB. Comparative expression of the line-1 p40 protein in human breast carcinomas and normal breast tissues. Oncol Res. 1996;8:239–47. https://doi.org/10.1373/clinchem.2016.257444.

53. Su Y, Davies S, Davis M, Lu H, Giller R, Krailo M, et al. Expression of LINE-1 p40 protein in pediatric malignant germ cell tumors and its association with clinicopathological parameters: a report from the Children's Oncology Group. Cancer Lett. 2007;247:204–12. https://doi.org/10.1016/j.canlet.2006.04.010.

54. Ikeda K, Shiraishi K, Eguchi A, Shibata H, Yoshimoto K, Mori T, et al. Long interspersed nucleotide element 1 hypomethylation is associated with poor prognosis of lung adenocarcinoma. Ann Thorac Surg. 2013;96:1790–4. https://doi.org/10.1016/j.athoracsur.2013.06.035.

55. Saito K, Kawakami K, Matsumoto I, Oda M, Watanabe G, Minamoto T. Long interspersed nuclear element 1 hypomethylation is a marker of poor prognosis in stage IA non-small cell lung cancer. Clin Cancer Res. 2010;16:2418–26. https://doi.org/10.1158/1078-0432.CCR-09-2819.

56. Guerra S, Vasquez MM, Bojang P, Ramos IN, Sherrill DL, Martinez FD, et al. Serum levels of LINE1-ORF1p and airflow limitation. Eur Respir J Open. 2019;5:00247-2018. https://openres.ersjournals.com/content/5/4/00247-2018. Accessed 1 Sept 2020.

57. Hogg JC. Why does airway inflammation persist after the smoking stops. Thorax. 2006;61:96–7. https://doi.org/10.1136/thx.2005.049502.

58. Martin SJ. The ORF1 protein encoded by LINE-1: structure and function during L1 retrotransposition. J Biomed Biotechnol. 2006;2006:45621. https://doi.org/10.1155/JBB/2006/45621.

59. Truebestein L, Leonard TA. Coiled-coils: the long and short of it. BioEssays. 2016;38:903–16. https://doi.org/10.1002/bies.201600062.

60. Bowers EC, Cavalcante AM, McKay BS, Ramos KS. The LINE-1 ORF1 protein content of extracellular vesicles mirrors cellular expression profiles in Non-Small Cell Lung Cancer cell lines. Submitted for publication, 2020.

61. Martin SL, Bushman FD. Nucleic acid chaperone activity of the ORF1 protein from the mouse LINE-1 retrotransposon. Mol Cell Biol. 2001;2:467–75. https://doi.org/10.1128/MCB.21.2.467-475.2001.

62. Naufer MN, Furano AV, Williams MC. Protein-nucleic acid interactions of LINE-1 ORF1p. Semin Cell Dev Biol. 2019;86:140–9. https://doi.org/10.1016/j.semcdb.2018.03.019.

63. Naufer NM, Callahan KE, Cook PR, Perez-Gonzalez CE, Williams MC, Furano AV. L1 retrotransposition requires rapid ORF1p oligomerization, a novel coiled coil-dependent property conserved despite extensive remodeling. Nucleic Acids Res. 2016;44:281–93. https://doi.org/10.1093/nar/gkv1342.

64. Goodier JL, Cheung LE, Kazazian HH. Mapping the LINE1 ORF1 protein interactome reveals associated inhibitors of human retrotransposition. Nucleic Acids Res. 2013;41(15):7401–19. https://doi.org/10.1093/nar/gkt512.

65. Abdelmohsen K, Goroscope M. RNA-binding protein nucleolin in disease. RNA Biol. 2012;9(6):799–808. https://doi.org/10.4161/rna.19718.
66. Piazzi M, Bavelloni A, Gallo A, Faenza I, Blalock WL. Signal transduction in ribosome biogenesis: a recipe to avoid disaster. Int J Mol Sci. 2019;20(11):2718. https://doi.org/10.3390/ijms20112718.
67. Jia W, Yao Z, Zhao J, Guan Q, Gao L. New perspectives of physiological and pathological functions of nucleolin (NCL). Life Sci. 2017;186:1–10. https://doi.org/10.1016/j.lfs.2017.07.025.
68. Huang F, Wu Y, Tan H, Guo T, Zhang K, Li D, et al. Phosphorylation of nucleolin is indispensable to its involvement in the proliferation and migration of non-small cell lung cancer cells. Oncol Rep. 2019;41:590–8. https://doi.org/10.3892/or.2018.6787.
69. Xu J-Y, Lu S, Xu X-Y, Hu S-L, Li B, Li W-X, et al. Prognostic significance of nuclear or cytoplasmic nucleolin expression in human non-small cell lung cancer and its relationship with DNA-PKcs. Tumor Biol. 2016;37(8):10349–56. https://doi.org/10.1007/s13277-016-4920-6.
70. Ramos KS, Moore S, Rogue I, Courty J, Reyes-Reyes EM. The nucleolin antagonist N6L inhibits LINE1 retrotransposon expression in non-small cell lung cancer cells. J Cancer. 2019;11:733–40. https://doi.org/10.7150/jca.37776.

Open Access   This chapter is licensed under the terms of the Creative Commons Attribution 4.0 International License (http://creativecommons.org/licenses/by/4.0/), which permits use, sharing, adaptation, distribution and reproduction in any medium or format, as long as you give appropriate credit to the original author(s) and the source, provide a link to the Creative Commons license and indicate if changes were made.

The images or other third party material in this chapter are included in the chapter's Creative Commons license, unless indicated otherwise in a credit line to the material. If material is not included in the chapter's Creative Commons license and your intended use is not permitted by statutory regulation or exceeds the permitted use, you will need to obtain permission directly from the copyright holder.

Part VI
Engaging Latinos in Cancer Research

Chapter 9
Optimizing Engagement of the Latino Community in Cancer Research

Lourdes Baezconde-Garbanati, Bibiana Martinez, Carol Ochoa,
Sheila Murphy, Rosa Barahona, Carolina Aristizabal,
and Yaneth L. Rodriguez

Overview

To optimize engagement of Latino communities in cancer research, we are working with communities in multiple areas of cancer prevention and control. Our purpose is to increase inclusion in life-saving programs, provide targets for precision medicine that are best suited for Latino populations, and accelerate the translation of scientific cancer discoveries into public health policy. Through research participation of Latinos, we have been able to generate focused and culturally grounded interventions in language for Latinos that resonate with communities and help save lives. As the population of Latinos in the United States continues to grow and is an emergent majority group, we are called to invest in this population's health, ensure Latinos are represented in research, understand barriers to implementation of public health guidelines, and encourage involvement in clinical trials. This will result in enhancements to precision medicine, providing better treatment options to this heterogeneous group as well as better focused precision public health measures for prevention.

L. Baezconde-Garbanati (✉) · R. Barahona · C. Aristizabal
USC Norris Comprehensive Cancer Center and Department of Population and Public Health Sciences, Keck School of Medicine, University of Southern California,
Los Angeles, CA, USA
e-mail: Baezcond@usc.edu

B. Martinez · C. Ochoa · Y. L. Rodriguez
Division of Health Behavior, Institute for Prevention Research, Department of Population and Public Health Sciences, Keck School of Medicine of USC, University of Southern California,
Los Angeles, CA, USA

S. Murphy
Annenberg School for Communication and Journalism, University of Southern California,
Los Angeles, CA, USA

© The Author(s) 2023
A. G. Ramirez, E. J. Trapido (eds.), *Advancing the Science of Cancer in Latinos*, https://doi.org/10.1007/978-3-031-14436-3_9

Demographics of the Latino Population

According to the Pew Research Center [1], the Latino population reached 60.6 million in 2019, representing 18% of the US population. Latinos make up a very heterogeneous group and tend to define themselves by nativity or country of origin. Seventy-one percent of Latinos 5 years or older speak English proficiently, even if they speak another language other than English at home. Over 60% of Latinos in the United States are of Mexican origin, followed by those of Puerto Rican origin. Recently, Puerto Rico has been devastated by hurricanes and earthquakes, resulting in large migration to the mainland. Puerto Ricans are US citizens, allowed to vote once in the US mainland. The fastest growth among Latinos is among people from Venezuela, Dominican Republic, Guatemala, and Honduras, who are scattered throughout the United States. Four in five Latinos are US citizens, representing over 32 million Latinos who were eligible to vote in 2020.

Catchment Area

The catchment area for our USC Norris Comprehensive Cancer Center is Los Angeles County, which has a population of 10,105,518. According to the 2020 US Bureau of the Census, that population is 48.7% Latino, 26.1% White alone, 14.0% Asian alone, and 8.1% African American alone. In Los Angeles County, 34.2% are foreign born and 14.2% are people in poverty. Latinos make up 35% of Los Angeles County's homeless population. Much of our outreach and engagement concentrates in the Eastern side of Los Angeles, which is predominantly Latino. The ethnic breakdown of the East side consists of 91.2% Latino, 5.2% Asian, 2.3% White, 0.7% African American, and 0.6% other. In this region, 5.1% of residents aged 25 and older have a four-year college degree and 14.2% of these residents are high school dropouts. More than two-thirds of the residents in the region, approximately 66.8%, live in shared housing.

Cancer Burden in the Catchment Area

Although cancer rates are declining overall for all populations, cancer disparities still exist among some groups. Cancer is the leading cause of death among Latinos, followed by heart disease. Latino men and women have a lower lifetime probability of developing cancer than non-Hispanic White men and women (This varies however, by cancer type and by foreign born versus the U.S. born. It may in part be due to cultural factors (acculturation, language); social factors (low levels of educational attainment, low socioeconomic status, low literacy and numeracy levels); environmental factors (exposure to pesticide, exposure to chemicals); clinical factors (lack of knowledge in navigating the system of care); psychological factors (fear of diagnosis, fatalism); biological and genetic factors (family history of disease); behavioral factors (sedentary lifestyles, obesity); and a variety of other factors that may impact these disparities [2]. The priority cancers in the catchment area selected by our Comprehensive Cancer Center (not just for Latinos but all population groups) include breast cancer, prostate cancer, lung cancer, colorectal cancer, liver cancer, and acute lymphoblastic leukemia. Our focus is also on associated cancer risk behaviors and factors that include tobacco, energy balance and obesity, diet and physical activity, cervical cancer screening, HPV vaccinations, and environmental pollutants. We work in particular on cervical cancer, as it has one of the highest rates of all cancers among Latinas in Los Angeles and is one of the most treatable and preventable cancers today.

Human Papillomavirus (HPV) Infections and Cervical Cancer

Cervical cancer is highly preventable and treatable, and although deaths from cervical cancer have declined over the past 40 years, Latinas in general have not benefitted equally. HPV is the most common sexually transmitted infection in the United States. It is one of the major causes of infection-related cancers worldwide. Current guidelines for HPV vaccination in the United States call for three vaccine doses for children who receive their first dose after their 15th birthday. If children are vaccinated earlier, before initiating sexual activity, they are protected with only two doses. Unfortunately, Latinos have the lowest rates of initiation and completion of the HPV vaccine series and thus have higher rates of HPV-associated cervical cancer than non-Hispanic Whites.

Latinas have higher incidence and mortality from HPV-related cervical cancer than any other major racial/ethnic group in the United States, at a time when a vaccine against human papillomavirus (HPV) is available and strong screening guidelines are in place around the nation. Incidence rates for cervical cancer among low-income women in Los Angeles County are as high as 14.3 per 100,000 for Latina women compared to 9.3 per 100,000 for Asian/Pacific Islander women, 7.6 per 100,000 among black women, and 7.5 per 100,000 among non-Hispanic white women [3]. Women at the lowest levels of socioeconomic status (SES) have the highest age-adjusted rate of cervical cancer (20 per 100,000) compared with those at the highest levels of SES (7 per 100,000). Identifiable social determinants of health affect women's participation in research. Yet, there is an obvious need to reduce morbidity and mortality from HPV-related cancers in this population.

Intersectionality

Intersectionality contributes to lack of participation in cancer research among Latinos and is a focal point for understanding the high rates of cervical cancer. A series of factors come together to create a complex situation that combines low socioeconomic status, lack of health insurance, cultural and personal fears, and cancer-specific beliefs, which may deter women from going in for screening in a timely fashion. The excess morbidity and mortality from cervical cancer among Latinas may be also due in part to a significant education gap in this population when compared to other groups. Information often is lacking in language and requires it be delivered in culturally appropriate ways. Research has also shown that Latinas often do not know where to go for low to no-cost screenings or how to obtain the HPV vaccine for them or their children [4]. Some older women who have never had a Pap test may not know how one is done. Multiple situations may come together in the same individual making it more difficult for them to participate in clinical trials, as well as comply with treatment and properly adhere to medical guidelines. To address these issues, we developed specific strategies and programs that facilitate inclusion in order to increase: (1) research participation, (2) compliance with cancer screening guidelines, (3) clinical follow-up to abnormal test results, and (4) the number of Latino girls and boys vaccinated against HPV. This has allowed us to recruit Latinas into our studies and foster sustained participation in longitudinal research efforts.

Service Programs that Enhance Participation in Cancer Research

Our team from the USC Norris Comprehensive Cancer Center's (USC NCCC) Office of Community Outreach and Engagement (COE) has developed interventions and service programs that are culturally specific, account for literacy and numeracy, engage community residents, and use patient advocates and *promotores de salud*. These support programs reduce barriers to treatment compliance, as well as to participation in clinical trials. These programs also help to promote research in the community while tending to individual patient needs. Since 2015, our Lippin Navigation project, funded by the Tower Cancer Foundation, has navigated over 600 patients mostly Spanish speaking, and reduced the number of cultural barriers. Our Lazarex Cancer Foundation financial assistance program has allowed us to alleviate the financial toxicity, which may prevent individuals from participating in clinical trials. Our California-Florida Cancer Research, Education and Engagement Health Equity Center (CaRE2), funded by the National Cancer Institute (NCI) has facilitated the development of educational materials to reduce cancer disparities. Our National Outreach Network Community Health Educator (NON CHE), funded by the Center to Reduce Cancer Health Disparities (NCI) program facilitates the offering of workshops at the community level with follow-up on clinical trial participation in general and on HPV trials in particular. Hundreds of patients have been served through these support programs, reducing barriers to participation in cancer research.

Along with these service and intervention programs in place, we have identified strategies that help increase community-based and participatory engagement of Latinos in all aspects of cancer research. These strategies provide a foundation for culturally grounded, patient-centered implementation efforts. From our research and services, we have found that these strategies are critical in making the behavioral, attitudinal, knowledge-based changes necessary to engage the population in health seeking behaviors, such as regular screening and vaccination, as well as participation in cancer clinical trials. Our evidence-based interventions and educational materials to inform communities on cancer in the Latino population have been successful in mobilizing communities to take action for their health, and descriptions can be found in our website (https://uscnorriscancer.usc.edu/community-outreach-engagement/).

Examples of Innovative Cancer Research Engagement

We have successfully utilized strategies for inclusion described below successfully in our *Es Tiempo*—Jacaranda Initiative—and in our *Tamale Lesson* award-winning films and related interventions. Several projects and programs have resulted from these cervical cancer and HPV vaccination campaigns, helping to increase screening rates among Latinas, as well as examining barriers and hesitancy to HPV vaccination.

We present here two recent studies that illustrate the situation in the Latino community regarding HPV vaccination and cervical cancer screening. These studies were conducted with inclusion of *promotores de salud* and lay community workers who assisted us in conceptualization, recruitment, translations, cultural adaptation, and other important aspects of the research, making it more relevant and of greater interest to the community.

Promotores de Salud

An essential element to our work is the engagement of *promotores de salud (lay community health workers (CHWs)*. Our *promotores* tend to be part of *Vision y Compromiso*, a network of over 5,000 individuals who support health education efforts and community-based research. The *promotores de salud* are trusted individuals who come from the communities they work in. They are trained in the research enterprise and help implement research programs and objectives at the community level. In particular, we have worked with *promotores de salud* in our clinical interventions at *Clinicas Monsenor Oscar A. Romero*. Other programs also have contributed *promotores de salud* supporting these efforts at the community level.

Sample Intervention I—Reducing Barriers to Completing HPV Vaccinations and Cervical Cancer Screening Among Latinos

Our *Es Tiempo* campaign—the Jacaranda Initiative described elsewhere [5]—has been instrumental in engaging Latinas in cervical cancer research via recruitment by community health workers and community intercept surveys conducted by *promotores de salud*. A 2019 study from the Jacaranda Initiative [6] helped us better understand barriers to completion of the HPV vaccine doses and Pap tests screening among Latinas and their children. Seven hundred and forty five (n=745) women participated in a community sample for *Es Tiempo* between July and September 2019, another 1,428 women participated in a controlled experiment with Clinicas Monsenor Oscar A. Romero regarding compliance with cervical cancer screening guidelines. Two clinics (one in Boyle Heights and another in Pico Union) participated as intervention vs control in the testing of the Es Tiempo campaign. All participants in the community sample were foreign born, and 89% reported having some form of health insurance; 11% had at least one child between the ages of 9 and 26 years, and the women had a mean age of 49.

Findings revealed the following regarding HPV vaccinations in the community sample: (1) 83% of women did not understand the purpose of the HPV vaccine; (2) the most common response when asked about barriers to HPV vaccination was "I do not think it's necessary"; (3) 53% reported they had not heard about the HPV vaccine; and (4) over 50% of the women in the sample reported having received the HPV vaccine. Identified barriers to receiving the HPV vaccine included "not thinking it was necessary" to "not knowing why it was important." When asked about cervical cancer screening via Pap smears, responses were as follows: (1) 92% percent of the women reported knowing what a Pap smear exam detected. An overwhelming majority (94%) reported getting tested was "very important"; (2) 81% of the children of women in the sample had been vaccinated; (3) 62% of the children had received the full vaccination schedule according to guidelines; and (4) almost all (96%) women in the sample reported having received a Pap smear exam in the last 3 years. In the clinic sample, post intervention, when assessed about Pap tests, more women in the intervention clinic (Boyle Heights) (65%) were in compliance with screening guidelines, vs 34% in the control clinic (Pico Union). This was a significant difference (Chi Square <.001) of 13 percentage points. This study concluded that while Pap smear knowledge and screening were relatively high, HPV vaccine knowledge was low and attitudes differed about receiving information regarding the HPV vaccine. This study pointed to a need to continue our education for HPV vaccinations, particularly among foreign-born Latinas. Culturally and language specific materials displayed in billboards and other outdoor media along with educational materials sent to the home, made a difference in screening for Latinas in the Boyle Heights area of Los Angeles.

Sample Intervention II—Effectiveness of Storytelling in Educating and Changing Attitudes About the HPV Vaccine

Our award-winning Tamale Lesson cervical cancer intervention yielded tremendous results among English-speaking Latinas. However, we did not test its impact among mostly monolingual Spanish-speaking women. To do so, the films Tamale Lesson and It's Time [7] were translated into Spanish and culturally adapted by a team of *promotores de salud* from *Vision y Compromiso* (VyC) with funding from the Clinical Translation Science Institute (CTSI). We thus tested the effectiveness of two films in educating and changing attitudes about the uptake of the HPV vaccine among Spanish-speaking, Mexican American women [8]. We utilized narrative (storytelling) to convey crucial health information on cervical cancer and HPV vaccination. The sample consisted of 300 women who were randomly assigned to either the storytelling narrative (Tamale Lesson) or a non-narrative (It's Time) created by our team of investigators and described elsewhere [7]. All information was delivered in Spanish and accounted for literacy and numeracy levels. Data were collected by telephone. We conducted pre- and posttests using random digit dialing. Following the same methodology as our studies with English-speaking Latinas, posttests were conducted within 2 weeks of having viewed either film.

Findings for Spanish-speaking women showed that at baseline, women assigned to the narrative film (Tamale Lesson) were less likely to have heard of the HPV than women assigned to the non-narrative film (It's Time) (54% vs. 78%, $P = 0.008$). They were, however, more likely to know that the HPV vaccine was for both males and females (66.1% vs. 48.9%, $P = 0.008$). A total of 109 Spanish-speaking women completed all waves of the surveys. They were between the ages of 25 and 45 years and had incomes less than $20,000 per household. Over half of the women had less than a high school education (59%). Most were married or living with a partner (91%); 77% had a daughter and 24% had a son. The majority (84%) had some form of health-care coverage. Although the average number of years in the United States was 25, only 25% reported speaking English very well or well. Results indicated that the average increase in knowledge was 41% for storytelling versus 52% for non-narrative with more facts. From pretest to posttest, there was also an increase in supportive attitudes, such as reporting less embarrassment, increased perception of HPV importance, and vaccine safety. While these findings revealed that both films produced an increase in knowledge and an increase in supportive attitudes, they also suggested a lack of awareness and knowledge of HPV and the HPV vaccine among Spanish-speaking, Mexican-born women. This signaled to us the importance of evaluating the effectiveness of health education delivery methods among lower income and less acculturated Hispanic women, in order to achieve needed changes in health behaviors.

Sample Intervention III—Engaging Latinos in Virtual Reality (VR) Experiences to Increase HPV Vaccination Rates and Enhance End-of-Life Experiences for Immigrant Cancer Patients

A newer area of research we are beginning to explore in cancer care is the use of virtual reality to examine HPV vaccine hesitancy among Latino parents and their children, and the potential role VR technologies can play in end-of-life enhancements for patients dying from cancer. The LAC+USC Medical Center, the USC Institute of Creative Technology, and the USC SensoriMotor Assessment and Rehabilitation Training in the Virtual Reality Center develop virtual technologies with the goal of improving health care. We are currently working on the development of studies that pattern themselves after the Family Reunions Project, which helps individuals return home or to familiar places through the use of virtual reality. The goal is to better understand potential use of these new and emerging technologies to improve HPV uptake among youth, and of enhancing the quality of life of hospice patients and their families. The use of technologies, including virtual reality experiences, allows the cancer patient the ability to return back home.

Data from the Pew Research Center [9] reveal that this area of research among Latinos is promising. Already, about three in ten US adults say they are almost constantly online. Over 80% of adults go online several times a day. Younger adults in particular are almost constantly connected (46%). Individuals 65 years of age or older are online less; only 7% go online almost constantly and 35% go online multiple times a day. For Latinos in particular, over 72% say they own a desktop or a laptop computer. Prior to the COVID-19 pandemic, 78% of Latinos stated they went online at least occasionally compared to 87% among whites. Given new shut down restrictions in schools with the Coronavirus Pandemic, these numbers are likely to have risen tremendously and may be at an all-time high among Latinos. Although previously in 2015, wide gaps in Internet use existed among Latinos when compared to other Americans. The pandemic has created a real shift in usage, bringing in more who are Spanish dominant into the use of new and emerging technologies. Issues of Internet connectivity, lack of equipment, proper WiFi access, and other factors are still recognized barriers for use of these technologies. However, in spite of these barriers, we still anticipate much higher usage of these technologies, especially among younger populations; so this technology would be useful in the development of interventions for the HPV vaccine hesitancy experienced by youth and young adults.

The COVID-19 pandemic has brought the need to stay connected, resulting in an increased use of technology, so people of all ages can still communicate with friends and family members, work, and school. There is thus promise for expanding the use of new and emerging technologies among older populations of Latinos, if the experiences are tailored to their unique cultural needs, provided in their preferred language, personalized, and utilized at critical stages in their lives. Examples of successful virtual reality experiences in other areas beyond cancer include the

Family Reunions Project aimed at virtual reunification of immigrant families, LAC+USC County Hospital, USC Institute for Creative Technology, Quality of Life of Cancer Patients, and *Rendever*—a program where seniors are able to check off their bucket list. Engaging Latinos via virtual reality may enhance their interest in participating in clinical and prevention trials that may save lives, especially as related to HPV reductions via vaccinations and increased cervical cancer screening.

Common Strategies for Inclusion of Latinos in Cancer Research

Principles for Optimizing Participation

In order to engage Latinos in cancer research, specifically in cervical cancer and HPV trials and research, we have utilized and adopted a variety of principles of engagement generated by Israel and colleagues [10] for inclusion in community-based participatory research. This includes participation from the beginning stages of the research enterprise all the way to the dissemination of research findings. We engage participants in a bidirectional manner, so we not only provide scientific information to the community, but we also appreciate community knowledge when training academic researchers in community issues and how to reduce barriers to participation. Hence, the community is able to participate in reciprocal learning throughout the research process. This also facilitates engagement of communities in research decision-making. When we are able to obtain community consent for conducting research, communities are more open to engaging in the research. Furthermore, we share power and purpose empowering Latino communities at the grass roots level to take action for their own health. Community members are able to influence the research process, as well as foster new research by directly expressing their ideas to investigators via town hall meetings, online communities, community advisory boards, and as patient advocates in the research. We work on common visions, goals, values, and priorities. We regularly remunerate community partners, *promotores de salud*, and cultural experts with whom we engage in the research, and we strategize jointly with our community members via focus groups, meetings, and engagement activities in multifaceted ways.

In addition to the established principles described, our strategies for increasing participation in cancer research among Latinos focuses on the key areas of information delivery (knowledge transfer), consultation with stakeholders and partners, and collaboration with community key opinion leaders. The overarching goal is to optimize engagement of Latinos in research to find more tailored therapeutics and accelerate information transfer to the community. Our efforts aim to optimize engagement and communication in a bidirectional manner in order to impact attitudes, beliefs, and behaviors that may place Latinos at risk for cancer and to engage in research topics that make sense in the community.

Information Delivery (Knowledge Transfer)

In participatory engagement, we inform our community partners of the various aspects of a study and discuss culturally grounded and specific areas of the content needed to increase Latino engagement in particular communities. This goes beyond presenting the nature of the problem (e.g., high rates of cervical cancer) to fostering a discussion about needs and priorities in these areas within the community. These discussions are very intentional with the goal of accelerating knowledge transfer to communities more quickly while focusing on their expressed needs. When informing Latinos of specific areas of cancer research or providing cancer-specific message regarding the latest scientific findings, we have found a strategy to be most effective.

Key strategies include designing messages according to different levels of acculturation, language, and channels. In order to engage the Latino community, various channels must be utilized depending on specific audiences: channels include social media, Twitter, Facebook, Instagram, and Spanish language TV and radio. Limiting to three messages and using those messages to appeal to Latino cultural values has been most effective. Other channels that can be used to engage Latinos include online communities created specifically for program purposes. These include websites, webinars, and list serves. Written methods that have been traditionally utilized for outreach may include, newsletters, flyers, pamphlets, press releases, reports, brochures, direct mailers, and magazines. Interpersonal communication is another effective channel that works in the Latino community. In addition to the traditional formats of knowledge transfer, such as workshops, conferences, topic meetings, association and coalition meetings, and neighborhood council meetings, these strategies have worked well in our research.

Engage Stakeholders in Responsive Communication and Consultation Efforts

While trying to pursue engagement in cancer research and clinical trials, attentive listening is essential to empower Latino community stakeholders in the research. To facilitate stakeholder engagement, we produce and provide translated material and interpretation services in Spanish and Mandarin (for a large Asian population in Los Angeles) and use lay language. Other channels of stakeholder engagement in responsive communication include the development of community advisory boards, patient advocates, and citizen scientists.

Collaborate with Partner Organizations

We can enhance Latino engagement in research by casting a wide net of partners. To capitalize on this aspect, we formed an HPV local Los Angeles Coalition in 2016 that previously did not exist. We were able to develop this coalition with a grant from the National Cancer Institute as a Supplement to our Cancer Center on HPV. This coalition now includes over 30 community providers among cancer centers, hospitals, immunization coalitions, and health corporations, and it is housed at the Los Angeles Department of Public Health. We work on projects together, including expanding research capacity of its various members, helping each other in recruitment, sharing ideas for retention, and engaging in research as appropriate. We meet on a quarterly basis and are able to participate and have a voice in discussions about the current situation in Los Angeles related to HPV and other immunization efforts. Coalition development and participation can also be expanded to include multiple stakeholders, including faith-based organizations, cancer support groups, local clinics, schools, pharmacies, retailers, local neighborhood councils, parent groups, and senior centers. Critical audiences for inclusion, especially recognizing the need for physicians to make recommendations about the vaccine, are collaborations with community physicians, health professionals, associations, alliances, other coalitions, and other groups that would be interested in the research.

Conclusions

We have presented here sample support services programs that enhance participation by reducing barriers toward inclusion; presented research examples that utilize common strategies that have been proven to be effective in engaging Latinos in cancer research, particularly cervical cancer and other HPV-related research. One project on virtual reality seems promising. Our overarching goal for engagement has been to optimize Latino participation, so more tailored therapeutics can be found and more effective public health educational interventions can be developed. These strategies for engagement also maximize the potential for accelerating the transfer of research findings into the community. It takes an average of 8 years for research to make it into the community. Given the importance of life-threatening diseases such as cancer, that is too long for discoveries to reach society. Furthermore, lack of engagement of Latinos and other population groups in clinical trials hinders the ability to develop therapeutics with targeted precision that can benefit this population. Yet, barriers still exist and mistrust is frequently found in our communities, especially from efforts that may entail providing vital information or biological samples, for which there is fear of how these might be utilized to identify individuals or that may have a potential to do harm. Through the engagement of *promotores de salud*, we have bridged some of these trust factors, securing and retaining participants. However, to retain them, principles of participatory research need to be implemented where participant communities feel they are an essential and important part of the research. Mechanisms identified have been utilized successfully in the implementation of our research signature initiatives (*Tamale Lesson* and *Es Tiempo* campaigns) and serve as the backdrop to enhance participation in cancer research and provide opportunities for saving lives.

Acknowledgments We wish to acknowledge the USC Norris Comprehensive Cancer Center, NCI-NIH grant number P30CA014089 (Lerman), CTSI, award NIH grant number UL1TR00130 (Buchanan), NCI—TR01, R01CA144052 (Murphy/Baezconde-Garbanati), CaRE2 Program on health disparities (Carpten/Stern et al.) (1U54CA233465-01), and the USC Center for Health Equity in the Americas (CenHealth) for their contributions. In particular, we wish to acknowledge Dr. Lauren Frank at the University of Portland; Dr. Meghan Moran at John's Hopkins University, Dr. Joyee Chaterjee at the Asian Institute of Technology, and Paula Amezola, project manager. We also wish to thank our patient navigators: Ghecemy Lopez, Priscilla Marin, and Elena Nieves; and community health educators Bianca Rosales, Eduardo Ibarra, Juan Carmen, and *promotores de salud* from *Vision y Compromiso* at the Office of Community Outreach and Engagement of the Norris Comprehensive Cancer Center at the University of Southern California. We also wish to thank Dr. Mariantina Gotsis at the USC Annenberg School for Communication and Journalism on her contributions to our virtual reality and animation initiatives, and Dr. Jennifer Tsui and Dr. Jennifer Unger in the Department of Population and Public Health Sciences at the Keck School of Medicine of USC for their contributions to our programs on HPV vaccine hesitancy. We also want to acknowledge the National Cancer Institute supplemental grant from the NCI Center to Reduce Cancer Health Disparities, National Outreach Network (CRCHD, 3P30-CA014089-44S2) that supports our NON CHE program to increase participation in cancer and HPV clinical trials. Our gratitude as well to our Lazarex Cancer Foundation—Neighborhood program that facilitates participation through reductions in financial toxicity and the Lippin Program, Tower Cancer Research Foundation that supports our patient navigation. Our *promotores de salud* are part of *Vision y Compromiso* (VyC), *Clinicas Monsenor Oscar A. Romero*, and were trained in part by a grant for CA4SPA4 from UniHealth to the University of Southern California.

References

1. Noe-Bustamante L LM, Krogstad JM. U.S. Hispanic population surpassed 60 million in 2019, but growth has slowed. In: FactTank news in the numbers. Pew Research Center. 2020. https://www.pewresearch.org/fact-tank/2020/07/07/u-s-hispanic-population-surpassed-60-million-in-2019-but-growth-has-slowed/. Accessed 11 Nov 2020.
2. Elk R, Landrine H, editors. Cancer disparities: causes and evidence-based solutions. Atlanta: Springer Publ; American Cancer Society; 2012.
3. Liu L, Wang Y, Sherman RL, Cockburn M, Deapen D. Cancer in Los Angeles County: trends by race/ethnicity 1976–2016. Los Angeles: Los Angeles Cancer Surveillance Program, University of Southern California; 2016.
4. Baezconde-Garbanati L, Murphy ST, Moran MB, Cortessis VK. Reducing the excess burden of cervical cancer among Latinas: translating science into health promotion initiatives. Calif J Health Promot. 2013;11(1):45–57.
5. Baezconde-Garbanati L, Ochoa C, Murphy ST, Moran MB, Rodriguez YL, Barahona R, et al. Es Tiempo: engaging Latinas in cervical cancer research. In: Rodriguez AG, Trapido EJ, editors. Advancing the science of cancer in Latinos. 1st ed. Cham: Springer International Publishing; 2020.

6. Martinez BOC, Barahona R, Aristizabal C, Rodriguez Y, Murphy S, Baezconde-Garbanati L. Barriers to completing HPV vaccination schedule among Latinas: examining the results of a community intercept survey in Los Angeles. In: Advancing the science of cancer in Latinos. San Antonio; 2020.
7. Murphy ST, Frank LB, Chatterjee JS, Moran MB, Zhao N, Amezola de Herrera P, et al. Comparing the relative efficacy of narrative vs nonnarrative health messages in reducing health disparities using a randomized trial. Am J Public Health. 2015;105(10):2117–23. https://doi.org/10.2105/AJPH.2014.302332.
8. Ochoa C, Martinez B, Murphy S, Frank L, Baezconde-Garbanati L, editors. The effectiveness of two films in educating and changing attitudes about the uptake of the HPV vaccine among Spanish speaking Mexican American women. In: Advancing the science of cancer in latinos. San Antonio; 2020.
9. Lopez H, Gonzalez-Barrera A, Patten E. Closing the digital divide: Latinos and technology adoption. Hispanic Trends Pew Research Center; 2013. https://www.pewresearch.org/hispanic/2013/03/07/closing-the-digital-divide-latinos-and-technology-adoption/. Accessed 11 Nov 2020.
10. Israel BA, Schulz AJ, Parker EA, Becker AB. Review of community-based research: assessing partnership approaches to improve public health. Annu Rev Public Health. 1998;19:173–202. https://doi.org/10.1146/annurev.publhealth.19.1.173.

Open Access   This chapter is licensed under the terms of the Creative Commons Attribution 4.0 International License (http://creativecommons.org/licenses/by/4.0/), which permits use, sharing, adaptation, distribution and reproduction in any medium or format, as long as you give appropriate credit to the original author(s) and the source, provide a link to the Creative Commons license and indicate if changes were made.

The images or other third party material in this chapter are included in the chapter's Creative Commons license, unless indicated otherwise in a credit line to the material. If material is not included in the chapter's Creative Commons license and your intended use is not permitted by statutory regulation or exceeds the permitted use, you will need to obtain permission directly from the copyright holder.

Part VII
Emerging Policies Impacting Latino Care

Chapter 10
Latino Population Growth and the Changing Demography of Cancer

Rogelio Sáenz

Introduction

The growth of the Latino population over the last half century has been phenomenal. The Latino population shifted from a relatively small homogeneous group concentrated in selected parts of the country to a large diverse population found throughout the nation [1]. Latinos became the nation's largest minority population in 2003. Even though the pace at which the Latino population grew in the last couple of decades has decreased somewhat, Latinos continue to account for the majority of growth in the United States today and in the coming decades [1].

In the process, the prominent growth of Latinos has been associated with their impact on changes taking place in societal institutions and a wide variety of national trends. For example, higher education institutions in considering their futures need to incorporate Latino students into their student recruitment plans as the number of White students in the traditional college-attending ages has plummeted alongside recent declines among Black students [2]. In addition, business leaders have devoted a growing amount of attention to Latino consumers as their population and purchasing power have grown [3, 4]. Furthermore, the significant augmentation of the Latino population is linked to changes in other settings as well. One of these domains is in the area of health outcomes, including the incidence and mortality associated with cancer. As is the case with other groups, cancer is the leading cause of death of Latinos today [5]. Nonetheless, consistent with the Latino paradox, Latinos have lower death rates from cancer compared to Whites and other racial and ethnic groups [6, 7], the exception being certain types of cancers associated with infectious disease, including liver, stomach, and uterine cervix cancer [5, 8]. Even though Latinos are relatively more protected from cancer than other groups, their disproportionate growth is likely to contribute to the shifting demography of cancer [8].

R. Sáenz (✉)
University of Texas at San Antonio, San Antonio, TX, USA
e-mail: rogelio.saenz@utsa.edu

© The Author(s) 2023
A. G. Ramirez, E. J. Trapido (eds.), *Advancing the Science of Cancer in Latinos*, https://doi.org/10.1007/978-3-031-14436-3_10

This chapter examines the relative growth of Latinos among persons who developed cancer and those who died from it in the recent past and in the future. The next section illustrates the demographic context that serves as the backdrop for the rising importance of Latinos in the shifting demography of cancer. The chapter concludes with a discussion of the public policy implications of the results.

The Demographic Context

We highlight here the dynamics that produced the major growth of Latinos over the last several decades. Between 1980 and 2019, the Latino population more than quadrupled from 14.6 to 60.6 million [9, 10]. Over the same period, the White population rose by only 9.5%. Latinos increased their percentage share of the nation's population from 6.4% in 1980 to 18.5% in 2019 while that of Whites fell from 79.6% to 60.1%. The disparate growth of Latinos and Whites has been driven by a youthful Latino (median age of 22 in 1980) and an older White (median age of 31 in 1980) population. Furthermore, during the period of examination below (1999–2016) regarding the analysis of changes in cancer cases and deaths, Latinos primarily drove the nation's demographic change. Indeed, of the 46.8 million people that the United States added to its population between 2000 and 2019, Latinos accounted for the majority (54.0% or 25.3 million) and Whites constituted only a sliver of the growth (5.9% or nearly 2.8 million) [10, 11].

Latinos today continue to be a younger population than Whites. For example, in 2018 the median age of the Latino population was 29 compared to 43 for the White population; persons less than 18 years of age accounted for 31% of the Latino population compared to 19% of the White population; and persons 65 years of age and older made up 7% of Latinos but 20% of Whites [12]. The youthfulness of the Latino population will again impel future change in the US population. For example, the latest population projections from the US Census Bureau show that the Latino population is projected to almost double from about 57.5 million in 2016 to 111.2 million in 2016. In contrast, the White population is projected to decline from 198 to 179.2 million, a 9.5% decrease [13]. Undoubtedly, the dominating growth of the Latino population will shift the demography of people who develop cancer or die from it.

Data and Methods

The analysis conducted is based on two time periods—a look at the past between 1999 and 2016 and a look into the future between 2016 and 2060. First, the analysis uses information from the US Cancer Statistics public data [14] to obtain the number of cancer cases and deaths alongside the respective age-adjusted cancer incidence rates (number of persons with cancer per 100,000 persons) and age-adjusted death rates (number of deaths from cancer per 100,000 persons) for each year between 1999 and 2016 for Latinos and for two comparison groups: non-Hispanic Whites and non-Hispanic Blacks (referred to as simply "White" and "Black" below). These data were used to assess variations across Latinos, Whites, and Blacks in the growth of cancer cases and deaths between 1996 and 2016.

Second, the analysis subsequently turns to the projection of cancer cases and deaths into the future (2016–2060) to examine the impact of the projected growth of the Latino population on the changing demography of cancer over the next four decades. This exercise involves two sets of data: the latest 2016 age-specific cancer incident rates (CIRs) and cancer death rates (CDRs) per 100,000 for Latinos and the total population obtained from the US Census Statistics public data [14] and the US Census Bureau's age–sex-specific population projections for Latinos and the total population [15]. Essentially, the projected cancer cases and deaths for Latinos and the total population assume that the CIRs and CDRs observed in 2016 remain constant over time between 2016 and 2060 and these are applied to the projected Latino population and the total population for 2020, 2030, 2040, 2050, and 2060. The projected Latino cancer cases and deaths for each specific year are obtained from the following formulas:

$$PRJCI_i = (CIR_i / 100,000) * PRJPOP_i$$
$$PRJCD_i = (CDR_i / 100,000) * PRJPOP_i$$

where i represents a given age category (0–14, 15–24, 25–34, 35–44, 45–54, 55–64, 65–74, 75–84, and 85 and older). The projected number of age-specific cancer cases ($PRJCI_i$) and cancer deaths ($PRJCD_i$) are obtained by multiplying the age-specific proportion format of the cancer incidence rate ($CIR_i/100,000$) and the cancer death rate ($CDR_i/100,000$), respectively, by the age-specific population projections ($PRJPOP_i$). The same formulas are used to generate the projections for the total cancer cases and deaths to determine the percentage share of future growth in cancer cases and deaths that would likely be Latino. Obviously, it is unlikely that the age-specific cancer incidence and death rates would remain unchanged over the course of the next 44 years (2016–2060). However, we use the latest rates to illustrate how the demography of cancer could change over the next four decades given the growing Latino population.

Results

An Examination of the Recent Past

The incidence of cancer changed significantly between 1999 and 2016. While the age-adjusted cancer incidence rates (AACIRs) declined for all three racial and ethnic groups, the number of cancer cases increased across all of the groups. Yet,

Table 10.1 Demographic changes in cancer cases and deaths between 1999 and 2016 [14]

Indicators	Latino	White	Black
Percentage change between 1999 and 2016:			
Cancer cases	106.0	17.5	50.0
Cancer deaths	94.1	2.2	13.5
Percentage of total increase between 1999 and 2016:			
Cancer cases	18.8	50.3	16.2
Cancer deaths	39.5	21.1	17.3
Percentage of all cancer cases by year:			
1999	5.1	82.7	9.3
2016	8.2	75.5	10.9
Percentage of all cancer deaths by year:			
1999	3.7	83.0	11.2
2016	6.6	78.0	11.7

consistent with the demographic context illustrated above, the number of cancer cases more than doubled for Latinos from 67,955 in 1999 to 139,976 with those of Blacks rising by 50% and by 17.5% for Whites (Table 10.1). The overall number of cancer cases in the nation increased by 382,545 between 1999 and 2016. Of the total national growth, Latinos made up approximately 19% of the total increase in the incidence of cancer between 1999 and 2016, with Whites responsible for 50% of the growth and Blacks for 16%. Overall, the share of the incidence of cancer in a given year increased somewhat for Latinos from 5.1% in 1999 to 8.2% in 2016, while it decreased for Whites from 82.7% to 75.5%.

As is the case with the incidence of cancer, cancer death rates declined between 1996 and 2016, but the absolute number of deaths increased across the three groups. The relative increase of cancer deaths, however, was less for cancer deaths (9%) than for cancer cases (29%). As such, the increase in the volume of deaths among Latinos stands out, nearly doubling from 20,233 in 1999 to 39,263 in 2016. In contrast, the number of cancer deaths increased by only 2% for Whites and 14% for Blacks. Overall, there was an increase of 48,202 cancer deaths in the country between 1999 and 2016 with Latinos accounting for about 40% of the growth compared to 21% for Whites and 17% for Blacks.

Several observations to note include:

- Latinos have the lowest age-adjusted cancer incidence rate and cancer death rate compared to Whites and Blacks.
- The incidence of cancer more than doubled and the number of cancer deaths nearly doubled between 1999 and 2016 among Latinos largely due to their major population growth.
- Latinos disproportionately accounted for the nation's growth in cancer cases (one-fifth) and cancer deaths (two-fifths) between 1999 and 2016.
- Latinos continued to comprise only a fraction of all cancer cases (8.2%) and deaths (6.6%) in 2016. These trends are expected to intensify with the major population growth that Latinos will experience over the coming decades.

An Examination of the Future

The growth of the Latino population will have a mark on the changing face of people with cancer in the coming decades. The projected incidence of cancer among Latinos is expected to grow 3.5-fold from 139,000 in 2016 to 480,000 in 2060, with their projected deaths more than quadruple from 39,000 to 168,000 (Fig. 10.1). The respective growth is more gradual among non-Latinos at 43% in projected cancer cases and 68% in deaths. It is expected that Latinos would account for one-third of the US-projected increase in cancer cases and one-fourth of that in cancer deaths.

The Latino percentage share of the nation's incidence and deaths associated with cancer annually is likely to more than double between 2016 and 2060, with the portion of cases that are Latino rising from 8.1% in 2016 to 17.6% in 2060 and that of deaths climbing from 6.5% to 15.2% (Table 10.2). The doubling of the percentage share of Latinos among persons with cancer is expected at ages 45 and older, reflecting the aging of Latinos in the coming decades. By 2060, roughly one of six persons with cancer or who die from it are expected to be Latino. As Latinos will continue to be younger than other groups, they will make up a larger share—approximately one in four—of cancer cases and deaths among persons less than 45 years of age in 2060.

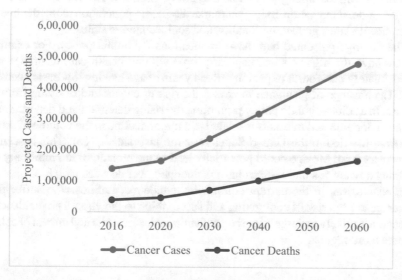

Fig. 10.1 Projected Latino cancer cases and deaths, 2016–2060 [14, 15]

Table 10.2 Percentage share of Latinos of all projected cancer cases and deaths by age group, 2016 and 2060 [14, 15]

Age category	Percentage of projected cancer cases Latinos		Percentage of projected cancer deaths Latino	
	2016	2060	2016	2060
0–14	24.6	31.0	25.3	32.0
15–24	20.3	28.9	25.4	36.2
25–34	16.5	24.4	18.4	27.2
35–44	15.7	21.7	16.4	22.6
45–54	11.3	20.6	10.4	18.9
55–64	8.0	19.0	7.1	16.9
65–74	6.5	17.2	5.7	15.0
75–84	6.1	16.4	5.8	15.6
85 and older	5.4	13.9	5.0	13.0
Total	8.1	17.6	6.5	15.2

Conclusions

As Latinos have driven the nation's changing demography, they are also playing a disproportionate role in the changing demography of cancer over the last 18 years and will do so even more in the next four decades. Cancer researchers, medical personnel, and health providers will need to devote more attention to the growing presence of Latinos among the people they study, treat, and care for. There is a need to better understand the diversity that marks the Latino population along the lines of generational status, gender, nationality, and socioeconomic status.

The findings presented here have implications for public policy. For example, Latinos have the highest percentage of people without health-care insurance with approximately one-fourth of persons 18–64 years of age lacking this basic necessity [12]. The absence of insurance increases the risk of cancer and of dying from the disease. In addition, public policy promoting the rising detention and deportation of Latino undocumented migrants is related to a major decline in the volume of migration from Mexico to the United States over the last decade [16]. This descent of newcomers from Mexico could potentially lead to the erosion of the morbidity and mortality advantages that Latinos have maintained over decades [6, 7].

In conclusion, in the current coronavirus pandemic, Latinos who suffer from cancer are at high risk of contracting and succumbing to the virus. The incidence of cancer is also likely to surge after the pandemic as doctor visits and annual checkups become more regular.

References

1. Sáenz R, Morales MC. Latinos in the United States: diversity and change. Cambridge, UK: Polity Press; 2015.
2. Sáenz R. Latino continual demographic growth: implications for educational practices and policy. J Hisp High Educ. 2020;19:134–48. https://doi.org/10.1177/1538192719900383.
3. Korzenny F, Korzenny BA, Chapa S. Hispanic marketing: the power of the new Latino consumer. 3rd ed. London: Routledge; 2017.
4. Dolliver MUS. Hispanics 2019: a big population poised for greater buying power. New York: eMarketer; 2019.
5. Ramirez AG, Trapido EJ. Advancing the science of cancer in Latinos. In: Ramirez AG, Trapido EJ, editors. Advancing the science of cancer in Latinos. Cham: Springer; 2019. https://doi.org/10.1007/978-3-030-29286-7_1.
6. Pinheiro PS, Williams M, Miller EA, Easterday S, Moonie S, Trapido EJ. Cancer survival among Latinos and the Hispanic paradox. Cancer Causes Control. 2011;22:553–61. https://doi.org/10.1007/s10552-011-9727-6.
7. Goldman N. Will the Latino mortality advantage endure? Res Aging. 2016;38:263–82. https://doi.org/10.1177/0164027515620242.
8. Miller KD, Sauer AG, Ortiz AP, Fedewa SA, Pinheiro PS, Tortolero-Luna G, et al. Cancer statistics for Hispanics/Latinos, 2018. CA Cancer J Clin. 2018;68:425–45. https://doi.org/10.3322/caac.21494.
9. Hobbs F, Stoops N. Demographic trends in the 20th century. 2000 special reports, series CENSR-4. Washington, DC: U.S. Government Printing Office; 2002. https://www.census.gov/prod/2002pubs/censr-4.pdf. Accessed 29 June 2020.
10. U.S. Census Bureau. Annual estimates of the resident population by sex, race, and Hispanic origin: April 1, 2020 to July 1, 2019. National population by characteristics: 2010–2019. 2019. https://www.census.gov/data/tables/time-series/demo/popest/2010s-national-detail.html#par_textimage_1537638156. Accessed 29 June 2020.
11. U.S. Census Bureau. Hispanic or Latino and not Hispanic or Latino by race. 2000 Decennial census summary file 1. 2000. https://data.census.gov/cedsci/table?g=0100000US & y=2000 & tid=DECENNIALSF12000.P004 & t=Hispanic%20or%20Latino & hidePreview=false & vintage=2000 & layer=VT_2018_040_00_PP_D1 & cid=H009001. Accessed 30 June 2020.
12. Ruggles S, Flood S, Goeken R, Grover J, Meyer E, Pacas J, Sobek M. 2018 American community survey 1-year estimates. IPUMS USA: version 10.0. Minneapolis, MN: Integrated Public Use Microdata Series; 2020. https://doi.org/10.18128/D010.V10.0. Accessed 29 June 2020.
13. U.S. Census Bureau. Projected race and Hispanic origin. 2017 National population projections tables: main series. 2017. https://www.census.gov/data/tables/2017/demo/popproj/2017-summary-tables.html. Accessed 29 June 2020.
14. Centers for Disease Control and Prevention. U.S. cancer statistics: public information data. CDC WONDER. 2020. https://wonder.cdc.gov/cancer.html. Accessed 28 June 2020.
15. U.S. Census Bureau. Projected population by single year of age, sex, race, and Hispanic origin for the United States: 2016 to 2060 [Main Series]. 2017 National Population Projections Datasets 2017. https://www.census.gov/data/datasets/2017/demo/popproj/2017-popproj.html. Accessed 29 June 2020.
16. Sáenz R. Far fewer Mexican migrants are coming to the US—and those who do are more educated. The Conversation. 9 Sept 2015. https://theconversation.com/far-fewer-mexican-immigrants-are-coming-to-the-us-and-those-who-do-are-more-educated-122524. Accessed 2 July 2020.

Open Access   This chapter is licensed under the terms of the Creative Commons Attribution 4.0 International License (http://creativecommons.org/licenses/by/4.0/), which permits use, sharing, adaptation, distribution and reproduction in any medium or format, as long as you give appropriate credit to the original author(s) and the source, provide a link to the Creative Commons license and indicate if changes were made.

The images or other third party material in this chapter are included in the chapter's Creative Commons license, unless indicated otherwise in a credit line to the material. If material is not included in the chapter's Creative Commons license and your intended use is not permitted by statutory regulation or exceeds the permitted use, you will need to obtain permission directly from the copyright holder.

Chapter 11
Financial Hardship, Food Insecurity, and Forgone Medical Care

Jean A. McDougall, Shoshana Adler Jaffe, Dolores D. Guest,
V. Shane Pankratz, Charles L. Wiggins, Angela L. W. Meisner,
and Andrew L. Sussman

Introduction

Tremendous progress has been made in the fight against cancer. From its peak in 1991, cancer mortality in the United States has declined by 29% [1]. From 2007 to 2016, cancer mortality declined by 1.6% and 1.0% annually for Latino males and females, respectively [2]. However, socioeconomic disparities in cancer mortality

J. A. McDougall (✉) · D. D. Guest · V. S. Pankratz
University of New Mexico Comprehensive Cancer Center, Albuquerque, NM, USA

Department of Internal Medicine, University of New Mexico, Albuquerque, NM, USA
e-mail: jamcdougall@salud.unm.edu; dguest@salud.unm.edu; VPankratz@salud.unm.edu

S. A. Jaffe
University of New Mexico Comprehensive Cancer Center, Albuquerque, NM, USA
e-mail: sadlerjaffe@salud.unm.edu

C. L. Wiggins
University of New Mexico Comprehensive Cancer Center, Albuquerque, NM, USA

Department of Internal Medicine, University of New Mexico, Albuquerque, NM, USA

New Mexico Tumor Registry, Albuquerque, NM, USA
e-mail: CWiggins@salud.unm.edu

A. L. W. Meisner
University of New Mexico Comprehensive Cancer Center, Albuquerque, NM, USA

New Mexico Tumor Registry, Albuquerque, NM, USA
e-mail: AWMeisner@salud.unm.edu

A. L. Sussman
University of New Mexico Comprehensive Cancer Center, Albuquerque, NM, USA

Department of Community and Family Medicine, University of New Mexico,
Albuquerque, NM, USA
e-mail: ASussman@salud.unm.edu

© The Author(s) 2023
A. G. Ramirez, E. J. Trapido (eds.), *Advancing the Science of Cancer in Latinos*, https://doi.org/10.1007/978-3-031-14436-3_11

are widening [3]. Progress has come at a considerable cost to society, the health-care system, and to patients and their families.

In 2020, it was projected that as much as $200 billion dollars will be spent on cancer care in the United States [4]. The average price of new cancer drugs on the market today is $14,000 per month, and cancer patients can expect to pay approximately $5000 out-of-pocket in the first year following a cancer diagnosis [5, 6]. The high costs of cancer care contribute to widening socioeconomic disparities in cancer mortality. The age-adjusted cancer mortality rate is now 80% higher for males living in poverty and 55% higher for females living in poverty than for those with incomes that are 600% of the federal poverty level [3].

As the costs of cancer care skyrocketed over the past decade, new terms emerged to define the problems a patient may experience in relation to the cost of medical care: *financial toxicity* and *financial hardship*. Akin to physical toxicities, like nausea, neutropenia, and fatigue, financial toxicity makes it difficult for cancer patients to complete treatment [7]. Numerous studies have described financial hardships experienced by cancer survivors including debt, inability to pay medical bills, bankruptcy, and other financial sacrifices [8]. To cope with the high costs of cancer care, patients make financial sacrifices, shifting money that might have previously been budgeted for food to pay for medical care. In a study by Zafar et al., 46% of cancer patients reporting financial hardship stated that they coped with the cost of care by reducing spending on basic necessities, including food [9], raising concerns that cancer survivors may be at risk of food insecurity.

Food insecurity, defined as an inability to acquire enough food because of insufficient money or other resources, befell 37.2 million people in the United States in 2018 [10]. In 2020, the economic ramifications of the novel coronavirus (COVID-19) pandemic are projected to increase the number of people experiencing food insecurity by over 17 million, to approximately 54 million people [11]. Inextricably linked to income, the prevalence of food insecurity is highest among households with annual incomes below the official poverty line (35.3%); among households with children headed by a single woman (27.8%); and among households with non-Hispanic Black (21.2%) and Hispanic (16.2%) heads of household [10]. Food insecurity is increasingly recognized as a social determinant of health, with numerous studies finding strong associations between food insecurity and diabetes, hypertension, and hyperlipidemia [12–16]. Evidence from cross-sectional studies also suggests a high prevalence of food insecurity among cancer patients [13, 17–19]. In a small ($n = 115$) sample of predominantly non-Hispanic white (85%) cancer patients in an academic medical center in Kentucky, Simmons et al. found 17% of patients to be food insecure [19]. Among a cohort of underserved oncology patients at New York City cancer clinics ($n = 404$), Gany et al. reported a 56% prevalence of food insecurity and found that women were significantly more likely to be food insecure than men [17]. Food insecurity may be an early indicator of financial problems, as individuals make daily or weekly choices about purchasing food, whereas other bills can often be delayed longer [20]. Moreover, financial sacrifices made to cope with the high cost of cancer care may exacerbate existing food insecurity or cause new food insecurity for cancer patients. The precarious balance between having enough to eat and affording medical care has been described in cancer patients [9, 13, 17, 19], and evidence supports a strong association between food insecurity and poor treatment adherence [19, 21, 22], inadequate symptom control [23, 24], and increased utilization of high-cost services [25].

Emerging evidence suggests that cancer-related financial hardship disproportionately affects Latinos. In a study of the Health and Retirement Study Cohort, a nationally representative longitudinal survey of more than 37,000 individuals over age 50, 60% of Latinos reported at least one financial hardship compared to 16% of non-Latinos [26]. Importantly, those in the study who reported at least one financial hardship had a higher risk of mortality than those who were financially stable, providing evidence of a link between financial hardship and disparities in mortality that has also been observed in cancer survivors filing for bankruptcy [27]. Data from the Cancer Care Outcomes Research and Surveillance (CanCORS) Consortium showed similar findings among cancer survivors, with 58% of Latinos and 45% of non-Hispanic whites reported financial hardship [28].

The purpose of this chapter is to describe financial hardship and food insecurity, and their relationships to accessing cancer care, using data from the recently completed Comprehensive History of Individual Cancer Experiences (CHOICE) Project with cancer survivors in New Mexico. Among New Mexicans, the term "Hispanic" is frequently chosen as a self-defined social identity term and will be used throughout the rest of this chapter to refer to individuals reporting Hispanic ethnicity in the CHOICE Project survey [29]. The research on financial hardship and food insecurity among Hispanic cancer survivors is limited. To address these gaps, we reflect on our own research and propose directions for future study.

Methods

The CHOICE Project used a cross-sectional survey to quantify the prevalence of financial hardship and food insecurity among population-based Hispanic and non-Hispanic cancer survivors. Individuals from 21 through 64 years of age, diagnosed with a first primary, invasive breast, colorectal, or prostate cancer between 2008 and 2016 were identified from the population-based New Mexico Tumor Registry (NMTR). To be eligible for the study, cancer survivors at the time of their cancer diagnosis had to have private insurance, Medicaid, or have been uninsured with an income that was greater than $24,000 (approximately 200% of the Federal Poverty Level for an individual [30]). In addition, they had to be able to speak English or Spanish and provide informed consent.

Participants were asked to complete a survey measuring their financial experiences. Available in both English and Spanish, surveys were web-based, computer-assisted telephone interviews or paper versions. Material financial hardship was measured using four questions from the Medical Expenditure Panel Survey Experiences with Cancer Supplement (MEPS-ECS) that asked participants: whether they had to borrow money or go into debt; make financial sacrifices (e.g., reduced spending on vacation or leisure activities, delayed large purchases, reduced spending on basics, used savings set aside for other purposes, or made a change to living situation); whether they were unable to cover the cost of medical visits; or filed for bankruptcy because of their cancer, its treatment, or the lasting effects of treatment [31]. Food insecurity was measured using the two-item Hunger VitalSign™ food insecurity screening tool [32]. Participants responding "often true" or "sometimes true" to either of the following statements were classified as food insecure: (1) "Within the past 12 months, we worried whether our food would run out before we got money to buy more"; (2) "Within the past 12 months, the food we bought just didn't last and we didn't have money to get more." In the survey, participants were asked to recall their situation at two timepoints: the 12 months prior to their cancer diagnosis and the 12 months after diagnosis. Food security status at each timepoint was combined to characterize participants as persistently food secure (i.e., food secure at both timepoints); newly food insecure (i.e., food secure prior to diagnosis and food insecure after diagnosis); persistently food insecure (i.e., food insecure at both timepoints); or newly food secure (i.e., food insecure prior to diagnosis and food secure after diagnosis). A single question from the MEPS-ECS was used to measure access to care, asking participants whether they ever had to delay, forego, or have to make other changes to any of the following cancer care because of cost: prescription medicine, visit to specialist, treatment (other than prescription medicine), follow-up care, or mental health services [31]. In addition, participants' sociodemographic information was ascertained from the survey, and tumor type, stage, and treatments received were collected from NMTR records. Ethnicity was classified using survey data, indicating whether a participant self-identified as Hispanic.

Data were summarized with descriptive statistics including means, standard deviations, frequencies, and proportions. Differences between Hispanic and non-Hispanic participants were compared using t-tests for continuous variables, Pearson's chi-square tests for nominal categorical variables, and nonparametric tests of trend across ordinal categorical variables. Polytomous logistic regression was used to estimate odds ratios (OR) and 95% confidence intervals (CI) that assessed the relationship between Hispanic ethnicity and food insecurity. Multivariable logistic regression models were developed to assess the association between Hispanic ethnicity and forgoing, delaying, or making changes to each type of medical care, adjusting for sociodemographic and clinical characteristics that differed between Hispanic and non-Hispanic cancer survivors at the $P < 0.20$ level. Adjustment variables in the final models included food insecurity status, age at diagnosis, education, annual household income, insurance type at diagnosis, marital status, and cancer type. All analyses were conducted using STATA v.15.

Results

Of the 1211 eligible individuals identified from the NMTR, 394 completed the survey (response rate 33%). Forty-two percent ($n = 164$) of study participants identified as Hispanic (Table 11.1). Ninety-seven percent of both Hispanic and non-Hispanic cancer survivors identified as White race. Cancer survivors identified as Hispanic tended to be diagnosed with cancer at a younger age (mean 49.7 vs. 51.6, $P = 0.01$), were less likely to have a college or professional degree (30% vs. 59%, $P < 0.01$), were more likely to have an annual household income <\$30,000 (44% vs. 24%, $P < 0.01$), and were less likely to have private insurance (65% vs. 77%, $P = 0.01$) compared with non-Hispanic cancer survivors.

Material Financial Hardship

Hispanic cancer survivors were more likely to report being unable to cover the cost of their medical bills (32% vs. 21%, $P = 0.02$) and more likely to reduce spending on basics such as food and clothing (40% vs. 30%, $P = 0.04$) than non-Hispanic cancer survivors (Fig. 11.1). Hispanic cancer survivors were also slightly, though not significantly, more likely than non-Hispanics to make a change to their living situation (18% vs. 13%, $P = 0.21$), delay large purchases (46% vs. 43%, $P = 0.46$), and borrow money or go into debt (29% vs. 23%, $P = 0.19$). Four percent of cancer survivors filed for bankruptcy, while more than half of all cancer survivors reported reducing spending on vacation or leisure activities, and no difference was observed by ethnicity for these types of financial hardship.

Food Insecurity

Both new and persistent food insecurity were significantly more common among Hispanic cancer survivors than non-Hispanics (Table 11.2). Thirteen percent of Hispanic cancer survivors and 7% of non-Hispanic cancer survivors were newly food insecure in the 12 months after their diagnosis (OR = 2.59, 95% CI: 1.29–5.19), while 34% of Hispanic cancer survivors were persistently food insecure compared to 20% of non-Hispanics (OR = 2.61, 95% CI: 1.61–4.21). Combining both newly and persistently food insecure individuals, the overall prevalence of food insecurity in the 12 months after cancer diagnosis was 47% for Hispanic cancer survivors and 27% for non-Hispanic cancer survivors in this study.

Table 11.1 Characteristics of survey participants by ethnicity, $N = 394$

	Hispanic ($n = 164$)		Non-Hispanic ($n = 230$)		
	n or mean	% or SD	n or mean	% or SD	p-value
Age at diagnosis (years)	49.7	7.3	51.6	6.3	0.01
Time since diagnosis (years)	5.7	2.2	5.9	2.5	0.44
Sex					0.38
Female	118	72%	156	68%	
Male	46	28%	74	32%	
Race					0.81
White	159	97%	222	97%	
Non-White	5	3%	8	3%	
Education					<0.01
≤High School	113	70%	93	41%	
≥College	49	30%	132	59%	
Annual household income					<0.01
Less than $30,000	71	44%	56	24%	
$30,000–$69,999	33	20%	35	15%	
$70,000 or more	59	36%	139	60%	
Marital status					0.11
Married	64	40%	72	32%	
Not Married	97	60%	154	68%	
County of residence					0.87
Urban	109	67%	152	66%	
Rural	54	33%	78	34%	
Insurance type at diagnosis					0.01
Private	107	65%	176	77%	
Medicaid	43	26%	47	20%	
Uninsured	14	9%	7	3%	
Cancer type					0.14
Breast	104	63%	134	58%	
Colorectal	34	21%	41	18%	
Prostate	26	16%	55	24%	
Cancer stage					0.52
I	66	40%	105	46%	
II	69	47%	91	40%	
III	29	18%	34	15%	
Cancer directed surgery					0.17
Yes	149	91%	197	86%	
No	15	9%	31	13%	
Radiation therapy					0.65
Yes	56	34%	84	37%	
No	105	64%	144	63%	
Chemotherapy					0.78
Yes	69	42%	90	39%	
No	93	57%	138	60%	

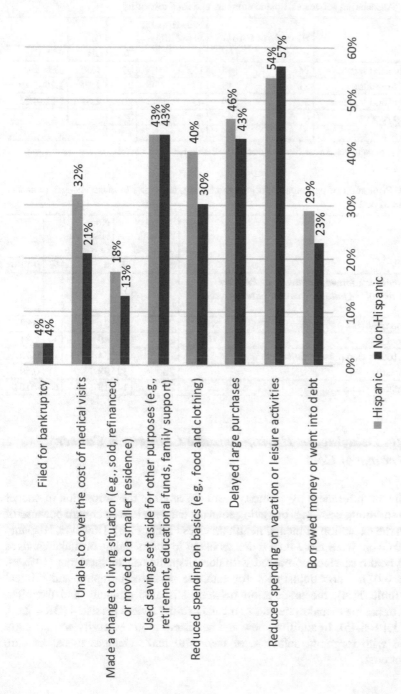

Fig. 11.1 Proportion of individuals experiencing material financial hardship

Table 11.2 Association between Hispanic ethnicity and food insecurity

	Hispanic (n = 164)		Non-Hispanic (n = 230)			
	n	%	n	%	OR	95% CI
Persistently food secure	74	45	155	67	1.00	Reference
Newly food insecure	21	13	17	7	**2.59**	**1.29–5.19**
Persistently food insecure	56	34	45	20	**2.61**	**1.61–4.21**
Newly food secure	6	4	7	3		
Missing	7	4	6	3		

Bold values represent statistical significance at the 2-sided $P < 0.05$ level

Table 11.3 Proportion of participants forgoing, delaying, or having to make changes to cancer care because of cost

	Hispanic (n = 164)		Non-Hispanic (n = 230)		
	n	%	n	%	p-value
Did you ever delay, forego, or have to make other changes to any of the following cancer care because of cost?					
Prescription medicine	23	14	31	13	0.88
Visit to specialist	27	16	40	17	0.81
Treatment (other than prescription medicine)	19	12	24	10	0.72
Follow-up care	28	17	38	17	0.89
Mental health services	23	14	13	6	<0.01

Forgoing, Delaying, or Having to Make Changes to Cancer Care Because of Cost

No significant differences by ethnicity were observed in the proportion of cancer survivors forgoing, delaying, or having to make changes to cancer care because of cost, with the exception of mental health services (Table 11.3). However, Hispanic cancer survivors were more than twice as likely to forgo, delay, or make changes to mental health services compared with non-Hispanic cancer survivors (14% vs. 6%, $P < 0.01$). Upon adjustment for multiple sociodemographic and clinical factors (Table 11.4), the association between Hispanic ethnicity and forgoing, delaying, or having to make changes to mental health services persisted (OR = 2.67, 95% CI: 1.11–6.45). In addition, new and persistent food insecurity was strongly associated with forgoing, delaying, or having to make changes to cancer care because of cost.

Table 11.4 Multivariable models for the association between Hispanic ethnicity and forgoing, delaying, or making changes to medical care because of cost

	Prescription medication		Treatment other than prescription medication		Specialist visits		Follow-up care		Mental health services	
	OR	95% CI	OR	95% CI	OR	95% CI	OR	95% CI	OR	95% CI
Ethnicity										
Non-Hispanic	1.00	Reference	1.00	Reference	1.00	Reference	1.00	Reference	1.00	Reference
Hispanic	0.68	0.32–1.40	0.97	0.44–2.15	0.62	0.32–1.21	0.77	0.40–1.48	**2.67**	**1.11–6.45**
Food security status										
Persistently food secure	1.00	Reference	1.00	Reference	1.00	Reference	1.00	Reference	1.00	Reference
Newly food insecure	2.37	0.80–7.05	**5.54**	**1.79–17.1**	**4.45**	**1.67–11.9**	**4.45**	**1.72–11.5**	**3.90**	**1.15–13.3**
Persistently food insecure	**3.14**	**1.34–7.33**	**6.23**	**2.38–16.3**	**3.90**	**1.78–8.55**	**4.45**	**2.04–9.72**	**5.13**	**1.82–14.4**
Age at diagnosis (years)	1.00	0.95–1.05	1.04	0.98–1.09	1.00	0.96–1.04	1.00	0.96–1.05	0.98	0.93–1.04
Education										
≤High School	1.00	Reference	1.00	Reference	1.00	Reference	1.00	Reference	1.00	Reference
≥College	0.60	0.28–1.29	**3.19**	**1.32–7.69**	0.92	0.46–1.83	1.61	0.80–3.21	**3.12**	**1.16–8.40**
Income										
Less than $30,000	1.00	Reference	1.00	Reference	1.00	Reference	1.00	Reference	1.00	Reference
$30,000–$69,999	1.99	0.70–5.67	1.46	0.48–4.44	**2.78**	**1.10–7.05**	2.06	0.81–5.22	2.68	0.83–8.73
$70,000 or more	2.38	0.74–7.66	1.13	0.34–3.82	1.86	0.65–5.33	1.73	0.62–4.84	1.65	0.40–6.84
Insurance										
Private	1.00	Reference	1.00	Reference	1.00	Reference	1.00	Reference	1.00	Reference
Medicaid	1.05	0.39–2.83	0.39	0.12–1.28	0.97	0.39–2.37	0.79	0.32–1.96	1.06	0.34–3.35
Uninsured	**4.96**	**1.20–20.6**	2.62	0.56–12.3	2.09	0.49–8.93	2.42	0.61–9.63	2.01	0.35–11.7
Marital status										
Married	1.00	Reference	1.00	Reference	1.00	Reference	1.00	Reference	1.00	Reference
Not married	0.52	0.25–1.09	0.82	0.37–1.81	1.21	0.61–2.41	1.09	0.56–2.14	0.67	0.27–1.62
Cancer type										

(continued)

Table 11.4 (continued)

	Prescription medication		Treatment other than prescription medication		Specialist visits		Follow-up care		Mental health services	
	OR	95% CI	OR	95% CI	OR	95% CI	OR	95% CI	OR	95% CI
Breast	1.00	Reference	1.00	Reference	1.00	Reference	1.00	Reference	1.00	Reference
Colorectal	1.06	0.45–2.49	1.14	0.45–2.89	1.64	0.78–3.45	1.58	0.77–3.24	0.87	0.31–2.46
Prostate	0.73	0.27–1.97	0.49	0.15–1.56	0.80	0.33–1.95	0.38	0.14–1.06	–	–

Bold values represent statistical significance at the $P < 0.05$ level

OR odds ratio, *CI* confidence interval

Discussion

The results of the CHOICE Project highlight important differences in the prevalence of financial hardship and food insecurity between Hispanic and non-Hispanic cancer survivors. Hispanic cancer survivors were significantly more likely to report being unable to cover the cost of their medical bills and to reduce spending on food and clothing because of their cancer, its treatment, or the lasting effects of treatment. The struggle to afford medical care and food contributed to the substantially higher prevalence of both new and persistent food insecurity among Hispanic cancer survivors. Overall, 47% of Hispanic cancer survivors in the CHOICE Project experienced food insecurity in the year following their cancer diagnosis. This is alarmingly high compared to the overall prevalence of food insecurity in the CHOICE Project of 36% and far exceeds the 11% prevalence of food insecurity for US adults [10, 18]. Although few prior studies of financial hardship have had large numbers of Hispanic cancer survivors, those that report on the prevalence of financial hardship by ethnicity find similar disparities [27, 28]. These results provide justification for the need to develop interventions designed to address social needs, including financial hardship and food insecurity, among all cancer survivors.

The factors influencing the development of financial hardship and food insecurity following a cancer diagnosis occur within a dynamic system comprising multiple levels of contextual influence, including the individual patient, provider, social support networks, and the local community, state and national environments [33]. Sociodemographic characteristics of the individual, such as age, income, education, occupation, health literacy, and insurance, are all strongly associated with financial hardship [34–37]. To the extent that these characteristics differ between Hispanic and non-Hispanic cancer survivors, these factors may explain the high prevalence of financial hardship observed in the CHOICE Project. The interplay between the individual and the other levels of the socioecological framework often determines the degree to which financial hardship contributes to negative health outcomes. Communication between patients and providers, social support from family and larger social networks, availability of culturally appropriate patient support services within oncology clinics, and state and national policies shaping insurance, reimbursement, and access to financial and food resources can all serve as barriers to, or facilitators of, receiving timely appropriate cancer care among patients experiencing financial hardship. Factors at each of these levels thus contribute both to the risk of financial hardship and to the downstream negative effects of financial hardship, including food insecurity.

A cyclic model exists to explain the relationship between food insecurity and chronic disease in which the inability to access enough healthy food leads to compensatory strategies, including skipping meals and reducing caloric intake in times of food shortage and systematic overconsumption in times of food adequacy [23]. Stress, constrained dietary options, and eating patterns of food insecure individuals lead to medication nonadherence, postponement of needed health care, and impaired self-management capacity, ultimately increasing health-care expenditures for food insecure individuals [23, 25, 38]. In the CHOICE Project, the relationship between food insecurity and forgoing, delaying, or making changes to medical care was strong, and did not appear to differ for Hispanic and non-Hispanic cancer survivors. While little research has directly addressed the problem of food insecurity among cancer survivors, there is a rich body of literature documenting the experience of food insecurity and health disparities among Hispanic communities in the United States [20, 39, 40]. Issues of food access and agency among Hispanic households are intertwined with structural inequality and economic development, but the inter-section with personal experience often reveals nuanced cultural meanings and prac-tices around food and times of food shortage [20]. Given the disproportionate burden of food insecurity among Hispanic cancer survivors identified in the CHOICE Project, strategies to address food insecurity will likely benefit from community-based approaches that seek to understand the lived experience of food insecurity in Hispanic households.

Evidence-based financial hardship and food insecurity screening tools exist. The COST-FACIT Measure of Financial Toxicity has demonstrated reliability and valid-ity for identifying financial hardship in cancer patients [41]. The Hunger VitalSign™ food insecurity screening tool is also widely endorsed for the use in clinical settings [32]. Integrating these tools into oncology practice in a culturally appropriate, sus-tainable, and effective way to improve cancer outcomes remains a critical area of future research.

In summary, the CHOICE Project highlights persisting ethnic disparities in financial hardship and food insecurity. The strong relationship between food insecu-rity and cancer care access supports future research to address this social determi-nant of health to address cancer disparities and achieve health equity.

References

1. Siegel RL, Miller KD, Jemal A. Cancer statistics, 2020. CA Cancer J Clin. 2020;70(1):7–30. https://doi.org/10.3322/caac.21590.
2. American Cancer Society. Cancer facts and figures for Hispanics/Latinos 2018–2020. Atlanta: American Cancer Society, Inc.; 2018.
3. Singh GK, Jemal A. Socioeconomic and racial/ethnic disparities in cancer mortality, inci-dence, and survival in the United States, 1950-2014: over six decades of changing pat-terns and widening inequalities. J Environ Public Health. 2017;2017:2819372. https://doi.org/10.1155/2017/2819372.
4. Mariotto AB, Yabroff KR, Shao Y, Feuer EJ, Brown ML. Projections of the cost of cancer care in the United States: 2010-2020. J Natl Cancer Inst. 2011;103(2):117–28. https://doi.org/10.1093/jnci/djq495.
5. Dieguez G, Ferro C, Pyenson BS. A multi-year look at the cost burden of cancer care. Milliman Research Report. 2017.
6. Dusetzina SB, Huskamp HA, Keating NL. Specialty drug pricing and out-of-pocket spending on orally administered anticancer drugs in Medicare Part D, 2010 to 2019. JAMA. 2019;321(20):2025–7. https://doi.org/10.1001/jama.2019.4492.
7. Zafar SY, Abernethy AP. Financial toxicity, Part I: a new name for a growing problem. Oncology (Williston Park). 2013;27(2):80–1, 149.

8. Altice CK, Banegas MP, Tucker-Seeley RD, Yabroff KR. Financial hardships experienced by cancer survivors: a systematic review. J Natl Cancer Inst. 2017;109(2):1–17. https://doi.org/10.1093/jnci/djw205.
9. Zafar SY, Peppercorn JM, Schrag D, Taylor DH, Goetzinger AM, Zhong X, et al. The financial toxicity of cancer treatment: a pilot study assessing out-of-pocket expenses and the insured cancer patient's experience. Oncologist. 2013;18(4):381–90. https://doi.org/10.1634/theoncologist.2012-0279.
10. Coleman-Jensen A, Rabbitt MP, Gregory CA, Singh A. Household food security in the United States in 2018, ERR-2702019.
11. Hake M, Dewey A, Engelhard E, Gallagher A, Summerfelt T, Malone-Smolla C, et al. The impact of the coronavirus on local food insecurity. Published online at https://www.feedingamerica.org/sites/default/files/2020-05/Brief_Local%20Impact_5.19.2020.pdf2020. Accessed 19 May 2020.
12. Seligman HK, Laraia BA, Kushel MB. Food insecurity is associated with chronic disease among low-income NHANES participants. J Nutr. 2010;140(2):304–10. https://doi.org/10.3945/jn.109.112573.
13. Charkhchi P, Fazeli Dehkordy S, Carlos RC. Housing and food insecurity, care access, and health status among the chronically ill: an analysis of the behavioral risk factor surveillance system. J Gen Intern Med. 2018;33(5):644–50. https://doi.org/10.1007/s11606-017-4255-z.
14. Decker D, Flynn M. Food insecurity and chronic disease: addressing food access as a healthcare issue. R I Med J (2013). 2018;101(4):28–30.
15. Gregory CA, Coleman-Jensen A. Food insecurity, chronic disease, and health among working age adults. Published online at https://www.ers.usda.gov/webdocs/publications/84467/err-235.pdf?v=02017. Accessed 1 Oct 2019.
16. Laraia BA. Food insecurity and chronic disease. Adv Nutr. 2013;4(2):203–12. https://doi.org/10.3945/an.112.003277.
17. Gany F, Lee T, Ramirez J, Massie D, Moran A, Crist M, et al. Do our patients have enough to eat?: food insecurity among urban low-income cancer patients. J Health Care Poor Underserved. 2014;25(3):1153–68. https://doi.org/10.1353/hpu.2014.0145.
18. McDougall JA, Anderson J, Adler Jaffe S, Guest DD, Sussman AL, Meisner ALW, et al. Food insecurity and forgone medical care among cancer survivors. JCO Oncol Pract. 2020:JOP1900736. https://doi.org/10.1200/JOP.19.00736.
19. Simmons LA, Modesitt SC, Brody AC, Leggin AB. Food insecurity among cancer patients in Kentucky: a pilot study. J Oncol Pract. 2006;2(6):274–9. https://doi.org/10.1200/JOP.2006.2.6.274.
20. Page-Reeves J. Women redefining the experience of food insecurity: life off the edge of the table. Lanham: Lexington Books; 2014.
21. Berkowitz SA, Seligman HK, Choudhry NK. Treat or eat: food insecurity, cost-related medication underuse, and unmet needs. Am J Med. 2014;127(4):303–10 e3. https://doi.org/10.1016/j.amjmed.2014.01.002.
22. Sattler EL, Lee JS. Persistent food insecurity is associated with higher levels of cost-related medication nonadherence in low-income older adults. J Nutr Gerontol Geriatr. 2013;32(1):41–58. https://doi.org/10.1080/21551197.2012.722888.
23. Seligman HK, Schillinger D. Hunger and socioeconomic disparities in chronic disease. N Engl J Med. 2010;363(1):6–9. https://doi.org/10.1056/NEJMp1000072.
24. Gany F, Leng J, Ramirez J, Phillips S, Aragones A, Roberts N, et al. Health-related quality of life of food-insecure ethnic minority patients with cancer. J Oncol Pract. 2015;11(5):396–402. https://doi.org/10.1200/JOP.2015.003962.
25. Berkowitz SA, Seligman HK, Meigs JB, Basu S. Food insecurity, healthcare utilization, and high cost: a longitudinal cohort study. Am J Manag Care. 2018;24(9):399–404.
26. Tucker-Seeley RD, Li Y, Subramanian SV, Sorensen G. Financial hardship and mortality among older adults using the 1996–2004 Health and Retirement Study. Ann Epidemiol. 2009;19(12):850–7. https://doi.org/10.1016/j.annepidem.2009.08.003.

27. Ramsey SD, Bansal A, Fedorenko CR, Blough DK, Overstreet KA, Shankaran V, et al. Financial insolvency as a risk factor for early mortality among patients with cancer. J Clin Oncol. 2016;34(9):980–6. https://doi.org/10.1200/JCO.2015.64.6620.
28. Pisu M, Kenzik KM, Oster RA, Drentea P, Ashing KT, Fouad M, et al. Economic hardship of minority and non-minority cancer survivors 1 year after diagnosis: another long-term effect of cancer? Cancer. 2015;121(8):1257–64. https://doi.org/10.1002/cncr.29206.
29. Hunley K, Edgar H, Healy M, Mosley C, Cabana GS, West F. Social identity in New Mexicans of Spanish-speaking descent highlights limitations of using standardized ethnic terminology in research. Hum Biol. 2017;89(3):217–28.
30. Office of the Assistant Secretary for Planning and Evaluation. 2017 poverty guidelines. In: U.S. Department of Health and Human Services, editor. Published Online at https://aspe.hhs.gov/2017-poverty-guidelines#threshholds. Accessed 6/5/192017.
31. Yabroff KR, Dowling E, Rodriguez J, Ekwueme DU, Meissner H, Soni A, et al. The Medical Expenditure Panel Survey (MEPS) experiences with cancer survivorship supplement. J Cancer Surviv. 2012;6(4):407–19. https://doi.org/10.1007/s11764-012-0221-2.
32. Hager ER, Quigg AM, Black MM, Coleman SM, Heeren T, Rose-Jacobs R, et al. Development and validity of a 2-item screen to identify families at risk for food insecurity. Pediatrics. 2010;126(1):e26–32. https://doi.org/10.1542/peds.2009-3146.
33. Taplin SH, Anhang Price R, Edwards HM, Foster MK, Breslau ES, Chollette V, et al. Introduction: understanding and influencing multilevel factors across the cancer care continuum. J Natl Cancer Inst Monogr. 2012;2012(44):2–10. https://doi.org/10.1093/jncimonographs/lgs008.
34. Shankaran V, Jolly S, Blough D, Ramsey SD. Risk factors for financial hardship in patients receiving adjuvant chemotherapy for colon cancer: a population-based exploratory analysis. J Clin Oncol. 2012;30(14):1608–14. https://doi.org/10.1200/JCO.2011.37.9511.
35. Veenstra CM, Regenbogen SE, Hawley ST, Griggs JJ, Banerjee M, Kato I, et al. A composite measure of personal financial burden among patients with stage III colorectal cancer. Med Care. 2014;52(11):957–62. https://doi.org/10.1097/MLR.0000000000000241.
36. Zafar SY, McNeil RB, Thomas CM, Lathan CS, Ayanian JZ, Provenzale D. Population-based assessment of cancer survivors' financial burden and quality of life: a prospective cohort study. J Oncol Pract. 2015;11(2):145–50. https://doi.org/10.1200/JOP.2014.001542.
37. Yabroff KR, Dowling EC, Guy GP Jr, Banegas MP, Davidoff A, Han X, et al. Financial hardship associated with cancer in the United States: findings from a population-based sample of adult cancer survivors. J Clin Oncol. 2016;34(3):259–67. https://doi.org/10.1200/JCO.2015.62.0468.
38. Berkowitz SA, Basu S, Meigs JB, Seligman HK. Food insecurity and health care expenditures in the United States, 2011-2013. Health Serv Res. 2018;53(3):1600–20. https://doi.org/10.1111/1475-6773.12730.
39. Page-Reeves J, Scott AA, Moffett M, Apodaca V, Apodaca V. "Is always that sense of wanting … never really being satisfied": women's quotidian struggles with food insecurity in a Hispanic community in New Mexico. J Hunger Environ Nutr. 2014;9(2):183–209. https://doi.org/10.1080/19320248.2014.898176.
40. Counihan C. A tortilla is like life: food and culture in the San Luis valley of Colorado. Louann Atkins Temple women & culture series. 1st ed., vol. bk 21. Austin: University of Texas Press; 2009.
41. de Souza JA, Yap BJ, Wroblewski K, Blinder V, Araujo FS, Hlubocky FJ, et al. Measuring financial toxicity as a clinically relevant patient-reported outcome: the validation of the COmprehensive Score for financial Toxicity (COST). Cancer. 2017;123(3):476–84. https://doi.org/10.1002/cncr.30369.

Open Access   This chapter is licensed under the terms of the Creative Commons Attribution 4.0 International License (http://creativecommons.org/licenses/by/4.0/), which permits use, sharing, adaptation, distribution and reproduction in any medium or format, as long as you give appropriate credit to the original author(s) and the source, provide a link to the Creative Commons license and indicate if changes were made.

The images or other third party material in this chapter are included in the chapter's Creative Commons license, unless indicated otherwise in a credit line to the material. If material is not included in the chapter's Creative Commons license and your intended use is not permitted by statutory regulation or exceeds the permitted use, you will need to obtain permission directly from the copyright holder.

Part VIII
Implementation Science, Innovative Technologies and the Future of Cancer Care

Chapter 12
Implementation Science to Enhance the Value of Cancer Research in Latinos: A Perspective from the National Cancer Institute

Gila Neta

Introduction

The goals of *Advancing the Science of Cancer in Latinos* as set forth by the conference chairs, Drs. Amelie Ramirez and Edward Trapido, are to "develop actionable goals to translate basic research into clinical best practices, effective community interventions, and professional training programs to eliminate cancer disparities in Latinos" [1]. Over the course of the meetings, a variety of clinical practices and effective community interventions were described, which can improve cancer outcomes in Latino populations. However, these programs are not sufficiently implemented in practice. In the proceedings from the first conference held in 2018 [1], Dr. Anna Napoles noted that clinical practices and effective interventions are not reaching Latino populations to the same degree as the general public. Furthermore, she indicated that although there are platforms for the dissemination of evidence-based interventions, they are primarily used by researchers. The goal of implementation science is to bridge the gap between research and practice by understanding methods to promote the adoption and integration of evidence into a variety of settings where people are seeking care, including clinical, public health, and community settings.

G. Neta (✉)
Division of Cancer Control and Population Sciences, National Cancer Institute, National Institutes of Health, Rockville, MD, USA
e-mail: Gila.Neta@nih.gov

© The Author(s) 2023
A. G. Ramirez, E. J. Trapido (eds.), *Advancing the Science of Cancer in Latinos*, https://doi.org/10.1007/978-3-031-14436-3_12

Implementation Science

Implementation science has been defined as the "scientific study of methods to promote the systematic uptake of research findings and other evidence-based practices into routine practice" [2]. At the National Cancer Institute (NCI), we describe implementation science as the study of "identifying, understanding, and developing strategies for overcoming barriers to the adoption, adaptation, integration, scale-up and sustainability of evidence-based interventions, tools, policies, and guidelines," highlighting the various aspects of implementation to ensure patient and population health benefit [3]. Within the scope of implementation science, NCI also highlights the value of studying strategies to stop or reduce ("de-implement") the use of practices that are ineffective, unproven, low value, or harmful.

Why focus explicitly on studying implementation? In a 2000 review, Balas and Boren [4] delineated the pathway from original research to the implementation of scientific findings in practice. They included research on health interventions for a variety of diseases and defined implementation as 50% uptake in eligible populations. They accounted for the various steps in the pathway from research to implementation, including the submission, acceptance, and publication of findings; the use of evidence in systematic reviews; the development of guidelines and recommendations; and the ultimate uptake of those guidelines and recommendations in practice. They estimated the time it takes for each of these steps, as well as ways that evidence is lost in the process (e.g., small studies not getting published or incorporated into reviews, poor indexing). They found that it takes approximately 17 years for 14% of original research to benefit patients. As a public health community addressing urgent health needs, implementation science can provide a valuable tool to bridge that research to practice gap.

To ensure that evidence and evidence-based interventions are used and reach the relevant populations, implementation efforts should:

1. Determine whether the intervention can be adopted by the different health systems or communities who can benefit. Is it feasible, acceptable, and appropriate for those settings and populations?
2. Identify and train practitioners who can deliver the intervention.
3. Make certain that trained practitioners can incorporate the intervention into their routine practice by providing the necessary supports, which might be technical assistance, clinical reminders, staff resources, or financial incentives.
4. Ensure that the intervention can reach everyone who could potentially benefit from it.

If we do not account for each of these steps (as well as challenges with equitable access, adequate adherence, appropriate dosage, and maintenance), our interventions are unlikely to benefit the populations we aim to serve [5]. Implementation science seeks to build the knowledge base on how best to address these critical steps.

In contrast to traditional clinical trials, which often focus on understanding *what* evidence or evidence-based intervention can improve specific health outcomes, implementation science focuses on understanding *how* those evidence-based interventions can be adopted, implemented, and sustained to ensure their value in practice [6]. Without understanding the strategies that will support the capacity for cancer control interventions to be delivered in a variety of settings, including health care and community settings, interventions cannot be guaranteed to have the intended health benefits. Implementation science focuses on understanding which strategies can ensure that our interventions are deemed *feasible* to be delivered, that they are *acceptable* to populations using them, that they *penetrate* into the systems and communities using them, that they can *reach* all eligible populations, that they are *sustained* over time, and that they have high rates of *uptake*. These implementation outcomes, defined by Proctor and colleagues [7], are what the field seeks to maximize. By focusing on the strategies to meet these implementation outcomes, we can ensure that our interventions have the intended population health impact.

Several reviews have been published about strategies [8, 9] that enhance the adoption, implementation, and sustainability of an intervention. Some examples include strategies to educate or train practitioners to effectively adopt and deliver an intervention; strategies to ensure practitioners can incorporate interventions into their work flow or integrate them into their community settings; evaluative and iterative strategies to ensure implementation fidelity; and strategies to adapt interventions for a specific context. Which strategy to select depends on the barriers to be overcome, the resources that can be leveraged, and the stakeholders who will be involved [10].

Implementation science hinges on understanding the multilevel context in which implementation occurs and engages stakeholders to ensure that strategies address the critical barriers; are feasible, acceptable, and appropriate; and are likely to be integrated, sustained, and scaled. We need to consider all the levels that may influence implementation beyond the interaction between a consumer and practitioner. The clinic, organization, system, or community where that practitioner works is critical to understanding and supporting implementation efforts. Without accounting for these broader contexts, we risk exacerbating disparities and health delivery gaps, potentially ignoring populations with less access to care and fewer resources. Strategies that support implementation at these broader levels should be used, including strategies to support organizational change and strategies to get communities and municipalities, states, and nations to support the implementation of evidence and evidence-based interventions.

Implementation science relies on several core components. First, theories and frameworks are used to help understand factors that influence implementation processes and how best to address challenges to the adoption, implementation, and sustainability of effective interventions. An interactive webtool (https://dissemination-implementation.org/) can help researchers and practitioners select and use appropriate theories or frameworks to address a given practice gap. Second, stakeholder engagement at multiple levels (i.e., clinic, organization, community, state) to address a practice problem can ensure that the development, selection, and implementation of an effective intervention will be a good fit for the relevant populations and settings. Furthermore, stakeholders can help to inform the necessary adaptations that may be needed, while still maintaining the integrity or "core" components of the intervention. Third, valid and reliable measures of implementation outcomes provide a means for evaluating the success of our efforts. These include measures of acceptability, adoption, appropriateness, costs, feasibility, fidelity, penetration, and sustainability [7], and they can be measured at multiple levels including at the provider, organization, community, and policy levels. Fourth, rigorous methods and study designs allow us to make generalizable observations about our implementation efforts. Brown et al. [11] have described a variety of study designs and methods used in the field.

NCI has been soliciting implementation studies since 2003 through a range of funding opportunity announcements. At first, NCI-funded grant supplements focused on the implementation of tobacco control programs. However, the challenges of implementing evidence-based interventions span across cancer control and other health areas. Thus, beginning in 2005, NCI worked with other institutes and centers across the National Institutes of Health (NIH) to issue funding opportunities in implementation science [3]. Given that implementation challenges are not unique to a specific area of health, these trans-NIH funding opportunities can help build solutions to overcome the limited use of evidence in practice.

To date, over 300 grants have been funded through these trans-NIH funding opportunities in implementation science, and over 90 of these by the NCI alone. NCI-funded grants span topic areas across the cancer control continuum, including studies of effective training models for implementing health-promoting practices afterschool; the use of technology to scale-up an occupational sun protection policy program; strategies to increase colorectal cancer screening rates in community health centers; and strategies to facilitate and maintain universal lynch syndrome screening programs in different organizational contexts [12]. Historically, most NCI-funded studies in implementation science have focused on the best ways to adopt and implement evidence-based practices in cancer prevention and screening. In recent years, more studies have focused on uptake of evidence-based interventions in cancer treatment and survivorship. However, gaps remain particularly in research on the best ways to sustain and scale evidence-based practices across the cancer continuum, as well as how to de-implement practices that are not evidence-based or are harmful or wasteful.

While implementation science is focused on studying how to implement evidence and effective interventions, researchers can also consider implementation science within the broader translational research continuum, and particularly in intervention development and effectiveness studies. For example, researchers could consider how to design an intervention that is more likely to be implemented. One way to do this is by incorporating research aims around implementation within effectiveness trials. As we design interventions, we can consider who will deliver and receive the intervention, and build in tests of the implementation strategies, alongside tests of their effectiveness, to see whether they can enable the interventions to be used in practice. Curran et al. [13] laid out a road map for how to incorporate implementation aims into effectiveness studies. These effectiveness–implementation hybrid designs include research aims on both the intervention's effectiveness as well as its implementation. They propose rationales for different types of hybrid studies depending on which aims are the main focus.

With the launch of the Cancer Moonshot in 2016, implementation science has become an increasingly important priority for the NCI. Various Moonshot initiatives have focused on implementation science and the uptake of colorectal cancer screening and follow-up [14], symptom management in cancer survivors [15], and genetic testing and cascade screening in cancer patients and their families [16]. Additionally, seven Implementation Science Centers in Cancer Control have been funded to build infrastructure, develop and improve measures, and support studies across a range of cancer control challenges [17]. And in 2020, NCI for the first time has included implementation science as a strategic priority to advance cancer research and population health in its annual plan [18]. In addition to investing in implementation science through research grants, the NCI also supports training opportunities and initiatives to foster collaborations. One of these, the Implementation Science Consortium in Cancer, seeks to address major gaps in the field, including the integration of a health equity lens into the frameworks, methods, and measures we use. By advancing implementation science and concentrating on the *how* in addition to the *what*, we can ensure that cancer discoveries are able to most effectively reduce the burden of cancer for Latinos.

References

1. Ramirez AG, Trapido EJ. Advancing the science of cancer in Latinos. Cham: Springer International Publishing; 2019.
2. Eccles MP, Mittman BS. Welcome to implementation science. Implement Sci. 2006;1(1):1. https://doi.org/10.1186/1748-5908-1-1.
3. National Institutes of Health. Dissemination and implementation research in health program announcement. 2019. https://grants.nih.gov/grants/guide/pa-files/PAR-19-274.html. Accessed 11 Aug 2020.
4. Balas EA, Boren SA. Managing clinical knowledge for health care improvement. Yearb Med Inform. 2000;1:65–70.
5. Glasgow RE, Harden SM, Gaglio B, Rabin B, Smith ML, Porter GC, et al. RE-AIM planning and evaluation framework: adapting to new science and practice with a 20-year review. Front Public Health. 2019;7:64. https://doi.org/10.3389/fpubh.2019.00064.
6. Proctor EK, Landsverk J, Aarons G, Chambers D, Glisson C, Mittman B. Implementation research in mental health services: an emerging science with conceptual, methodological, and training challenges. Admin Pol Ment Health. 2009;36(1):24–34. https://doi.org/10.1007/s10488-008-0197-4.
7. Proctor E, Silmere H, Raghavan R, Hovmand P, Aarons G, Bunger A, et al. Outcomes for implementation research: conceptual distinctions, measurement challenges, and research agenda. Admin Pol Ment Health. 2011;38(2):65–76. https://doi.org/10.1007/s10488-010-0319-7.
8. Powell BJ, Waltz TJ, Chinman MJ, Damschroder LJ, Smith JL, Matthieu MM, et al. A refined compilation of implementation strategies: results from the Expert Recommendations for Implementing Change (ERIC) project. Implement Sci. 2015;10:21. https://doi.org/10.1186/s13012-015-0209-1.
9. Waltz TJ, Powell BJ, Matthieu MM, Damschroder LJ, Chinman MJ, Smith JL, et al. Use of concept mapping to characterize relationships among implementation strategies and

assess their feasibility and importance: results from the Expert Recommendations for Implementing Change (ERIC) study. Implement Sci. 2015;10:109. https://doi.org/10.1186/s13012-015-0295-0.

10. Powell BJ, Beidas RS, Lewis CC, Aarons GA, McMillen JC, Proctor EK, et al. Methods to improve the selection and tailoring of implementation strategies. J Behav Health Serv Res. 2017;44(2):177–94. https://doi.org/10.1007/s11414-015-9475-6.

11. Brown CH, Curran G, Palinkas LA, Aarons GA, Wells KB, Jones L, et al. An overview of research and evaluation designs for dissemination and implementation. Annu Rev Public Health. 2017;38:1–22. https://doi.org/10.1146/annurev-publhealth-031816-044215.

12. National Cancer Institute. Sample grant applications. 2020. https://cancercontrol.cancer.gov/IS/sample-grant-applications.html. Accessed 11 Aug 2020.

13. Curran GM, Bauer M, Mittman B, Pyne JM, Stetler C. Effectiveness-implementation hybrid designs: combining elements of clinical effectiveness and implementation research to enhance public health impact. Med Care. 2012;50(3):217–26. https://doi.org/10.1097/MLR.0b013e3182408812.

14. National Cancer Institute. Accelerating colorectal cancer screening and follow-up through implementation science (ACCSIS) program. 2020. https://accsis.rti.org/about/. Accessed 11 Aug 2020.

15. National Cancer Institute. Improving the management of symptoms during and following cancer treatment (IMPACT). 2020. https://impactconsortium.org/. Accessed 11 Aug 2020.

16. National Cancer Institute. Prevention and early detection of hereditary cancers. 2018. https://www.cancer.gov/research/key-initiatives/moonshot-cancer-initiative/implementation/hereditary-cancers. Accessed 11 Aug 2020.

17. National Cancer Institute. Implementation science center in cancer control (ISC3). 2020. https://cancercontrol.cancer.gov/IS/initiatives/ISC3.html. Accessed 11 Aug 2020.

18. National Cancer Institute. NCI annual plan & budget proposal for fiscal year 2021. 2019. https://www.cancer.gov/about-nci/budget/plan/index. Accessed 11 Aug 2020.

Open Access This chapter is licensed under the terms of the Creative Commons Attribution 4.0 International License (http://creativecommons.org/licenses/by/4.0/), which permits use, sharing, adaptation, distribution and reproduction in any medium or format, as long as you give appropriate credit to the original author(s) and the source, provide a link to the Creative Commons license and indicate if changes were made.

The images or other third party material in this chapter are included in the chapter's Creative Commons license, unless indicated otherwise in a credit line to the material. If material is not included in the chapter's Creative Commons license and your intended use is not permitted by statutory regulation or exceeds the permitted use, you will need to obtain permission directly from the copyright holder.

Chapter 13
Advancing E-health Interventions in Cancer Control and Survivorship for Hispanic/Latina Breast Cancer Patients

Sharon H. Baik, Joanna Buscemi, Laura B. Oswald, Diana Buitrago, Judith Guitelman, Francisco Iacobelli, Melissa A. Simon, Frank J. Penedo, and Betina Yanez

E-health Interventions for Breast Cancer

Breast cancer is the most commonly diagnosed cancer among Hispanic/Latina women, and epidemiological data indicate that there are approximately 220,000 Hispanic/Latina breast cancer survivors (BCS) currently living in the United States

S. H. Baik · D. Buitrago
Department of Medical Social Sciences, Northwestern University Feinberg School of Medicine, Chicago, IL, USA

J. Buscemi
Department of Psychology, DePaul University, Chicago, IL, USA

Institute for Health Research and Policy, University of Illinois at Chicago, Chicago, IL, USA

L. B. Oswald
Department of Health Outcomes and Behavior, Moffitt Cancer Center, Tampa, FL, USA

J. Guitelman
ALAS-WINGS, Latina Association for Breast Cancer, Chicago, IL, USA

F. Iacobelli
Department of Computer Science, Northeastern Illinois University, Chicago, IL, USA

M. A. Simon
Department of Obstetrics and Gynecology, Northwestern University Feinberg School of Medicine, Chicago, IL, USA

Robert H. Lurie Comprehensive Cancer Center, Chicago, IL, USA

F. J. Penedo
Department of Psychology, University of Miami, Coral Gables, FL, USA

B. Yanez (✉)
Department of Medical Social Sciences, Northwestern University Feinberg School of Medicine, Chicago, IL, USA

Robert H. Lurie Comprehensive Cancer Center, Chicago, IL, USA
e-mail: betina.yanez@northwestern.edu

© The Author(s) 2023
A. G. Ramirez, E. J. Trapido (eds.), *Advancing the Science of Cancer in Latinos*, https://doi.org/10.1007/978-3-031-14436-3_13

[1]. Continued increases in the numbers of BCS are expected because of advancements in early detection and cancer treatments. As such, there has been a greater focus on health-related quality of life (HRQOL), which represents the impact of health on one's physical, functional, emotional, and social functioning. Compared to non-Hispanic/Latina BCS, Hispanics/Latinas report poorer HRQOL, worse symptom burden, and more cancer-related psychosocial needs [2–10]; Hispanic/Latina cancer survivors also report greater unmet needs than non-Hispanic/Latina White cancer survivors [11]. Furthermore, Hispanic/Latina BCS report greater unmet needs than both prostate and colorectal cancer survivors (OR 2.33–5.86 [1.27–14.01]), with the highest unmet needs existing in the domains of psychological, health system and information, patient care and support, and physical and daily living [11].

Despite these documented disparities, few psychosocial interventions [12–14] have specifically targeted Hispanic/Latina BCS [2, 8, 15]. Research has demonstrated the importance of culturally appropriate interventions, as they are more effective when tailored to a particular racial/ethnic group [16] and show moderate to large effects [17]. Specific Hispanic/Latina cultural beliefs and values such as *familismo*, *marianismo*, and *personalismo* may need to be considered, as they can indirectly impact health and well-being outcomes [18, 19]. Thus, there is a need for culturally and linguistically appropriate interventions that address the unique needs and specific concerns of Hispanic/Latina BCS.

E-health platforms are increasingly being used to deliver psychosocial and supportive care interventions to cancer survivors, with preliminary data indicating benefits for psychosocial outcomes and lifestyle behaviors [20, 21]. Broadly, e-health platforms refer to health services delivered through the use of information technology, including the Internet and mobile and wireless applications. Notably, Hispanic/Latino individuals in the United States seek health information online at similar or higher rates than other racial/ethnic groups [22], and the use of smartphone technologies has increased with eight out of ten Hispanics/Latinos now owning a smartphone [23]. E-health interventions reduce the need to travel for in-person cancer care and support, and they may be especially appealing to minority and underserved patients who may have more logistical barriers to accessing in-person cancer care. Therefore, harnessing technology-based interventions such as smartphone applications and additional e-health interventions has the potential to increase the accessibility of scalable, evidence-based supportive care interventions that are culturally and linguistically appropriate for Hispanic/Latina patient populations.

Despite the increasing use of e-health platforms to deliver programs for cancer patients and survivors, more studies are needed to evaluate their efficacy and effectiveness, especially for racial/ethnic minority and underrepresented cancer patients. A systematic review revealed that the majority of available smartphone applications for cancer patients still lack evidence for their effectiveness [24]. Another recent systematic review identified 24 e-health psychosocial interventions for improving HRQOL in BCS, including six e-health platforms for health management and four mobile applications for physical activity [25]. A majority of these studies demonstrated encouraging results, including improvement of health literacy, disease and treatment knowledge, coping abilities, and social support [25]. However, some results were inconclusive, negative, or mixed. Furthermore, the feasibility and effectiveness of e-health platforms among Hispanic/Latina BCS have not been established, as only a handful of e-health studies have focused on Hispanic/Latina cancer patients and survivors [26]. Given the increasing focus on e-health platforms in the delivery of supportive care interventions, evaluating whether and how Hispanics/Latina BCS benefit from these programs is an essential step toward reducing documented cancer disparities.

To address this gap in the literature, our research team developed a culturally informed, evidence-based psychosocial smartphone application called *My Guide* to improve the HRQOL and symptom burden among Hispanic/Latina BCS who completed active treatment within the past 2 years. In this chapter, we briefly describe the development and evaluation of *My Guide* and discuss future directions for culturally tailored e-health intervention platforms for Hispanic/Latina BCS and patients.

My Guide

Intervention Development

A key aspect of *My Guide* development was our existing partnership with the Latina Breast Cancer Association of Chicago [27]. This community organization provides educational and emotional support programs for Hispanic/Latina BCS and their families in the Chicagoland area. The goal of our partnership was to identify the highest priority needs of Hispanic/Latina BCS in the Chicagoland area and address those needs via a bilingual and culturally tailored smartphone application [27]. Guided by principles of community-engaged research [28], our team developed the *My Guide* smartphone-based intervention through an iterative process that began with meetings with our community partner to identify specific concerns of this population and relevant topics to include within *My Guide*.

Our team used an iterative process of developing *My Guide* to ensure that both the content and delivery of the material were relevant to Hispanic/Latina BCS. Our first step was to conduct field interviews with nine Hispanic/Latina BCS to obtain thematic information on the experiences of Hispanic/Latina BCS, specifically related to aspects of emotional and physical HRQOL during the transition from active breast cancer treatment to breast cancer survivorship. Important themes identified included managing symptoms and side effects, coping with cancer, impact of cancer on friends and family, financial concerns, and additional cancer-related resources for Hispanic/Latina survivors. These themes were used to inform the content development within the *My Guide* application. Cultural issues such as the importance of family values within the Hispanic/Latina communities, perceived stigma regarding illness perceptions and cancer, and language barriers were also integrated within the application.

The second step in our iterative design process was to evaluate the usability of the initial prototypes of the *My Guide* application to ensure the appeal and ease of use among Hispanic/Latina BCS. We conducted two rounds of usability testing with 28 college students and 9 Hispanic/Latina BCS. Results indicated high usability feedback among the Hispanic/Latina BCS with an average response of 4.23 out of a maximum of 5 (SD = 0.9) on the usability questionnaire. Additionally, Hispanic/Latina BCS expressed a preference to be able to listen to the content within the application and to have less content or text in each section. Before transitioning to the next stage of development, participant feedback was integrated within application development [29]. Specifically, our team developed audio content that was embedded throughout the application, which allowed participants to choose to read or listen to the content in each section. The audio content also helped address concerns related to low literacy.

Our third step was to finalize the programming through a brief 4-week, single-arm field trial of the *My Guide* application with 25 Hispanic/Latina BCS [30]. Consistent with previous e-health intervention studies, we incorporated a weekly telecoaching protocol to enhance supportive accountability in using *My Guide*. From the initial trial, recruitment and retention rates exceeded 70%, participants used *My Guide* for an average of 9.25 hours across the 4 weeks (2.31 hours/week), and the mean score on the satisfaction survey was 65.91 out of a possible 70 points (range: 42–70), in which higher scores reflect greater satisfaction. Breast cancer knowledge significantly improved across time ($d = 0.59$), and there was a trend for improved HRQOL over the course of 4 weeks that did not reach statistical significance. There were several key lessons learned from our field trial. For example, we observed that most eligible patients had their own smartphones, with less than 20% of study participants relying on a study-issued smartphone. Additionally, approximately half of the study participants engaged with *My Guide* at the recommended levels of weekly use (2 hours/week). Based on this observation, our team recommended future use of a stepped-care telecoaching protocol to minimize calls for those meeting adherence goals and to provide more support for those struggling to meet study usage goals.

Pilot Randomized Controlled Trial (RCT)

Following the single-arm field trial, our team conducted a pilot RCT to evaluate the feasibility, acceptability, and preliminary efficacy of *My Guide* relative to an attention-control condition. Thus, we developed a second smartphone application titled *My Health* [31]. Both *My Guide* and *My Health* were web-based applications accessible on smartphones as well as computers and tablets, and available in English and Spanish. Similar to attention-control content used in other psychosocial intervention studies among cancer populations [32, 33], we designed *My Health* to provide easy-to-understand and evidence-based recommendations for promoting healthy lifestyles (e.g., nutrition, physical activity, prevention of chronic illness).

Study Procedures Participants completed a baseline (T1) survey of sociodemo-graphic information, primary intervention outcomes (i.e., symptom burden, HRQOL), and secondary intervention outcomes (i.e., nutrition, physical activity). Participants were randomized 1:1 to *My Guide* or *My Health* for 6 weeks and were encouraged to use their assigned smartphone application for 2 hours/week. Follow-up surveys were administered immediately post-intervention (T2) and 2 weeks after the T2 assessment (T3). Similar to the single-arm field trial, we used a telecoaching protocol to encourage participants' weekly use of their assigned application [30, 34]. All participants received telecoaching calls in their preferred language before Week 1, Week 2, and Week 6 of the intervention. In the remaining weeks, a stepped-care approach informed the need for additional telecoaching, with 90 minutes of application use in a given week (out of the recommended 2 hours) used as the threshold.

Results and Discussion Of 80 participants enrolled and randomized, 2 were lost to follow-up (one from each condition) and 78 were analyzed (*My Guide*: $n = 39$, *My Health*: $n = 39$). Sociodemographic and clinical characteristics did not differ between study conditions. Participants were an average of 52.54 years old (SD = 11.36). Most participants were born outside the United States (71%), reported Mexican ancestry (64%) and preferred to communicate in Spanish (64%). More than half of the participants had a high school education or less (54%) and an annual household income of <$25,000 (53%). Most participants had stage II disease (41%) and received chemotherapy (58%) and/or radiation therapy (71%).

Consistent with prior studies [32, 35–37], we considered a 70% recruitment rate and an 80% retention rate feasible. We also considered 90 minutes of application use per week feasible based on our single-arm field trial [30]. In this pilot RCT, we successfully recruited 79% of eligible women and retained 95% of enrolled partici-pants through the T3 assessment, indicating good feasibility [38]. On average, par-ticipants used the *My Guide* and *My Health* smartphone applications for 86.58 minutes/week (SD = 66.08) and 72.80 minutes/week (SD = 62.57), respec-tively, neither of which reached the 90 minutes/week threshold to indicate feasibil-ity. However, average use exceeded 1 hour/week for both applications, which is more time than a patient might expect to spend individually with an in-person coun-selor (typically 50-minute appointments once a week or less) [38]. Acceptability was evaluated at T2 with a survey assessing participant satisfaction with each smart-phone application. The vast majority of participants were satisfied (*My Guide* = 97%, *My Health* = 92%) and would recommend their assigned application to another woman with breast cancer (*My Guide* = 100%, *My Health* = 95%). Specifically, one participant stated, "I would recommend *My Guide* because I no longer feel alone. It helped with my side effects and helped me realize that others are going through the same thing," and another said, "Of course I would recommend *My Guide*! While using *My Guide* you learn so much about everything and things that you didn't even realize you didn't know. I would love if everyone could have access to this informa-tion." Participants expressed that "*My Guide* is a form of support..." and "the videos of other survivors and learning how to relax was so helpful to deal with my anxiety. How to manage my symptoms was very helpful as well." In addition, most participants indicated that they would like to continue using the application for longer than the 6-week study period (*My Guide* = 92%, *My Health* = 84%) [38].

In terms of preliminary efficacy, we evaluated breast cancer symptom burden and HRQOL (primary outcomes) with the Breast Cancer Prevention Trial symptom questionnaire [39] and the Functional Assessment of Cancer Therapy-Breast [40, 41], respectively. We assessed differences in symptom burden and HRQOL domains between study conditions over time using linear mixed-effects models controlling for language preference, education, and application use (i.e., whether or not the participant used their assigned application for an average 90 minutes/week). Across both study conditions, breast cancer symptom burden declined from T1 to T2 (d = 0.08), breast cancer well-being improved from T1 to T2 (d = 0.20), and improvements in breast cancer well-being were maintained at T3 (d = 0.17) [38]. We also evaluated nutrition and physical activity (secondary outcomes) with the Brief Dietary Assessment Tool for Hispanics [42] and the International Physical Activity Questionnaire Short Form (IPAQ-SF) [43, 44], respectively. *My Health* participants reported a greater decrease in daily fat sources from T1 to T2 compared to *My Guide* participants (d = 0.30), and this was maintained at T3 (d = 0.47). In addition, participants in both conditions reported increased time spent walking from T1 to T2 (d = 0.31) [45].

To our knowledge, this was the first study to design and evaluate two culturally informed smartphone applications for Hispanic/Latina BCS, *My Guide* (intervention) and *My Health* (control). Results demonstrated that the study procedures were feasible and acceptability was high for both applications. Both *My Guide* and *My Health* reported improvements in breast cancer symptom burden and breast cancer well-being over time; however, there were no differential effects between study conditions. Additionally, improvements in symptom burden were not sustained at the two-week follow-up assessment. These results suggest that technology-based interventions may facilitate engagement in care post-treatment among Hispanic/Latina BCS.

My Guide for Breast Cancer Treatment

Throughout the field trial [30] and pilot RCT [38], many women reported that it would have been even more beneficial if they had access to their assigned application during active breast cancer treatment. Additionally, *My Guide* participants expressed wanting more information about general health and lifestyle behaviors, while *My Health* participants wanted more information specific to breast cancer and coping strategies. To address this feedback, our team developed a new smartphone application, *My Guide for Breast Cancer Treatment* [46], for Hispanic/Latina women in active treatment for breast cancer.

Given the high use of *My Guide* and *My Health*, both smartphone applications [31] were combined and content was adapted to be more relevant for Hispanic/Latina women currently receiving treatment for breast cancer. Notably, the *My Guide for Breast Cancer Treatment* intervention includes information specific to breast cancer and its treatment and symptom and stress management strategies, as well as content promoting healthy diet and physical activity for breast cancer patients during treatment. Additional notable differences between *My Guide* and *My Guide for Breast Cancer Treatment* include a longer study period of 12 weeks versus 6 weeks, tailored content, and gamification features. A 12-week intervention timeframe was selected as it is the expected length of adjuvant treatments, and prior behavioral interventions reported benefits in symptom burden and HRQOL after 10 weeks [47–49]. Additionally, this revised intervention highlights targeted content based on the participants' concerns and needs, which are assessed every 2 weeks. Finally, participant adherence and motivation to use the *My Guide for Breast Cancer Treatment* application are reinforced by virtual awards based on different levels of weekly use (e.g., ribbon for 30 minutes/week, medal for 45 minutes/week, and trophy for 60 minutes/week).

My Guide for Breast Cancer Treatment is currently undergoing evaluation among a sample of 60 Hispanic/Latina women in active treatment for breast cancer. Participants are randomized 1:1 to the intervention or enhanced usual care control condition, which in addition to care as usual includes educational materials regarding breast cancer and survivorship from the National Cancer Institute [50] and a list of supportive care resources and organizations in the Chicagoland area. Control participants will be given access to *My Guide for Breast Cancer Treatment* after the study completion.

Conclusion

With increasing technology access and use among Hispanics/Latinos in the United States [22, 23], e-health platforms provide an innovative opportunity to deliver more easily accessible, scalable, and tailored psychosocial and symptom management interventions to those with limited access to culturally and linguistically appropriate supportive care resources. Growing evidence indicates high acceptability of technology-based interventions among Hispanic/Latino cancer patients [26, 51, 52]. However, few e-health interventions have been developed specifically for Hispanic/Latina BCS [2, 8, 15] despite documented disparities in HRQOL and psychosocial outcomes [2–10]. Additionally, cultural and linguistic factors should be considered in terms of the design and delivery of e-health interventions for the Hispanic/Latino population [53]. For example, aside from language barriers, a number of cultural attitudes and beliefs may impact health behaviors and should be included in the intervention such as importance of family values, taking care of others, gender roles, and relationship with the provider [53]. And given their high use, smartphones may be the optimal technology platform to deliver English and Spanish evidence-based resources to address the unmet psychosocial needs of this under-served population.

Using community-engaged approaches, our team developed a culturally informed, evidence-based psychosocial intervention, the *My Guide* smartphone application, which demonstrated feasibility, acceptability, and preliminary efficacy in improving breast cancer symptom burden and HRQOL over time. However, of note, there were no differential effects in outcomes between *My Guide* and the attention-control *My Health* application. Participants expressed wanting to have used their assigned application during active breast cancer treatment in addition to post-treatment. As such, our team expanded the scope and focus of *My Guide* to be relevant for Hispanic/Latina women in active breast cancer treatment. To the best of our knowledge, both smartphone applications (*My Guide* and *My Guide for Breast Cancer Treatment*) are among the first bilingual and culturally informed supportive care interventions for Hispanic/Latina women who completed or are currently undergoing active treatment for breast cancer. Technology-based supportive and behavioral interventions that focus on breast cancer treatment and self-management may improve patient engagement as well as patient-reported outcomes during active treatment for breast cancer and into survivorship. Additionally, the self-guided *My Guide* and *My Guide for Breast Cancer Treatment* applications may offer much needed patient support to Hispanic/Latina BCS. During patient interviews, some of our study participants expressed feelings of loneliness and difficulties obtaining or asking for support from their families, and often noted concerns of burdening their loved ones. Findings from other qualitative studies with Hispanic/Latina BCS have indicated family as the main source of support, but some have similarly noted feeling alone and wanting more emotional support [2].

Our studies are expected to contribute to the limited cancer survivorship research in Hispanic/Latino communities and establish whether e-health interventions are feasible and effective for delivering supportive oncology interventions to this under-represented patient population. Future studies should consider the inclusion of a social networking component, especially given the importance of and desire for more social support, as well as the integration of evidence-based, patient-centered tools into electronic health records. In addition, given the multiple components of these psychosocial interventions, the effect of each component should be individually evaluated in order to identify the most effective intervention elements on study outcomes. Finally, an additional area for future directions includes establishing the efficacy of *My Guide* and *My Guide for Breast Cancer Treatment* across a nation-wide, diverse sample of Hispanic/Latina BCS. If found efficacious, future efforts will focus on disseminating the applications to Hispanic/Latino communities across the United States, increasing the public health impact among Hispanic/Latina women with breast cancer. And future research focused on implementing culturally appropriate interventions for Hispanic/Latina BCS should evaluate the cultural nuances at the system level as well. Given the lack of culturally tailored, evidence-based, e-health psychosocial interventions for Hispanic/Latina BCS, *My Guide* and *My Guide for Breast Cancer Treatment* may help bridge a gap in cancer care and have the potential to reduce disparities in psychosocial outcomes among Hispanic/Latina BCS.

References

1. National Cancer Institute. Cancer of the breast (invasive). United States cancer prevalence estimates. SEER Cancer Statistics Review 1975–2017 [database on the Internet]. Available from: https://seer.cancer.gov/csr/1975_2017/browse_csr.php?sectionSEL=4&pageSEL=sect_04_table.24#b. Accessed 1 June 2020.
2. Ashing-Giwa KT, Padilla GV, Bohorquez DE, Tejero JS, Garcia M. Understanding the breast cancer experience of Latina women. J Psychosoc Oncol. 2006;24(3):19–52.
3. Eversley R, Estrin D, Dibble S, Wardlaw L, Pedrosa M, Favila-Penney W. Post-treatment symptoms among ethnic minority breast cancer survivors. Oncol Nurs Forum. 2005;32(2):250–6.
4. Spencer SM, Lehman JM, Wynings C, Arena P, Carver CS, Antoni MH, et al. Concerns about breast cancer and relations to psychosocial well-being in a multiethnic sample of early-stage patients. J Cancer Educ. 1999;18(2):159–68.
5. Yoon J, Malin JL, Tisnado DM, Tao ML, Adams JL, Timmer MJ, et al. Symptom management after breast cancer treatment: is it influenced by patient characteristics? Breast Cancer Res Treat. 2008;108(1):69–77.
6. Fu O, Crew K, Jacobson J, Greenlee H, Yu G, Campbell J, et al. Ethnicity and persistent symptom burden in breast cancer survivors. J Cancer Surviv. 2009;3(4):241–50.
7. Sammarco A, Konecny L. Quality of life, social support, and uncertainty among Latina and Caucasian breast cancer survivors: a comparative study. Oncol Nurs Forum. 2010;37(1):93–9.
8. Yanez B, Thompson EH, Stanton AL. Quality of life among Latina breast cancer patients: a systematic review of the literature. J Cancer Surviv. 2011;5(2):191–207.
9. Luckett T, Goldstein D, Butow PN, Gebski V, Aldridge LJ, McGrane J, et al. Psychological morbidity and quality of life of ethnic minority patients with cancer: a systematic review and meta-analysis. Lancet Oncol. 2011;12(13):1240–8.
10. Moadel AB, Morgan C, Dutcher J. Psychosocial needs assessment among an underserved, ethnically diverse cancer patient population. Cancer. 2007;109(S2):446–54.
11. Moreno PI, Ramirez AG, San Miguel-Majors SL, Castillo L, Fox RS, Gallion KJ, et al. Unmet supportive care needs in Hispanic/Latino cancer survivors: prevalence and associations with patient-provider communication, satisfaction with cancer care, and symptom burden. Support Care Cancer. 2019;27(4):1383–94.
12. Andersen BL, Yang HC, Farrar WB, Golden-Kreutz DM, Emery CF, Thornton LM, et al. Psychologic intervention improves survival for breast cancer patients: a randomized clinical trial. Cancer. 2008;113(12):3450–8. https://doi.org/10.1002/cncr.23969.
13. Antoni MH, Lechner SC, Kazi A, Wimberly SR, Sifre T, Urcuyo KR, et al. How stress management improves quality of life after treatment for breast cancer. J Consult Clin Psychol. 2006;74(6):1143–52. https://doi.org/10.1037/0022-006X.74.6.1152.
14. Antoni MH, Wimberly SR, Lechner SC, Kazi A, Sifre T, Urcuyo KR, et al. Reduction of cancer-specific thought intrusions and anxiety symptoms with a stress management intervention among women undergoing treatment for breast cancer. Am J Psychiatry. 2006;163(10):1791–7. https://doi.org/10.1176/appi.ajp.163.10.1791.
15. Molina Y, Thompson B, Espinoza N, Ceballos R. Breast cancer interventions serving US-based Latinas: current approaches and directions. Women's Health (Lond Engl). 2013;9(4):335–50. https://doi.org/10.2217/whe.13.30.
16. Griner D, Smith TB. Culturally adapted mental health intervention: a meta-analytic review. Psychother Theory Res Pract Train. 2006;43(4):531–48.

17. Rathod S, Gega L, Degnan A, Pikard J, Khan T, Husain N, et al. The current status of culturally adapted mental health interventions: a practice-focused review of meta-analyses. Neuropsychiatr Dis Treat. 2018:165–78.
18. Nápoles-Springer A, Ortíz C, O'Brien H, Díaz-Méndez M. Developing a culturally competent peer support intervention for Spanish-speaking Latinas with breast cancer. J Immigr Minor Health. 2009;11(4):268–80. https://doi.org/10.1007/s10903-008-9128-4.
19. Interian A, Díaz-Martínez AM. Considerations for culturally competent cognitive-behavioral therapy for depression with Hispanic patients. Cogn Behav Pract. 2007;14(1):84–97. https://doi.org/10.1016/j.cbpra.2006.01.006.
20. Duncan M, Moschopoulou E, Herrington E, Deane J, Roylance R, Jones L, et al. Review of systematic reviews of non-pharmacological interventions to improve quality of life in cancer survivors. BMJ Open. 2017;7(11):e015860.
21. Seiler A, Klaas V, Tröster G, Fagundes CP. eHealth and mHealth interventions in the treatment of fatigued cancer survivors: a systematic review and meta-analysis. Psycho-Oncology. 2017;26(9):1239–53.
22. Lopez MH, Gonzalez-Barrera A, Patten E. Closing the digital divide: Latinos and technology adoption. Washington, DC: Pew Research Center; 2013. http://www.pewhispanic.org/2013/03/07/closing-the-digital-divide-latinos-and-technology-adoption/. Accessed 1 Oct 2014.
23. Pew Research Center. Mobile fact sheet. Pew Research Internet & Technology Project 2019. http://www.pewinternet.org/fact-sheet/mobile/. Accessed 28 June 2020.
24. Bender JL, Yue RYK, To MJ, Deacken L, Jadad AR. A lot of action, but not in the right direction: systematic review and content analysis of smartphone applications for the prevention, detection, and management of cancer. J Med Internet Res. 2013;15(12):e287.
25. Triberti S, Savioni L, Sebri V, Pravettoni G. eHealth for improving quality of life in breast cancer patients: a systematic review. Cancer Treat Rev. 2019;74:1–14.
26. Nápoles AM, Santoyo-Olsson J, Chacón L, Stewart AL, Dixit N, Ortiz C. Feasibility of a mobile phone app and telephone coaching survivorship care planning program among Spanish-speaking breast cancer survivors. JMIR Cancer. 2019;5(2):e13543.
27. Oswald LB, Guitelman J, Buitrago D, Buscemi J, Iacobelli F, Perez-Tamayo A, et al. Community perspectives: developing and implementing a smartphone intervention for Latina breast cancer survivors in Chicago. Prog Community Health Partnersh. 2019;13(5):131–6.
28. Michener L, Cook J, Ahmed SM, Yonas MA, Coyne-Beasley T, Aguilar-Gaxiola S. Aligning the goals of community-engaged research: why and how academic health centers can successfully engage with communities to improve health. Acad Med. 2012;87(3):285–91.
29. Iacobelli F, Adler RF, Buitrago D, Buscemi J, Corden ME, Perez-Tamayo A, et al. Designing an mHealth application to bridge health disparities in Latina breast cancer survivors: a community-supported design approach. Des Health. 2018;2(1):58–76.
30. Buscemi J, Buitrago D, Iacobelli F, Penedo F, Maciel C, Guitleman J, et al. Feasibility of a smartphone-based pilot intervention for Hispanic breast cancer survivors: a brief report. Transl Behav Med. 2018;9(4):8. https://doi.org/10.1093/tbm/iby058.
31. Yanez BR, Buitrago D, Buscemi J, Iacobelli F, Adler RF, Corden ME, et al. Study design and protocol for my guide: an e-health intervention to improve patient-centered outcomes among Hispanic breast cancer survivors. Contemp Clin Trials. 2018;65:61–8. https://doi.org/10.1016/j.cct.2017.11.018.
32. Yanez B, McGinty HL, Mohr DC, Begale MJ, Dahn JR, Flury SC, et al. Feasibility, acceptability, and preliminary efficacy of a technology-assisted psychosocial intervention for racially diverse men with advanced prostate cancer. Cancer. 2015;9. https://doi.org/10.1002/cncr.29658.
33. Penedo FJ, Fox RS, Oswald LB, Moreno PI, Boland CL, Estabrook R, et al. Technology-based psychosocial intervention to improve quality of life and reduce symptom burden in men with advanced prostate cancer: results from a randomized controlled trial. Int J Behav Med. 2020. https://doi.org/10.1007/s12529-019-09839-7.

34. Mohr DC, Cuijpers P, Lehman K. Supportive accountability: a model for providing human support to enhance adherence to eHealth interventions. J Med Internet Res. 2011;13(1):e30. https://doi.org/10.2196/jmir.1602.
35. Bowen DJ, Kreuter M, Spring B, Cofta-Woerpel L, Linnan L, Weiner D, et al. How we design feasibility studies. Am J Prev Med. 2009;36(5):452–7. https://doi.org/10.1016/j.amepre.2009.02.002.
36. Campbell LC, Keefe FJ, Scipio C, McKee DC, Edwards CL, Herman SH, et al. Facilitating research participation and improving quality of life for African American prostate cancer survivors and their intimate partners. Cancer. 2007;109(S2):414–24. https://doi.org/10.1002/cncr.22355.
37. Kissane DW, Grabsch B, Clarke DM, Smith GC, Love AW, Bloch S, et al. Supportive-expressive group therapy for women with metastatic breast cancer: survival and psychosocial outcome from a randomized controlled trial. Psycho-Oncology. 2007;16(4):277–86. https://doi.org/10.1002/pon.1185.
38. Yanez B, Oswald LB, Baik SH, Buitrago D, Iacobelli F, Perez-Tamayo A, et al. Brief culturally informed smartphone interventions decrease breast cancer symptom burden among Latina breast cancer survivors. Psychooncology. 2020;29(1):195–203. https://doi.org/10.1002/pon.5281.
39. Stanton AL, Bernaards CA, Ganz PA. The BCPT symptom scales: a measure of physical symptoms for women diagnosed with or at risk for breast cancer. JNCI: J Natl Cancer Inst. 2005;97(6):448–56. https://doi.org/10.1093/jnci/dji069.
40. Brady MJ, Cella DF, Mo F, Bonomi AE, Tulsky DS, Lloyd SR, et al. Reliability and validity of the functional assessment of cancer therapy-breast quality-of-life instrument. J Clin Oncol. 1997;15(3):974–86.
41. Cella D, Hernandez L, Bonomi AE, Corona M, Vaquero M, Shiomoto G, et al. Spanish language translation and initial validation of the functional assessment of cancer therapy quality-of-life instrument. Med Care. 1998;36(9):1407–18.
42. Wakimoto P, Block G, Mandel S, Medina N. Development and reliability of brief dietary assessment tools for Hispanics. Prev Chronic Dis. 2006;3(3):A95.
43. Craig CL, Marshall AL, Sjostrom M, Bauman AE, Booth ML, Ainsworth BE, et al. International physical activity questionnaire: 12-country reliability and validity. Med Sci Sports Exerc. 2003;35(8):1381–95. https://doi.org/10.1249/01.MSS.0000078924.61453.FB.
44. Lee PH, Macfarlane DJ, Lam TH, Stewart SM. Validity of the International Physical Activity Questionnaire Short Form (IPAQ-SF): a systematic review. Int J Behav Nutr Phys Act. 2011;8:115. https://doi.org/10.1186/1479-5868-8-115.
45. Buscemi J, Oswald LB, Baik SH, Buitrago D, Iacobelli F, Phillips SM, et al. My health smartphone intervention decreases daily fat sources among Latina breast cancer survivors. J Behav Med. 2020. https://doi.org/10.1007/s10865-020-00136-3.
46. Yanez B, Baik SH, Oswald LB, Buitrago D, Buscemi J, Iacobelli F, et al. An electronic health intervention for Latina women undergoing breast cancer treatment (My Guide for Breast Cancer Treatment): protocol for a randomized controlled trial. JMIR Res Protoc. 2019;21(12):e14339.
47. Wagner LI, Duffecy J, Penedo F, Mohr DC, Cella D. Coping strategies tailored to the management of fear of recurrence and adaptation for E-health delivery: the FoRtitude intervention. Cancer. 2017;123(6):906–10. https://doi.org/10.1002/cncr.30602.
48. Yanez B, McGinty HL, Mohr DC, Begale MJ, Dahn JR, Flury SC, et al. Feasibility, acceptability, and preliminary efficacy of a technology-assisted psychosocial intervention for racially diverse men with advanced prostate cancer. Cancer. 2015;121(24):4407–15. https://doi.org/10.1002/cncr.29658.
49. Antoni MH, Lechner SC, Kazi A, Wimberly SR, Sifre T, Urcuyo KR, et al. How stress management improves quality of life after treatment for breast cancer. J Consult Clin Psychol. 2006;74(6):1143–52. https://doi.org/10.1037/0022-006X.74.6.1143.
50. National Cancer Institute. Facing forward: life after cancer treatment. 2018.

51. Banas JR, Victorson D, Gutierrez S, Cordero E, Guitleman J, Haas N. Developing a peer-to-peer mHealth application to connect Hispanic cancer patients. J Cancer Educ. 2017;32(1):158–65.
52. Yanez B, Oswald LB, Baik SH, Buitrago D, Iacobelli F, Perez-Tamayo A, et al. Brief culturally informed smartphone interventions decrease breast cancer symptom burden among Latina breast cancer survivors. Psycho-Oncology. 2019:1–9. https://doi.org/10.1002/pon.5281.
53. Victorson D, Banas J, Smith J, Languido L, Shen E, Gutierrez S, et al. eSalud: designing and implementing culturally competent ehealth research with Latino patient populations. Am J Public Health. 2014;104(12):2259–65.

Open Access   This chapter is licensed under the terms of the Creative Commons Attribution 4.0 International License (http://creativecommons.org/licenses/by/4.0/), which permits use, sharing, adaptation, distribution and reproduction in any medium or format, as long as you give appropriate credit to the original author(s) and the source, provide a link to the Creative Commons license and indicate if changes were made.

The images or other third party material in this chapter are included in the chapter's Creative Commons license, unless indicated otherwise in a credit line to the material. If material is not included in the chapter's Creative Commons license and your intended use is not permitted by statutory regulation or exceeds the permitted use, you will need to obtain permission directly from the copyright holder.

Part IX
Latino Lifestyles: Acculturation, Nutrition, and Health

Chapter 14
Impact of Obesity and Related Factors in Breast Cancer Survivorship Among Hispanic Women

Elisa V. Bandera, Chi-Chen Hong, and Bo Qin

Introduction

Breast cancer is the leading cause of cancer death among US Hispanic women [1]. In Hispanic women, breast cancer tends to be diagnosed at an earlier age, at a more advanced stage, and with more aggressive phenotypes, compared to non-Hispanic Whites (NHW) [1], similar to what has been reported for African American/Black (referred to hereafter as Black) women [2]. Because Hispanics are the fastest growing group in the United States [3] and cancer survival is improving [4], the population of Hispanic breast cancer survivors is increasing. However, this is an understudied population that is more vulnerable to cancer inequities as they tend to have lower socioeconomic status (SES) and poorer access to care [1]. Hispanic breast cancer survivors are also likely to experience increasing rates of obesity and related comorbidities, such as diabetes [5], which place further burden in their cancer care and survivorship.

Both Hispanic and Black women have a high prevalence of obesity [6] but have distinct patterns of obesity-related comorbidities and biomarkers [7–9]. Hispanic women are also more susceptible than other racial/ethnic groups to weight gain [10], which primarily results in abdominal accumulation of adipose tissue, with negative metabolic effects [11]. As a consequence, metabolic syndrome, insulin resistance, diabetes, and dyslipidemia are common among Hispanics [12, 13]. They have the highest prevalence of central obesity and metabolic syndrome of any racial/ethnic group [10], which has been linked to an increased risk of aggressive breast cancer subtypes [14, 15]. Obesity and related comorbidities can impact breast

E. V. Bandera (✉) · B. Qin
Rutgers Cancer Institute of New Jersey, New Brunswick, NJ, USA
e-mail: elisa.bandera@rutgers.edu

C.-C. Hong
Roswell Park Comprehensive Cancer Center, Buffalo, NY, USA

© The Author(s) 2023
A. G. Ramirez, E. J. Trapido (eds.), *Advancing the Science of Cancer in Latinos*, https://doi.org/10.1007/978-3-031-14436-3_14

163

cancer treatment [16–18] but little is known about their independent impact on breast cancer treatment in Hispanic women. Obesity has also been shown to have a negative impact on patient-reported outcomes (PROs) including quality of life (QoL), fatigue, and lymphedema [19]; Hispanic women also experience poorer QoL after diagnosis [20, 21], but the role of obesity and related factors on PROs among Hispanic women is not well understood. Weight changes are common and a major cause of distress [22–24], with implications for comorbid conditions and potentially a factor in treatment adherence among cancer survivors.

Obesity and Breast Cancer Treatment

Receipt of guideline-concordant care is associated with more favorable breast cancer outcomes, but both Hispanic and Black breast cancer patients experience reductions in treatment intensity compared to NHW [25]. Obesity contributes to underdosing due to dose capping [26, 27], and breast cancer patients with comorbid conditions are less likely to receive surgery, radiotherapy, and adjuvant chemotherapy [28–31], and to be less adherent to hormonal therapy [32, 33]. The management and control of obesity-related conditions, such as diabetes and hypertension, may be particularly relevant since these conditions explain up to 30–50% of the survival disparity observed in Black breast cancer patients [10, 34–37]. Also, adherence to chronic disease medications, including statins for hyperlipidemia and oral medications for type 2 diabetes, declines during and after breast cancer treatment [38, 39]. Racial/ethnic differences exist in the prevalence and management of various comorbidities [40–42], treatments prescribed [41], and medication adherence [38, 43] and may have differential impacts on breast cancer treatment and PROs. The types of medications used to treat obesity-related conditions can also vary by racial/ethnic group. Hispanics are less likely than Black women to be prescribed a diuretic or calcium channel blocker for hypertension but are more likely to use a β-blocker [41]. To date, little is known about how management of comorbid conditions affects breast cancer treatment among breast cancer survivors, particularly in minority groups who have lower access to care [44, 45], but it is a key question given the clear link between comorbidities and poorer outcomes in breast cancer survivors [18].

Obesity and Patient-Reported Outcomes

Breast cancer survivors often develop symptoms and psychosocial effects related to their diagnosis and treatments. As a consequence, PROs such as cancer-related QoL, symptoms, and psychosocial factors are increasingly being considered key in cancer survivorship [46]. Because Hispanic women tend to have more advanced diagnoses and aggressive treatments [20], PROs are particularly important in this population. Hispanic breast cancer survivors generally report worse mental, physical, and social QoL than NHWs after diagnosis [20], but most studies had small sample sizes, used a cross-sectional design, and had limited scope. Obesity and related comorbidities have been shown to negatively impact PROs [47–49], but associations are not well understood, and few studies have focused on Hispanic breast cancer survivors. Being overweight has been shown to be associated with better QoL, but being obese was associated with lower physical, but not mental health in a study among 69 Hispanic long-term breast cancer survivors in New Mexico [21]. In the Women's Healthy Eating and Living Study, obesity was associated with both lower physical and mental health among Hispanic breast cancer survivors approximately 2 years after diagnosis ($n = 165$) [50]. These results are intriguing and warrant further research to fully evaluate the impact of obesity-related factors on PROs, with consideration of a range of key factors among Hispanic breast cancer survivors.

Feasibility of Assembling a Population-Based Hispanic Breast Cancer Survivors Cohort: The New Jersey Hispanic Breast Cancer Survivors Study (NJHBS) Pilot

With the long-term goal of evaluating the impact of obesity-related factors among Hispanic women after a breast cancer diagnosis, we conducted a pilot study to assess the feasibility of assembling a cohort study of Hispanic breast cancer survivors in New Jersey and their willingness to donate biological specimens and engage in follow-up activities. The methodology used in the New Jersey Hispanic Breast Cancer Survivors Study (NJHBS) pilot was similar to that used in our established cohort of Black breast cancer survivors in New Jersey, the Women's Circle of Health Follow-Up Study (WCHFS) [51], to allow direct comparisons of two populations vulnerable to cancer inequities.

Methods

The WCHFS, described in detail elsewhere [51], is a population-based cohort study of Black breast cancer survivors, identified in ten counties in New Jersey through rapid case ascertainment by the New Jersey State Cancer Registry. Self-identified Black or African American women with newly diagnosed, histologically confirmed ductal carcinoma in situ (DCIS) or invasive breast cancer, aged 20–75 years with no previous history of cancer other than non-melanoma skin cancer, and able to speak and read English, were eligible to participate. Pre-diagnosis data on established or suspected risk factors for breast cancer, as well as a saliva sample and detailed body measurements, were collected during a baseline in-person interview approximately

9 months after diagnosis. Follow-up was conducted by recontacting cases annually, including two post-treatment home visits at approximately 24 months and 36 months post-diagnosis and a phone interview at ~48 and ~60 months post-diagnosis to obtain information on survivorship factors of interest, as well as to update medical and lifestyle information and ascertain new breast cancer events or other cancers. Annual linkage with the New Jersey State Cancer Registry provides information on clinical characteristics, treatment and other cancer events, and mortality outcomes.

The NJHBS pilot study used a similar methodology to that used in WCHFS with some differences due to budget constraints, including a more limited target area (6 counties in New Jersey) and only one home visit for data collection. Because we were interested in assessing survivorship needs, the timing of the home visit for the pilot corresponded to the follow-up 1 visit in WCHFS (i.e., approximately 24 months after diagnosis). In the pilot, women who were proficient in English and/or Spanish were able to participate.

Methods for recruitment and data collection were similar to those in WCHFS [51]. After confirming eligibility, we scheduled a home visit to obtain informed consent, administered questionnaires using computer-assisted interviewing, and obtained body measurements and a saliva sample for DNA extraction using WCHFS protocols [51].

Validated scales and validated Spanish versions of questionnaires were used when possible. Acculturation was assessed in the NJHBS pilot using the Short Acculturation Scale for Hispanics (SASH) [52, 53], which includes 12 items with 3 subscales: language use, media, and ethnic social relations. Responses to all items are given on a five-point Likert scale where 1 is "Only Spanish" and 5 is "Only English." Low acculturation is defined as a SASH average score below 2.99 [52]. We also asked questions on migration status (foreign/US born), age at migration, and generation (e.g., first, second generation).

Breast cancer-related QoL was assessed in both the WCHFS and NJHBS pilot using the Functional Assessment of Cancer Therapy, Breast scale (FACT-B+4) [54], which is available in English and Spanish and has been validated in Hispanic populations [55, 56].

Remaining questions (e.g., sociodemographic factors and reproductive and medical history) in the pilot questionnaire were translated by professional translators. Questionnaires were administered in the participants' choice of language (i.e., English or Spanish), with the Spanish version administered by a bilingual Spanish-speaking interviewer.

Results

Despite budget and time constraints in the NJHBS pilot study, we were able to recruit 102 Hispanic breast cancer survivors in approximately 5 months. This included time for New Jersey State Cancer Registry staff to identify potential participants; request physician permission by mail to contact the patient, allowing 3 weeks for response; seek patient permission to release contact information to Rutgers Cancer Institute of New Jersey staff; and schedule and carry out a home visit with the participant. Among those with confirmed eligibility, the cooperation rate was higher in Hispanic women than in Black women (92% vs. 83%). The majority of participants in the pilot donated saliva (98%, same as in WCHFS), 92% said they were willing to donate a blood sample, and 95% were interested in participating in future studies. These rates suggest that Hispanic breast cancer survivors have high interest and willingness to participate in research studies.

As expected, based on New Jersey demographics [57, 58], almost half of the population was Caribbean (Fig. 14.1), with wide heterogeneity in country of origin. Approximately 61% said they were White, 20% Black, 23% Indigenous, and 19% mixed race. Acculturation was low in the NJHBS pilot study based on SASH [52], with 87% being foreign-born, 79% moving to the United States as adults, and 86% speaking only Spanish (data not shown). Compared to Black breast cancer survivors, Hispanic breast cancer survivors were less educated (52.9% vs. 36.2% had a high school education or less), had lower income (50% vs. 36.2% with a household annual income <25K), were less likely to have health insurance (18% vs. 11%), and more likely to report that cancer had caused them financial hardship (61.7% vs. 43.2%) (Table 14.1).

When we compared treatment information from the New Jersey State Cancer Registry on participants in the NJHBS pilot study with Black women in WCHFS, we found that Hispanic breast cancer survivors were more likely to not have surgery than Black breast cancer survivors (13.7% vs. 6.5%) despite being more likely to have invasive cancer, and those who did were less likely to have breast-conserving surgery (49% vs. 61%) (Table 14.1).

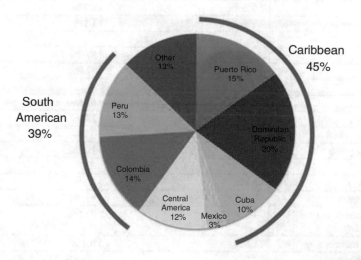

Fig. 14.1 Hispanic origin in the New Jersey Hispanic Breast Cancer Survivors Study (NJHBS) Pilot (*n* = 102)

Table 14.1 Demographic, clinical, and treatment characteristics of participants in the New Jersey Hispanic Breast Cancer Survivors Study (NJHBS) pilot and the Women's Circle of Health Follow-Up Study (WCHFS)

	Hispanic breast cancer survivors in NJHBS pilot	Black breast cancer survivors in WCHFS
	$n = 102$	$n = 720$
Age at diagnosis (years)		
20–40	8.8%	9.0%
41–60	57.8%	55.4%
61–75	33.3%	35.4%
Mean ± SD, years	53.6 ± 10.6	55.4 ± 10.8
Education		
≤High school graduate	52.9%	36.2%
≥Some college	47.1%	63.8%
Household income <$25,000	50.0%	32.2%
No insurance since diagnosis	17.6%	10.7%
Marital status		
Married	56.9%	34.4%
Widowed	6.9%	9.3%
Divorced/separated	31.4%	24.6%
Single/never married	4.9%	30.7%
Financial burden caused by cancer		
Not at all/A little	38.2%	56.7%
Some/A lot	61.7%	43.2%
Stage		
0 (DCIS)	12.5%	19.0%
I	43.2%	37.0%
II	34.1%	34.2%
III	7.9%	8.7%
IV	2.3%	1.1%
Grade		
I/II	50.6%	57.2%
III/IV	45.2%	42.8%
Subtype		
Luminal A	73.7%	61.8%
Luminal B	8.7%	13.9%
HER2-enriched	5.0%	5.2%
Triple-negative	12.5%	19.1%
Surgery		
No surgery	13.7%	6.5%
Lumpectomy	49.0%	61.2%
Subcutaneous or total mastectomy	24.5%	21.5%
Radical mastectomy	11.8%	9.3%
Chemotherapy	52.0%	45.4%
Radiation therapy	54.9%	48.5%
Endocrine therapy	56.9%	43.5%

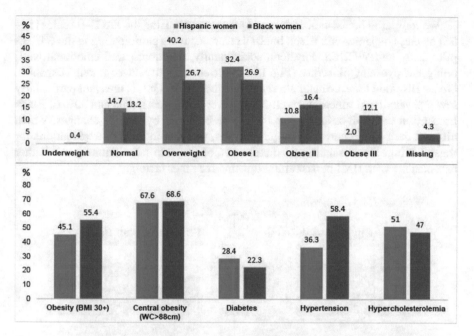

Fig. 14.2 Comparing Participants in the New Jersey Hispanic Breast Cancer Survivors Study Pilot versus Black Breast Cancer Survivors in the Women's Circle of Health Follow-Up Study. 1A (top): Distributions of weight status based on body mass index (BMI); 1B (bottom): Prevalence of obesity and related comorbidities. BMI was calculated by measured weight and height at approximately 24 months after diagnosis in both populations

Hispanic and Black breast cancer survivors were shown to have different patterns of obesity and obesity-related comorbidities. As shown in Fig. 14.2, Hispanics were more likely to be overweight or obese overall (85% vs. 82%), but Black women were more likely to be severely obese. Central obesity (waist circumference > 88 cm) was higher in Hispanic women at every level of body mass index (BMI) (data not shown). Overall, excess body fat was high in both groups, with 77.4% of Hispanic and 85% of Black breast cancer survivors having >35% percent body fat, and 68% of both Black and Hispanic women having central obesity (waist-to-hip ratio > 0.85) (data not shown). Hispanics were more likely to have diabetes (28.4% vs. 22.3%) and hypercholesterolemia (51% vs. 47%), while Black women were more likely to have hypertension (58.4% vs. 36.3%), but all these obesity-related comorbidities were highly prevalent in both groups. These differences may result in different metabolic consequences relevant to disease prognosis. Further work is needed to understand the complex impact of obesity on various breast cancer subtypes and the mechanistic pathways relevant to disease prognosis that may be differentially affected by obesity and related comorbidities across different racial/ethnic populations [59].

We compared breast cancer-related QoL measures using the FACT-B scales [54–56] among Hispanics and Black breast cancer survivors participating in the NJHBS pilot study and WCHFS. Physical, social/family, functional, and emotional well-being, and overall QoL scores (Fig. 14.3) were consistently lower among Hispanics. Obese Hispanic breast cancer survivors had the lowest QoL scores and particularly lower physical and functional well-being. Over 50% of Hispanic and 33% of Black breast cancer survivors said that they were bothered by weight changes, which affected their QoL scores. In future analyses, we plan to explore explanations for these findings by evaluating predictors of QoL in both populations and whether associations with BMI persist after adjusting for other factors.

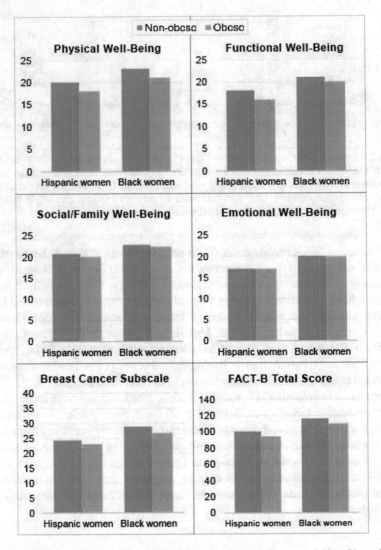

Fig. 14.3 Health-Related Quality of Life Measures Among Obese and Non-Obese Women Comparing Participants in the New Jersey Hispanic Breast Cancer Survivors Study Pilot versus Black Breast Cancer Survivors in the Women's Circle of Health Follow-Up Study

Summary

Our feasibility study among Hispanic breast cancer survivors demonstrated that Hispanic breast cancer survivors are very willing to participate in cohort studies and to donate biospecimens, consistent with what has been reported by others [60, 61]. We also found high financial distress due to cancer and intriguing treatment differences between Hispanic and Black breast cancer survivors. Obesity, central obesity, and comorbidities were highly prevalent in both populations, with Hispanic breast cancer survivors having higher rates of central obesity at each BMI category and higher rates of diabetes. Consistent with the few studies addressing QoL in Hispanic breast cancer survivors [20], we found lower overall breast cancer-related QoL scores for Hispanic breast cancer survivors, particularly for obese women.

Hispanics are a genetically admixed population with European, Indigenous American, and African Ancestry [62]. Historical factors account for the wide variations in admixture, with Puerto Ricans and Dominicans showing the largest proportion of African ancestry, while Mexicans show large proportions of Indigenous ancestry [63]. Genetic ancestry has been correlated with obesity-related physiologic measurements, adiposity, and risk of obesity-related comorbidities, including diabetes and hypertension among Hispanic and Black populations [64–70]. African admixture has been associated with BMI in Black women, but among Hispanic women, Indigenous American ancestry was strongly associated with waist-to-hip ratio, but not BMI [71]. Given this heterogeneity in obesity phenotypes and genetic ancestry, future studies need to address how genetic ancestry, obesity phenotypes, and related comorbidities affect aggressive breast cancer presentation, treatment, and survivorship factors by race/ethnicity.

Unfortunately, the heterogeneity of Hispanics is often raised by reviewers as a significant weakness when evaluating research in this population, as a single study is unlikely to have statistical power to evaluate associations by subgroups based on country of origin. However, there are unifying cultural themes across different subgroups (e.g., family values, religion/spirituality, perception of health and sickness), and only by starting to collect data on Hispanic breast cancer survivors, we will be able to dissect if indeed there are differences in the way breast cancer affects patient-reported outcomes and prognosis by Hispanic origin in the future and the complex interactions between race/ethnicity, culture, and ancestry. Despite increased interest in survivorship research, there is still a critical need to understand and address the needs of Hispanic breast cancer survivors, a growing and vulnerable population.

Acknowledgments This work was funded by the National Cancer Institute (R01CA185623) and the Rutgers Cancer Institute of New Jersey. We thank all the investigators and staff at the Rutgers Cancer Institute of New Jersey, the New Jersey State Cancer Registry, the Rutgers School of Public Health, and Roswell Park Comprehensive Cancer Center for their contribution to both studies. In particular, we would like to thank Dhanya Chanumolu and Baichen Xu for their technical support of this chapter. The project was supported by the Rutgers Cancer Institute of New Jersey Population Science Research Support Shared Resource.

References

1. Miller KD, Goding Sauer A, Ortiz AP, Fedewa SA, Pinheiro PS, Tortolero-Luna G, et al. Cancer statistics for Hispanics/Latinos, 2018. CA Cancer J Clin. 2018;68(6):425–45. https://doi.org/10.3322/caac.21494.
2. DeSantis CE, Miller KD, Goding Sauer A, Jemal A, Siegel RL. Cancer statistics for African Americans, 2019. CA Cancer J Clin. 2019;69(3):211–33. https://doi.org/10.3322/caac.21555.
3. Dominguez K, Penman-Aguilar A, Chang MH, Moonesinghe R, Castellanos T, Rodriguez-Lainz A, et al. Vital signs: leading causes of death, prevalence of diseases and risk factors, and use of health services among Hispanics in the United States – 2009–2013. MMWR Morb Mortal Wkly Rep. 2015;64(17):469–78.
4. Jemal A, Ward EM, Johnson CJ, Cronin KA, Ma J, Ryerson B, et al. Annual report to the nation on the status of cancer, 1975–2014, featuring survival. J Natl Cancer Inst. 2017;109(9):djx030. https://doi.org/10.1093/jnci/djx030.
5. Greenlee H, Shi Z, Sardo Molmenti CL, Rundle A, Tsai WY. Trends in obesity prevalence in adults with a history of cancer: results from the US National Health Interview Survey, 1997 to 2014. J Clin Oncol. 2016;34(26):3133–40. https://doi.org/10.1200/JCO.2016.66.4391.
6. Flegal KM, Kruszon-Moran D, Carroll MD, Fryar CD, Ogden CL. Trends in obesity among adults in the United States, 2005 to 2014. JAMA. 2016;315(21):2284–91. https://doi.org/10.1001/jama.2016.6458.
7. Morimoto Y, Conroy SM, Ollberding NJ, Kim Y, Lim U, Cooney RV, et al. Ethnic differences in serum adipokine and C-reactive protein levels: the multiethnic cohort. Int J Obes. 2014;38(11):1416–22. https://doi.org/10.1038/ijo.2014.25.
8. Goran MI. Ethnic-specific pathways to obesity-related disease: the Hispanic vs. African-American paradox. Obesity (Silver Spring). 2008;16(12):2561–5. https://doi.org/10.1038/oby.2008.423.
9. Romero-Corral A, Somers VK, Sierra-Johnson J, Thomas RJ, Collazo-Clavell ML, Korinek J, et al. Accuracy of body mass index in diagnosing obesity in the adult general population. Int J Obes. 2008;32(6):959–66. https://doi.org/10.1038/ijo.2008.11.
10. Lopez R, Agullo P, Lakshmanaswamy R. Links between obesity, diabetes and ethnic disparities in breast cancer among Hispanic populations. Obes Rev. 2013;14(8):679–91. https://doi.org/10.1111/obr.12030.
11. Keum N, Greenwood DC, Lee DH, Kim R, Aune D, Ju W, et al. Adult weight gain and adiposity-related cancers: a dose-response meta-analysis of prospective observational studies. J Natl Cancer Inst. 2015;107(2):djv088. https://doi.org/10.1093/jnci/djv088.
12. Velasco-Mondragon E, Jimenez A, Palladino-Davis AG, Davis D, Escamilla-Cejudo JA. Hispanic health in the USA: a scoping review of the literature. Public Health Rev. 2016;37:31. https://doi.org/10.1186/s40985-016-0043-2.
13. Cortes-Bergoderi M, Goel K, Murad MH, Allison T, Somers VK, Erwin PJ, et al. Cardiovascular mortality in Hispanics compared to non-Hispanic whites: a systematic review and meta-analysis of the Hispanic paradox. Eur J Intern Med. 2013;24(8):791–9. https://doi.org/10.1016/j.ejim.2013.09.003.
14. Agresti R, Meneghini E, Baili P, Minicozzi P, Turco A, Cavallo I, et al. Association of adiposity, dysmetabolisms, and inflammation with aggressive breast cancer subtypes: a cross-sectional study. Breast Cancer Res Treat. 2016;157(1):179–89. https://doi.org/10.1007/s10549-016-3802-3.
15. Davis AA, Kaklamani VG. Metabolic syndrome and triple-negative breast cancer: a new paradigm. Int J Breast Cancer. 2012;2012:809291. https://doi.org/10.1155/2012/809291.
16. Lee K, Kruper L, Dieli-Conwright CM, Mortimer JE. The impact of obesity on breast cancer diagnosis and treatment. Curr Oncol Rep. 2019;21(5):41. https://doi.org/10.1007/s11912-019-0787-1.

17. Minicozzi P, Van Eycken L, Molinie F, Innos K, Guevara M, Marcos-Gragera R, et al. Comorbidities, age and period of diagnosis influence treatment and outcomes in early breast cancer. Int J Cancer. 2019;144(9):2118–27. https://doi.org/10.1002/ijc.31974.
18. Hong CC, Ambrosone CB, Goodwin PJ. Comorbidities and their management: potential impact on breast cancer outcomes. Adv Exp Med Biol. 2015;862:155–75. https://doi.org/10.1007/978-3-319-16366-6_11.
19. Sheng JY, Sharma D, Jerome G, Santa-Maria CA. Obese breast cancer patients and survivors: management considerations. Oncology (Williston Park). 2018;32(8):410–7.
20. Yanez B, Thompson EH, Stanton AL. Quality of life among Latina breast cancer patients: a systematic review of the literature. J Cancer Surviv. 2011;5(2):191–207. https://doi.org/10.1007/s11764-011-0171-0.
21. Connor AE, Baumgartner RN, Pinkston CM, Boone SD, Baumgartner KB. Obesity, ethnicity, and quality of life among breast cancer survivors and women without breast cancer: the long-term quality of life follow-up study. Cancer Causes Control. 2016;27(1):115–24. https://doi.org/10.1007/s10552-015-0688-z.
22. Vance V, Mourtzakis M, McCargar L, Hanning R. Weight gain in breast cancer survivors: prevalence, pattern and health consequences. Obes Rev. 2011;12(4):282–94. https://doi.org/10.1111/j.1467-789X.2010.00805.x.
23. Vance V, Mourtzakis M, Hanning R. Relationships between weight change and physical and psychological distress in early-stage breast cancer survivors. Cancer Nurs. 2019;42(3):E43–50. https://doi.org/10.1097/NCC.0000000000000612.
24. Pila E, Sabiston CM, Castonguay AL, Arbour-Nicitopoulos K, Taylor VH. Mental health consequences of weight cycling in the first-year post-treatment for breast cancer. Psychol Health. 2018;33(8):995–1013. https://doi.org/10.1080/08870446.2018.1453510.
25. Fedewa SA, Ward EM, Stewart AK, Edge SB. Delays in adjuvant chemotherapy treatment among patients with breast cancer are more likely in African American and Hispanic populations: a national cohort study 2004–2006. J Clin Oncol. 2010;28(27):4135–41. https://doi.org/10.1200/JCO.2009.27.2427.
26. Griggs JJ, Liu Y, Sorbero ME, Jagielski CH, Maly RC. Adjuvant chemotherapy dosing in low-income women: the impact of Hispanic ethnicity and patient self-efficacy. Breast Cancer Res Treat. 2014;144(3):665–72. https://doi.org/10.1007/s10549-014-2869-y.
27. Griggs JJ, Sorbero ME, Lyman GH. Undertreatment of obese women receiving breast cancer chemotherapy. Arch Intern Med. 2005;165(11):1267–73. https://doi.org/10.1001/archinte.165.11.1267.
28. Louwman WJ, Janssen-Heijnen ML, Houterman S, Voogd AC, van der Sangen MJ, Nieuwenhuijzen GA, et al. Less extensive treatment and inferior prognosis for breast cancer patient with comorbidity: a population-based study. Eur J Cancer. 2005;41(5):779–85. https://doi.org/10.1016/j.ejca.2004.12.025.
29. Vulto AJ, Lemmens VE, Louwman MW, Janssen-Heijnen ML, Poortmans PH, Lybeert ML, et al. The influence of age and comorbidity on receiving radiotherapy as part of primary treatment for cancer in South Netherlands, 1995 to 2002. Cancer. 2006;106(12):2734–42. https://doi.org/10.1002/cncr.21934.
30. Harlan LC, Klabunde CN, Ambs AH, Gibson T, Bernstein L, McTiernan A, et al. Comorbidities, therapy, and newly diagnosed conditions for women with early stage breast cancer. J Cancer Surviv. 2009;3(2):89–98. https://doi.org/10.1007/s11764-009-0084-3.
31. Land LH, Dalton SO, Jensen MB, Ewertz M. Influence of comorbidity on the effect of adjuvant treatment and age in patients with early-stage breast cancer. Br J Cancer. 2012;107(11):1901–7. https://doi.org/10.1038/bjc.2012.472.
32. Hershman DL, Kushi LH, Shao T, Buono D, Kershenbaum A, Tsai WY, et al. Early discontinuation and nonadherence to adjuvant hormonal therapy in a cohort of 8,769 early-stage breast cancer patients. J Clin Oncol. 2010;28(27):4120–8. https://doi.org/10.1200/JCO.2009.25.9655.
33. Neugut AI, Zhong X, Wright JD, Accordino M, Yang J, Hershman DL. Nonadherence to medications for chronic conditions and nonadherence to adjuvant hormonal therapy in

women with breast cancer. JAMA Oncol. 2016;2(10):1326–32. https://doi.org/10.1001/jamaoncol.2016.1291.

34. Tammemagi CM, Nerenz D, Neslund-Dudas C, Feldkamp C, Nathanson D. Comorbidity and survival disparities among black and white patients with breast cancer. JAMA. 2005;294(14):1765–72. https://doi.org/10.1001/jama.294.14.1765.

35. Braithwaite D, Tammemagi CM, Moore DH, Ozanne EM, Hiatt RA, Belkora J, et al. Hypertension is an independent predictor of survival disparity between African-American and white breast cancer patients. Int J Cancer. 2009;124(5):1213–9. https://doi.org/10.1002/ijc.24054.

36. Polednak AP. Racial differences in mortality from obesity-related chronic diseases in US women diagnosed with breast cancer. Ethn Dis. 2004;14(4):463–8.

37. Braithwaite D, Moore DH, Satariano WA, Kwan ML, Hiatt RA, Kroenke C, et al. Prognostic impact of comorbidity among long-term breast cancer survivors: results from the LACE study. Cancer Epidemiol Biomark Prev. 2012;21(7):1115–25. https://doi.org/10.1158/1055-9965.EPI-11-1228.

38. Calip GS, Boudreau DM, Loggers ET. Changes in adherence to statins and subsequent lipid profiles during and following breast cancer treatment. Breast Cancer Res Treat. 2013;138(1):225–33. https://doi.org/10.1007/s10549-013-2424-2.

39. Calip GS, Hubbard RA, Stergachis A, Malone KE, Gralow JR, Boudreau DM. Adherence to oral diabetes medications and glycemic control during and following breast cancer treatment. Pharmacoepidemiol Drug Saf. 2015;24(1):75–85. https://doi.org/10.1002/pds.3660.

40. Mensah GA, Mokdad AH, Ford ES, Greenlund KJ, Croft JB. State of disparities in cardiovascular health in the United States. Circulation. 2005;111(10):1233–41. https://doi.org/10.1161/01.cir.0000158136.76824.04.

41. Kramer H, Han C, Post W, Goff D, Diez-Roux A, Cooper R, et al. Racial/ethnic differences in hypertension and hypertension treatment and control in the multi-ethnic study of atherosclerosis (MESA). Am J Hypertens. 2004;17(10):963–70. https://doi.org/10.1016/j.amjhyper.2004.06.001.

42. Egan BM, Zhao Y, Axon RN. US trends in prevalence, awareness, treatment, and control of hypertension, 1988–2008. JAMA. 2010;303(20):2043–50. https://doi.org/10.1001/jama.2010.650.

43. Calip GS, Hubbard RA, Stergachis A, Malone KE, Gralow JR, Boudreau DM. Adherence to oral diabetes medications and glycemic control during and following breast cancer treatment. Pharmacoepidemiol Drug Saf. 2014;24(1):75–85. https://doi.org/10.1002/pds.3660.

44. Kyanko KA, Franklin RH, Angell SY. Adherence to chronic disease medications among New York City Medicaid participants. J Urban Health. 2013;90(2):323–8. https://doi.org/10.1007/s11524-012-9724-4.

45. 2015 National healthcare quality and disparities report and 5th Anniversary update on the national quality strategy. Rockville: Agency for Healthcare Research and Quality; 2016. Report No.: AHRQ Pub. No. 16-0015.

46. Gordon BE, Chen RC. Patient-reported outcomes in cancer survivorship. Acta Oncol. 2017;56(2):166–73. https://doi.org/10.1080/0284186X.2016.1268265.

47. Smith AW, Reeve BB, Bellizzi KM, Harlan LC, Klabunde CN, Amsellem M, et al. Cancer, comorbidities, and health-related quality of life of older adults. Health Care Financ Rev. 2008;29(4):41–56.

48. Storey S, Cohee A, Gathirua-Mwangi WG, Vachon E, Monahan P, Otte J, et al. Impact of diabetes on the symptoms of breast cancer survivors. Oncol Nurs Forum. 2019;46(4):473–84. https://doi.org/10.1188/19.ONF.473-484.

49. Schmitz KH, Neuhouser ML, Agurs-Collins T, Zanetti KA, Cadmus-Bertram L, Dean LT, et al. Impact of obesity on cancer survivorship and the potential relevance of race and ethnicity. J Natl Cancer Inst. 2013;105(18):1344–54. https://doi.org/10.1093/jnci/djt223.

50. Paxton RJ, Phillips KL, Jones LA, Chang S, Taylor WC, Courneya KS, et al. Associations among physical activity, body mass index, and health-related quality of life by race/ethnicity

in a diverse sample of breast cancer survivors. Cancer. 2012;118(16):4024–31. https://doi.org/10.1002/cncr.27389.

51. Bandera EV, Demissie K, Qin B, Llanos AAM, Lin Y, Xu B, et al. The women's circle of health follow-up study: a population-based longitudinal study of Black breast cancer survivors in New Jersey. J Cancer Surviv. 2020;14(3):331–46. https://doi.org/10.1007/s11764-019-00849-8.

52. Marin G, Sabogal F, Marin BV, Otero-Sabogal R, Perez-Stable E. Development of a short acculturation scale for Hispanics. Hisp J Behav Sci. 1987;9:183–205.

53. Hamilton AS, Hofer TP, Hawley ST, Morrell D, Leventhal M, Deapen D, et al. Latinas and breast cancer outcomes: population-based sampling, ethnic identity, and acculturation assessment. Cancer Epidemiol Biomark Prev. 2009;18(7):2022–9. https://doi.org/10.1158/1055-9965.EPI-09-0238.

54. Brady MJ, Cella DF, Mo F, Bonomi AE, Tulsky DS, Lloyd SR, et al. Reliability and validity of the functional assessment of cancer therapy-breast quality-of-life instrument. J Clin Oncol. 1997;15(3):974–86. https://doi.org/10.1200/JCO.1997.15.3.974.

55. Belmonte Martinez R, Garin Boronat O, Segura Badia M, Sanz Latiesas J, Marco Navarro E, Ferrer FM. Functional assessment of cancer therapy questionnaire for breast cancer (FACT-B+4). Spanish version validation. Med Clin. 2011;137(15):685–8. https://doi.org/10.1016/j.medcli.2010.11.028.

56. Augustovski FA, Lewin G, Elorrio EG, Rubinstein A. The Argentine-Spanish SF-36 health survey was successfully validated for local outcome research. J Clin Epidemiol. 2008;61(12):1279–84. https://doi.org/10.1016/j.jclinepi.2008.05.004.

57. New Jersey Department of Labor and Workforce Development. NJ labor market views. People from many nations form New Jersey's Hispanic population. LMDR Labor Market and Demographic Research; 2011.

58. Center for Puerto Rican Studies, Hunter College, CUNY. In the garden: the state of Puerto Ricans in New Jersey. 2014. http://centroweb.hunter.cuny.edu/centrovoices/current-affairs/garden-state-puerto-ricans-new-jersey. Accessed 1 Mar 2018.

59. Bandera EV, Maskarinec G, Romieu I, John EM. Racial and ethnic disparities in the impact of obesity on breast cancer risk and survival: a global perspective. Adv Nutr. 2015;6(6):803–19. https://doi.org/10.3945/an.115.009647.

60. Nodora JN, Komenaka IK, Bouton ME, Ohno-Machado L, Schwab R, Kim HE, et al. Biospecimen sharing among Hispanic women in a safety-net clinic: implications for the precision medicine initiative. J Natl Cancer Inst. 2017;109(2). https://doi.org/10.1093/jnci/djw201.

61. Wendler D, Kington R, Madans J, Van Wye G, Christ-Schmidt H, Pratt LA, et al. Are racial and ethnic minorities less willing to participate in health research? PLoS Med. 2006;3(2):e19. https://doi.org/10.1371/journal.pmed.0030019.

62. Stern MC, Fejerman L, Das R, Setiawan VW, Cruz-Correa MR, Perez-Stable EJ, et al. Variability in cancer risk and outcomes within US Latinos by national origin and genetic ancestry. Curr Epidemiol Rep. 2016;3:181–90. https://doi.org/10.1007/s40471-016-0083-7.

63. Bryc K, Velez C, Karafet T, Moreno-Estrada A, Reynolds A, Auton A, et al. Colloquium paper: genome-wide patterns of population structure and admixture among Hispanic/Latino populations. Proc Natl Acad Sci U S A. 2010;107(Suppl 2):8954–61. https://doi.org/10.1073/pnas.0914618107.

64. Fejerman L, Romieu I, John EM, Lazcano-Ponce E, Huntsman S, Beckman KB, et al. European ancestry is positively associated with breast cancer risk in Mexican women. Cancer Epidemiol Biomark Prev. 2010;19(4):1074–82. https://doi.org/10.1158/1055-9965.EPI-09-1193.

65. Meigs JB, Grant RW, Piccolo R, Lopez L, Florez JC, Porneala B, et al. Association of African genetic ancestry with fasting glucose and HbA1c levels in non-diabetic individuals: the Boston Area Community Health (BACH) Prediabetes Study. Diabetologia. 2014;57(9):1850–8. https://doi.org/10.1007/s00125-014-3301-1.

66. Lins TC, Pires AS, Paula RS, Moraes CF, Vieira RG, Vianna LG, et al. Association of serum lipid components and obesity with genetic ancestry in an admixed population of elderly women. Genet Mol Biol. 2012;35(3):575–82. https://doi.org/10.1590/s1415-47572012005000047.

67. Piccolo RS, Pearce N, Araujo AB, McKinlay JB. The contribution of biogeographical ancestry and socioeconomic status to racial/ethnic disparities in type 2 diabetes mellitus: results from the Boston Area Community Health Survey. Ann Epidemiol. 2014;24(9):648–54, 54.e1. https://doi.org/10.1016/j.annepidem.2014.06.098.

68. Hu H, Huff CD, Yamamura Y, Wu X, Strom SS. The relationship between Native American ancestry, body mass index and diabetes risk among Mexican-Americans. PLoS One. 2015;10(10):e0141260. https://doi.org/10.1371/journal.pone.0141260.

69. Goonesekera SD, Fang SC, Piccolo RS, Florez JC, McKinlay JB. Biogeographic ancestry is associated with higher total body adiposity among African-American females: the Boston Area Community Health Survey. PLoS One. 2015;10(4):e0122808. https://doi.org/10.1371/journal.pone.0122808.

70. Lai CQ, Tucker KL, Choudhry S, Parnell LD, Mattei J, Garcia-Bailo B, et al. Population admixture associated with disease prevalence in the Boston Puerto Rican health study. Hum Genet. 2009;125(2):199–209. https://doi.org/10.1007/s00439-008-0612-7.

71. Nassir R, Qi L, Kosoy R, Garcia L, Allison M, Ochs-Balcom HM, et al. Relationship between adiposity and admixture in African-American and Hispanic-American women. Int J Obes. 2012;36(2):304–13. https://doi.org/10.1038/ijo.2011.84.

Open Access This chapter is licensed under the terms of the Creative Commons Attribution 4.0 International License (http://creativecommons.org/licenses/by/4.0/), which permits use, sharing, adaptation, distribution and reproduction in any medium or format, as long as you give appropriate credit to the original author(s) and the source, provide a link to the Creative Commons license and indicate if changes were made.

The images or other third party material in this chapter are included in the chapter's Creative Commons license, unless indicated otherwise in a credit line to the material. If material is not included in the chapter's Creative Commons license and your intended use is not permitted by statutory regulation or exceeds the permitted use, you will need to obtain permission directly from the copyright holder.

Chapter 15
A Strength-Based Approach to Cancer Prevention in Latinxs

Marisa S. Torrez-Ruiz, Sandra Soto, Nanette V. Lopez, and Elva M. Arredondo

Latinxs in the United States

Latinxs make up 17.7% of the US population, and this percentage is projected to increase to 23% by 2035 [1]. The rapid growth of the Latinx population in the US highlights the need to understand the lifestyle practices associated with the burden of chronic diseases like cancer. An estimated 18% of cancer cases in the United States are related to physical inactivity, poor nutrition, alcohol consumption, and adiposity [2]. Despite having lower socioeconomic status (SES) compared to other racial/ethnic groups, many chronic diseases are observed to be lower in Latinxs, a pattern often referred to as the Hispanic Paradox [1, 3–5]. As Latinxs acculturate to US culture, their risk for chronic disease increases [6]. As such, understanding the cultural and behavioral patterns of recent immigrants may shed light on the protective behavioral practices that may explain the better-than-expected health outcomes in this community. This chapter highlights the core cultural values among Latinx

M. S. Torrez-Ruiz (✉)
Division of Health Promotion and Behavioral Science, School of Public Health, San Diego State University, San Diego, CA, USA

School of Public Health, University of California, San Diego, CA, USA
e-mail: mstorresruiz@sdsu.edu; m8torres@health.ucsd.edu

S. Soto
School of Nursing, University of North Carolina at Chapel Hill, Chapel Hill, NC, USA
e-mail: shsoto@email.unc.edu

N. V. Lopez
Department of Health Sciences, Northern Arizona University, Flagstaff, AZ, USA
e-mail: nanette.lopez@nau.edu

E. M. Arredondo
Division of Health Promotion and Behavioral Science, School of Public Health, San Diego State University, San Diego, CA, USA
e-mail: earredon@sdsu.edu

© The Author(s) 2023
A. G. Ramirez, E. J. Trapido (eds.), *Advancing the Science of Cancer in Latinos*, https://doi.org/10.1007/978-3-031-14436-3_15

177

populations that may buffer the impact of low SES on lifestyle behaviors like physical activity and diet. These values include *personalismo* (e.g., formal friendliness), *familismo* (e.g., strong family values), collectivism, and aspects of acculturation. The following sections describe the potential buffering effects of these cultural factors on health outcomes in Latinx communities.

Bidimensional Aspects of Acculturation and Their Influence on Health

Acculturation is the change in an individual's attitudes, behaviors, and values from the culture of origin to the dominant or host culture; acculturation can influence disease risk through stress-induced exposures and the adoption of unhealthy behaviors [7, 8]. Some behaviors related to acculturation, such as increased physical activity during leisure time, can also decrease the risk of disease [9]. The process of acculturation is multi-faceted and can occur at the physical, biological, political, economic, and societal levels [10]. Some argue that acculturation is not a linear process and that individuals can maintain elements of their own culture while simultaneously adopting elements of the dominant culture (e.g., biculturalism) [11]. Other bidimensional aspects of acculturation include assimilation into the dominant culture, maintenance of the traditional culture, and marginalization (e.g., rejection of both the traditional and dominant culture). These processes of cultural acquisition and other cultural aspects of the Latinx heritage can contextualize the health practices of Latinxs to inform interventions.

Reframing Latinx Health Using a Strength-Based Approach

Strength-based research posits that individuals, groups, and organizations have strengths, and researchers could use this information to inform the development of health programs that aim to protect communities from chronic diseases [12]. Strength-based research is a counterpoint to the more traditional approach where intervention/prevention strategies are informed by the deficits of participants (e.g., low education) or communities [13]. The advantage of strength-based research is that it can enhance individuals' agency and empower communities to achieve and maintain recommended health practices [14]. Originally implemented in the field of social work, strength-based approaches have been used with greater frequency in psychology and public health. Using a strength-based framework to inform intervention research can empower individuals and re-affirm their cultural identity. Cultural identity, which often includes an individual's racial/ethnic or geographic origins, is also hypothesized to be associated with health-protective behaviors [15].

Latinx culture has many positive aspects that promote health and serve as protective factors. Cultural elements such as collectivism, *personalismo*, and *familismo* can be considered strengths as opposed to deficits or risks to health. When cultural strengths are recognized, they can be leveraged to increase the relevancy for individuals to engage in research and health programs. The incorporation of Latinx cultural practices and values into patient care and public health interventions may also increase health management behaviors. For example, the inclusion of cultural components such as language, values, and beliefs can influence medical mistrust, patient-provider communication, and adherence behaviors for Latinxs [16].

Latinx Cultural Strengths

Collectivism

Latinxs living in the United States are a heterogeneous group, with diverse attitudes, values, and beliefs. Within the context of the overall group, Latinx populations are collectivistic and prioritize the welfare of the group over the well-being of individuals within the group. Distinguishing features of collectivism include interdependence within members of the group and fostering social relationships that establish reciprocal obligations [17]. Social organization within collectivism is typically hierarchical, with all members of the group fulfilling roles that support the goals of the group. Health programs that build on collectivism and are group based have demonstrated positive outcomes in Latinx communities [18, 19].

Familismo

Within the overarching system of collectivism is *familismo*, which stresses the importance of social cohesion among the family unit and is one of the core cultural values for Latinxs [20, 21]. *Familismo*, as it is referred to in Latinx culture, is a multidimensional system of beliefs and values that emphasizes the connection to family, group harmony, respect (*respeto*), and obedience. The family unit is considered the primary "in-group" and can include the nuclear and extended family. *Familismo* encompasses social cohesion behaviors and structural values including frequent socialization and consultation with members of the family. For Latinxs, *familismo* is hypothesized to be a protective factor that minimizes risks related to physical health and could help explain some of the positive health outcomes between foreign-born and US-born Latinxs [22]. Health programs can build on this cultural aspect by engaging family members when addressing an individual's health to increase support and reinforcement of health guidelines and recommendations.

Personalismo

Personalismo refers to the value of personal relationships with an emphasis on friendliness and trust [22, 23]. Valuing interpersonal relationships may be one of many reasons why the *promotora* model has been successful in influencing behavioral outcomes in Latinx communities. Because *promotoras* are integrated and trusted members of their community, they can motivate individuals to engage in behavioral change based on cultural understanding and social support [24]. *Promotoras* can facilitate the cultural currency needed to achieve desired results or health outcomes of an intervention.

Health Practices Evident in Recent Immigrants

The following sections describe the hypothesized protective role of cultural strengths on health practices for behaviors related to diet and physical activity.

Dietary Intake

Healthy dietary patterns are linked to reduced cancer risk [25, 26]. Among the three most common forms of cancer (breast, colorectal, and prostate), diets rich in fruits, vegetables, whole grains, fiber, and fish can reduce cancer incidence and increase survival [25]. The nutritional value of foods consumed by recent Latinx immigrants declines with acculturation to US culture [27–30]. Specifically, studies show that less acculturated Latinxs consume more fruits, vegetables, whole grains, seafood, and plant proteins, and less sodium than more acculturated Latinxs [31, 32]. These findings are consistent with those of a systematic review of the dietary intake of Latinxs showing that less acculturated Latinxs consumed fewer sugary foods and sugar-sweetened beverages; and more fruits, rice, and beans compared to their acculturated counterparts [30]. Described below are family-related behaviors that may contribute to healthier nutritional intake among less acculturated Latinxs, who exhibit an array of protective dietary behaviors that contribute to the quality of foods consumed, including the frequency of consuming away-from-home foods, home-cooked meals, grocery shopping, and meal sharing.

Away-from-Home Foods Away-from-home eating includes consuming foods purchased at fast food and full-service restaurants, pre-prepared foods from grocery stores, and foods obtained from friends or relatives [33]. Among Latinxs, consuming away-from-home foods less frequently is associated with higher diet quality [34]. More acculturated Latinxs also tend to consume more fast food than less acculturated Latinxs [30].

Home-Cooked Meals One potential reason for lower away-from-home food consumption among less acculturated Latinxs is their emphasis on cooking meals at home. In the time-use study by Sliwa et al., over 90% of first-generation Latina mothers prepared foods at home in the previous 24 hours, compared to approximately 75% of third-generation mothers [35, 36]. Increased time spent preparing a meal may indicate greater cooking skill and less reliance on ready-to-eat foods, both of which are related to healthier food intake [37–39].

Grocery Shopping Grocery shopping is also an important indicator of cooking at home, which is associated with lower consumption of daily calories, fat, and sugar [40]. Using language as a proxy for acculturation, findings from the National Health Nutrition Examination Survey (NHANES) study show that purchases at grocery stores over 30 days were higher among Spanish-only speakers ($450) versus English-only speakers ($369) [36]. These studies suggest greater grocery shopping behaviors among Latinxs who are less acculturated to the United States.

Sharing Meals Sharing meals as a family is a dietary practice evident in less acculturated Latinos [41]. This behavioral practice acts as a protective factor as family meals versus individual meals are more likely to be healthier (e.g., include a variety of fruits and vegetables), provide for emotional connection among family members, and enable parents to model healthy eating behaviors [42].

Gender and Family Influences on Dietary Practices

The role Latinas play in planning, purchasing, and preparing meals may be a key reason why less acculturated Latinx families eat healthier [43–45]. Many Latina immigrant mothers preserve their traditional dietary patterns after immigrating to the United States where they incorporate fresh produce into their meals [46]. As such, Latina mothers' healthy food practices can positively influence their children's eating and food preferences [35, 45, 47, 48]. Latinx children can also influence the dietary practices of family members. For example, Latino mothers who have a bicultural versus an assimilated child are more likely to eat vegetables and are less likely to consume sugary beverages and eat away-from-home meals [49]. These findings suggest that children can influence the dietary practices of their parents and the type of influence may be dependent on the acculturation status of children.

Culture and Physical Activity

Physical Activity

Physical inactivity has been linked to bladder, colon, esophageal, kidney (renal cell), and stomach (gastric) cancers [50]. Physical activity is a modifiable factor that can help to decrease the risk of obesity and other related comorbid diseases. Active individuals may experience a 10–25% reduction in relative cancer risk in comparison to minimally active individuals [51, 52].

Active Transportation

Levels of physical activity among Latinxs will vary by acculturation status [53]. Among less acculturated Latinxs, exposure to US culture may decrease behaviors that were commonly practiced in the country of origin [54]. Behaviors such as completing errands by foot and the use of public transportation are often replaced by increased automobile use through the process of acculturation. Dependency on a vehicle may also be associated with neighborhoods that have limited infrastructure and are less walkable or safe to engage in physical activity [55]. Given the benefits of physical activity against cancer risk, public health programs may want to consider active transport (e.g., walking school buses) as an appealing and viable intervention option for diverse communities [56, 57].

Interventions That Build on the Strengths of Latinx Culture

Figure 15.1 outlines the ways in which behavioral interventions can integrate Latinx cultural factors.

Harnessing the Positive Aspects of Familismo

Although stressors from work and education may impact the division of responsibilities among family members, *familismo* may increase support for engaging in healthy behaviors. Research indicates that family support improves Latinx women's self-management of diabetes care, including increased physical activity and healthy dietary behaviors [55]. Several obesity-prevention programs that draw on *familismo* and engage family members have been successful. For example, Active and Healthy Families (*Familias Activas y Saludables*) recruited parent-child dyads to participate in 10 weekly 2-hour-long group sessions that addressed culturally relevant topics

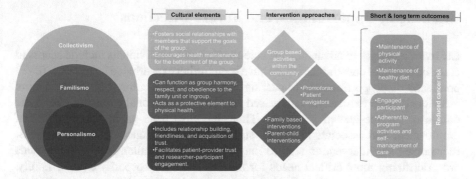

Fig. 15.1 Latinx cultural elements, intervention approaches, and outcomes. The first segment depicts a three-tiered socioecological model with ascending nested levels of *personalismo*, *familismo*, and collectivism. The second segment describes Latinx cultural elements at each level and their hypothesized protective factors. The third segment introduces intervention approaches for implementing the values into practice, and the fourth segment describes potential short- and long-term outcomes of Latinx practices

including parenting practices, dietary behaviors, immigration, and stress [55]. Another successful program that harnessed family relationships was *Entre Familia* [58]. This intervention was delivered by *promotoras* (community health workers) via home visits and telephone calls and was successful in increasing children's reported intake of a variety of vegetables and mothers' diet quality [58, 59]. Finding common ground through communication and shared experiences to engage family members in healthy practices may ultimately lead to increased familial bonds promoting family health.

Health Programs Embracing Collectivism and Personalismo

Studies that incorporate culturally specific values and beliefs, such as collectivism, may be more effective for their intended populations [60]. For Latinxs, the promotion of physical activity through group-based programs led by *promotores* in community settings has resulted in increased physical activity among Latinxs [61, 62]. The successes of these programs are, in large part, due to the *promotores*' ability to engage and interact with community members and participants receiving social support from and feeling connected to other group members.

Challenges, Opportunities, and Future Directions

Current challenges to advancing the science for Latinx individuals include access to care and financial constraints, which have been further exacerbated by the COVID-19 pandemic disproportionately impacting communities of color [63]. Many Latinx individuals have experienced increased risk and occupational exposure due to the nature of service-related jobs [61]. There has also been an increase in loss of employment and associated benefits, such as health insurance. For these reasons, recruitment for intervention studies may be especially challenging, as individuals are prioritizing more critical needs for the survival and prosperity of their family. Public health practice and research will also experience challenges due to the current political climate and social upheaval in our society related to the targeting and mistreatment of individuals of color [64]. This may contribute to health disparities already present among those with limited resources. Considering the challenges in front of us, it is essential that we connect with community groups to enforce the infrastructure and relationships that existed before the pandemic and to encourage their continued partnerships in health with providers, researchers, and healthcare systems.

Creating Future Opportunities Using Cultural Strengths to Advance the Science

To advance the health of Latinxs, health interventions need to build on the protective factors associated with Latinx health while recognizing the nuances specific to risk within the culture. The cultural aspects of *familismo*, collectivism, *personalismo*, and other shared values should be integrated into the design and practical application of research because they may serve as potential mechanisms of action related to health prevention, risk, and management behaviors. Community-based interventions that are implemented in churches, non-profit organizations, neighborhood clinics, and other community-endorsed establishments are effective because they are trusted sites for participants which align with the value of *personalismo*. With recruitment and participant engagement being the most challenging aspects of cancer prevention and treatment studies, community-based studies can be a key component to the advancement of health among Latinxs, especially now. Knowledge and understanding of the local community will also aid in the dissemination of information and the advancement of prevention efforts.

References

1. Dominguez K, Penman-Aguilar A, Chang MH, Moonesinghe R, Castellanos T, Rodriguez-Lainz A, et al. Vital signs: leading causes of death, prevalence of diseases and risk factors, and use of health services among Hispanics in the United States – 2009–2013. MMWR Morb Mortal Wkly Rep. 2015;64(17):469–78.
2. American Cancer Society. Diet and physical activity: what's the cancer connection? 2020. https://www.cancer.org/cancer/cancer-causes/diet-physical-activity/diet-and-physical-activity.html. Accessed 1 Sept 2020.
3. Franzini L, Ribble JC, Keddie AM. Understanding the Hispanic paradox. Ethn Dis. 2001;11(3):496–518.
4. Palloni A, Arias E. Paradox lost: explaining the Hispanic adult mortality advantage. Demography. 2004;41(3):385–415. https://doi.org/10.1353/dem.2004.0024.
5. Hiza HA, Casavale KO, Guenther PM, Davis CA. Diet quality of Americans differs by age, sex, race/ethnicity, income, and education level. J Acad Nutr Diet. 2013;113(2):297–306. https://doi.org/10.1016/j.jand.2012.08.011.
6. Goel MS, McCarthy EP, Phillips RS, Wee CC. Obesity among US immigrant subgroups by duration of residence. JAMA. 2004;292(23):2860–7. https://doi.org/10.1001/jama.292.23.2860.
7. Fox M, Thayer Z, Wadhwa PD. Acculturation and health: the moderating role of socio-cultural context. Am Anthropol. 2017;119(3):405–21. https://doi.org/10.1111/aman.12867.
8. Elder JP, Ayala GX, Parra-Medina D, Talavera GA. Health communication in the Latino community: issues and approaches. Annu Rev Public Health. 2009;30:227–51. https://doi.org/10.1146/annurev.publhealth.031308.100300.
9. Crespo CJ, Smit E, Carter-Pokras O, Andersen R. Acculturation and leisure-time physical inactivity in Mexican American adults: results from NHANES III, 1988–1994. Am J Public Health. 2001;91(8):1254–7. https://doi.org/10.2105/AJPH.91.8.1254.
10. Berry J. Acculturation and adaptation in a new society. Int Migr. 2009;30:69–85. https://doi.org/10.1111/j.1468-2435.1992.tb00776.x.
11. Berry J. Conceptual approaches to acculturation. In: Chun KM, Organista PB, Marin G, editors. Acculturation: advances in theory, measurement, and applied research. Washington, DC: American Psychological Association; 2003. p. 17–37.
12. Zhang A, Franklin C, Currin-McCulloch J, Park S, Kim J. The effectiveness of strength-based, solution-focused brief therapy in medical settings: a systematic review and meta-analysis of randomized controlled trials. J Behav Med. 2018;41(2):139–51. https://doi.org/10.1007/s10865-017-9888-1.
13. Coghlan D, Brydon-Miller M. Strengths-based approach. The SAGE encyclopedia of action research. SAGE Publications Ltd; Epub ahead of print 13 Oct 2014.
14. National Association of Social Workers. Standards and indicators for cultural competence in social work practice. 2015. https://www.socialworkers.org/LinkClick.aspx?fileticket=PonPTDEBrn4%3D&portalid=0. Accessed 5 Sept 2020.
15. Unger JB. Cultural identity and public health. In: Schwartz S, Luyckx K, Vignoles V, editors. Handbook of identity theory and research. New York: Springer; 2011. p. 811–25.
16. Yanez B, McGinty HL, Buitrago D, Ramirez AG, Penedo FJ. Cancer outcomes in Hispanics/Latinos in the United States: an integrative review and conceptual model of determinants of health. J Lat Psychol. 2016;4(2):114–29. https://doi.org/10.1037/lat0000055.
17. Raeff C, Greenfield PM, Quiroz B. Conceptualizing interpersonal relationships in the cultural contexts of individualism and collectivism. New Dir Child Adolesc Dev. 2000;87:59–74. https://doi.org/10.1002/cd.23220008706.
18. Darnell JS, Chang CH, Calhoun EA. Knowledge about breast cancer and participation in a faith-based breast cancer program and other predictors of mammography screening among African American women and Latinas. Health Promot Pract. 2006;7(3 Suppl):201s–12s. https://doi.org/10.1177/1524839906288693.

19. Penedo FJ, Molton I, Dahn JR, Shen B-J, Kinsinger D, Traeger L, et al. A randomized clinical trial of group-based cognitive-behavioral stress management in localized prostate cancer: development of stress management skills improves quality of life and benefit finding. Ann Behav Med. 2006;31(3):261–70. https://doi.org/10.1207/s15324796abm3103_8.

20. Sabogal F, Marín G, Otero-Sabogal R, Marín BV, Perez-Stable EJ. Hispanic familism and acculturation: what changes and what doesn't? Hisp J Behav Sci. 1987;9(4):397–412. https://doi.org/10.1177/07399863870094003.

21. Greenfield PM. The changing psychology of culture from 1800 through 2000. Psychol Sci. 2013;24(9):1722–31. https://doi.org/10.1177/0956797613479387.

22. Juckett G. Caring for Latino patients. Am Fam Physician. 2013;87(1):48–54. https://www.aafp.org/afp/2013/0101/p48.html. Accessed 4 Sept 2020.

23. Caballero AE. Understanding the Hispanic/Latino patient. Am J Med. 2011;124(10 Suppl):S10–5. https://doi.org/10.1016/j.amjmed.2011.07.018.

24. Shepherd-Banigan M, Hohl SD, Vaughan C, Ibarra G, Carosso E, Thompson B. "The promotora explained everything": participant experiences during a household-level diabetes education program. Diabetes Educ. 2014;40(4):507–15. https://doi.org/10.1177/0145721714531338.

25. Kerr J, Anderson C, Lippman SM. Physical activity, sedentary behaviour, diet, and cancer: an update and emerging new evidence. Lancet Oncol. 2017;18(8):e457–e71. https://doi.org/10.1016/s1470-2045(17)30411-4.

26. Harmon BE, Boushey CJ, Shvetsov YB, Ettienne R, Reedy J, Wilkens LR, et al. Associations of key diet-quality indexes with mortality in the Multiethnic Cohort: the Dietary Patterns Methods Project. Am J Clin Nutr. 2015;101(3):587–97. https://doi.org/10.3945/ajcn.114.090688.

27. Gerchow L, Tagliaferro B, Squires A, Nicholson J, Savarimuthu SM, Gutnick D, et al. Latina food patterns in the United States: a qualitative metasynthesis. Nurs Res. 2014;63(3):182–93. https://doi.org/10.1097/nnr.0000000000000030.

28. Pérez-Escamilla R. Acculturation, nutrition, and health disparities in Latinos. Am J Clin Nutr. 2011;93(5):1163s–7s. https://doi.org/10.3945/ajcn.110.003467.

29. Arandia G, Nalty C, Sharkey JR, Dean WR. Diet and acculturation among Hispanic/Latino older adults in the United States: a review of literature and recommendations. J Nutr Gerontol Geriatr. 2012;31(1):16–37. https://doi.org/10.1080/21551197.2012.647553.

30. Ayala GX, Baquero B, Klinger S. A systematic review of the relationship between acculturation and diet among Latinos in the United States: implications for future research. J Am Diet Assoc. 2008;108(8):1330–44. https://doi.org/10.1016/j.jada.2008.05.009.

31. Siega-Riz AM, Pace ND, Butera NM, Van Horn L, Daviglus ML, Harnack L, et al. How well do U.S. Hispanics adhere to the dietary guidelines for Americans? Results from the Hispanic Community Health Study/Study of Latinos. Health Equity. 2019;3(1):319–27. https://doi.org/10.1089/heq.2018.0105.

32. Marin G, Sabogal F, Marin BV, Otero-Sabogal R, Perez-Stable EJ. Development of a short acculturation scale for Hispanics. Hisp J Behav Sci. 1987;9(2):183–205. https://doi.org/10.1177/07399863870092005.

33. Guthrie JF, Lin BH, Frazao E. Role of food prepared away from home in the American diet, 1977–78 versus 1994–96: changes and consequences. J Nutr Educ Behav. 2002;34(3):140–50. https://doi.org/10.1016/s1499-4046(06)60083-3.

34. McClain AC, Ayala GX, Sotres-Alvarez D, Siega-Riz AM, Kaplan RC, Gellman MD, et al. Frequency of intake and type of away-from- home foods consumed are associated with diet quality in the Hispanic community health study/study of Latinos (HCHS/SOL). J Nutr. 2018;148(3):453–63. https://doi.org/10.1093/jn/nxx067.

35. Sliwa SA, Must A, Peréa F, Economos CD. Maternal employment, acculturation, and time spent in food-related behaviors among Hispanic mothers in the United States. Evidence from the American Time Use Survey. Appetite. 2015;87:10–9. https://doi.org/10.1016/j.appet.2014.10.015.

36. Langellier BA, Brookmeyer R, Wang MC, Glik D. Language use affects food behaviours and food values among Mexican-origin adults in the USA. Public Health Nutr. 2015;18(2):264–74. https://doi.org/10.1017/S1368980014000287.

37. Monsivais P, Aggarwal A, Drewnowski A. Time spent on home food preparation and indicators of healthy eating. Am J Prev Med. 2014;47(6):796–802. https://doi.org/10.1016/j. amepre.2014.07.033.
38. Cutler DM, Glaeser EL, Shapiro JM. Why have Americans become more obese? J Econ Perspect. 2003;17(3):93–118. https://doi.org/10.1257/089533003769204371.
39. Adams J, White M. Prevalence and socio-demographic correlates of time spent cooking by adults in the 2005 UK Time Use Survey. Cross-sectional analysis. Appetite. 2015;92:185–91. https://doi.org/10.1016/j.appet.2015.05.022.
40. Wolfson JA, Bleich SN. Is cooking at home associated with better diet quality or weight-loss intention? Public Health Nutr. 2015;18(8):1397–406. https://doi.org/10.1017/s1368980014001943.
41. Trofholz AC, Thao MS, Donley M, Smith M, Isaac H, Berge JM. Family meals then and now: a qualitative investigation of intergenerational transmission of family meal practices in a racially/ethnically diverse and immigrant population. Appetite. 2018;121:163–72. https://doi. org/10.1016/j.appet.2017.11.084.
42. Berge JM, Wall M, Hsueh T-F, Fulkerson JA, Larson N, Neumark-Sztainer D. The protective role of family meals for youth obesity: 10-year longitudinal associations. J Pediatr. 2015;166(2):296–301. https://doi.org/10.1016/j.jpeds.2014.08.030.
43. Martinez SM, Rhee K, Blanco E, Boutelle K. Maternal attitudes and behaviors regarding feeding practices in elementary school-aged Latino children: a pilot qualitative study on the impact of the cultural role of mothers in the US-Mexican border region of San Diego, California. J Acad Nutr Diet. 2015;115(5 Suppl):S34–41. https://doi.org/10.1016/j.jand.2015.02.028.
44. Portacio FG, Botero P, St. George SM, Stoutenberg M. Informing the adaptation and implementation of a lifestyle modification program in Hispanics: a qualitative study among low-income Hispanic adults. Hisp Health Care Int. 2018;16(4):204–12. https://doi. org/10.1177/1540415318808831.
45. Evans A, Chow S, Jennings R, Dave J, Scoblick K, Sterba KR, et al. Traditional foods and practices of Spanish-speaking Latina mothers influence the home food environment: implications for future interventions. J Am Diet Assoc. 2011;111(7):1031–8. https://doi.org/10.1016/j. jada.2011.04.007.
46. Sussner KM, Lindsay AC, Greaney ML, Peterson KE. The influence of immigrant status and acculturation on the development of overweight in Latino families: a qualitative study. J Immigr Minor Health. 2008;10(6):497–505. https://doi.org/10.1007/s10903-008-9137-3.
47. Diaz H, Marshak HH, Montgomery S, Rea B, Backman D. Acculturation and gender: influence on healthy dietary outcomes for Latino adolescents in California. J Nutr Educ Behav. 2009;41(5):319–26. https://doi.org/10.1016/j.jneb.2009.01.003.
48. Kittler PG, Sucher KP, Nelms M. Food and culture. 2011. https://books.google.com/books/ about/Food_and_Culture.html?id=R06H7WabJuMC. Accessed 20 Aug 2020.
49. National Cancer Institute. Physical activity and cancer. 2020. https://www.cancer.gov/about-cancer/causes-prevention/risk/obesity/physical-activity-fact-sheet. Accessed 24 Aug 2020.
50. Unger JB, Reynolds K, Shakib S, Spruijt-Metz D, Sun P, Johnson CA. Acculturation, physical activity, and fast-food consumption among Asian-American and Hispanic adolescents. J Community Health. 2004;29(6):467–81. https://doi.org/10.1007/s10900-004-3395-3.
51. Marquez DX, McAuley E. Gender and acculturation influences on physical activity in Latino adults. Ann Behav Med. 2006;31(2):138–44. https://doi.org/10.1207/s15324796abm3102_5.
52. Evenson KR, Sarmiento OL, Ayala GX. Acculturation and physical activity among North Carolina Latina immigrants. Soc Sci Med. 2004;59(12):2509–22. https://doi.org/10.1016/j. socscimed.2004.04.011.
53. Fisher L, Chesla CA, Skaff MM, Gilliss C, Mullan JT, Bartz RJ, et al. The family and disease management in Hispanic and European-American patients with type 2 diabetes. Diabetes Care. 2000;23(3):267–72. https://doi.org/10.2337/diacare.23.3.267.
54. Berrigan D, Dodd K, Troiano RP, Reeve BB, Ballard-Barbash R. Physical activity and acculturation among adult Hispanics in the United States. Res Q Exerc Sport. 2006;77(2):147–57. https://doi.org/10.1080/02701367.2006.10599349.

55. Falbe J, Cadiz AA, Tantoco NK, Thompson HR, Madsen KA. Active and healthy families: a randomized controlled trial of a culturally tailored obesity intervention for Latino children. Acad Pediatr. 2015;15(4):386–95. https://doi.org/10.1016/j.acap.2015.02.004.
56. Mendoza JA, Watson K, Baranowski T, Nicklas TA, Uscanga DK, Hanfling MJ. The walking school bus and children's physical activity: a pilot cluster randomized controlled trial. Pediatrics. 2011;128(3):e537–e44. https://doi.org/10.1542/peds.2010-3486.
57. Heelan KA, Abbey BM, Donnelly JE, Mayo MS, Welk GJ. Evaluation of a walking school bus for promoting physical activity in youth. J Phys Act Health. 2009;6(5):560–7. https://doi.org/10.1123/jpah.6.5.560.
58. Ayala GX, Ibarra L, Arredondo E, Horton L, Hernandez E, Parada H, et al. Promoting healthy eating by strengthening family relations: design and implementation of the *entre familia: feflejos de salud* intervention. In: Elk R, Landrine H, editors. Cancer disparities: causes and evidence-based solutions. New York: Springer; 2011. p. 237–52.
59. Horton LA, Ayala GX, Slymen DJ, Ibarra L, Hernandez E, Parada H, et al. A mediation analysis of mothers' dietary intake: the entre familia: *reflejos de salud* randomized controlled trial. Health Educ Behav. 2018;45(4):501–10. https://doi.org/10.1177/1090198117742439.
60. Arredondo EM, Haughton J, Ayala GX, Slymen DJ, Sallis JF, Burke K, et al. *Fe en accion*/faith in action: design and implementation of a church-based randomized trial to promote physical activity and cancer screening among churchgoing Latinas. Contemp Clin Trials. 2015;45(Pt B):404–15. https://doi.org/10.1016/j.cct.2015.09.008.
61. Ayala GX. Effects of a promotor-based intervention to promote physical activity: *Familias Sanas y Activas*. Am J Public Health. 2011;101(12):2261–8. https://doi.org/10.2105/ajph.2011.300273.
62. Arredondo EM, Elder JP, Haughton J, Slymen DJ, Sallis JF, Perez LG, et al. *Fe en acción*: promoting physical activity among churchgoing Latinas. Am J Public Health. 2017;107(7):1109–15. https://doi.org/10.2105/ajph.2017.303785.
63. Stokes EK, Zambrano LD, Anderson KN, Marder EP, Raz KM, Felix SEB, et al. Corona-virus disease 2019 case surveillance – United States, January 22-May 30, 2020. MMWR Morb Mortal Wkly Rep. 2020;69:759–65. https://doi.org/10.15585/mmwr.mm6924e2.
64. Quinnell K. Working people respond to the killing of George Floyd with nationwide protests. The American Federation of Labor and Congress of Industrial Organizations. 2020. https://aflcio.org/2020/6/2/working-people-respond-killing-george-floyd-nationwide-protests. Accessed 6 Sept 2020.

Open Access This chapter is licensed under the terms of the Creative Commons Attribution 4.0 International License (http://creativecommons.org/licenses/by/4.0/), which permits use, sharing, adaptation, distribution and reproduction in any medium or format, as long as you give appropriate credit to the original author(s) and the source, provide a link to the Creative Commons license and indicate if changes were made.

The images or other third party material in this chapter are included in the chapter's Creative Commons license, unless indicated otherwise in a credit line to the material. If material is not included in the chapter's Creative Commons license and your intended use is not permitted by statutory regulation or exceeds the permitted use, you will need to obtain permission directly from the copyright holder.

Part X
Advances in Cancer Therapy
and Clinical Trials

Chapter 16
Overcoming Clinical Research Disparities by Advancing Inclusive Research

Melissa Gonzales

Better Science and Better Medicine

To deliver the personalized medicine of tomorrow and advance better health outcomes for all, today's clinical research must reflect current demographic trends and include more underrepresented populations, including members of the Hispanic community. Currently, Hispanics are the youngest and largest minority group in the United States [1], yet they represent only 1–8% of patients enrolled in US clinical trials [2]. The lack of participation in clinical trial research, coupled with systemic factors such as higher unemployment rates [3] and higher likelihood to be uninsured [4], means that many Hispanic communities are being left behind and do not have equal opportunities to access investigational medicines and contribute to medical-scientific progress.

Throughout the COVID-19 pandemic, communities of color have experienced disproportionately negative outcomes compared to Whites. Data from the Centers for Disease Control and Prevention show that Hispanic and Black people are nearly three times as likely to become hospitalized by COVID-19 and are nearly twice as likely to die from the virus as non-Hispanic Whites [5]. Without significant participation in clinical research from underrepresented groups, it will be much more difficult to develop novel treatments and therapies that will be effective for all racial and ethnic backgrounds.

Improving health outcomes for our most vulnerable communities must be a coordinated effort among the healthcare industry, clinical researchers, academia, advocacy organizations, and policymakers. To make meaningful progress, the entire healthcare ecosystem needs to work together to reduce disparities in clinical research participation for underrepresented groups, improve patient access to

M. Gonzales (✉)
Genentech, San Francisco, CA, USA
e-mail: Sandoval.veronica@gene.com; mgonzales@adaptivebiotech.com

© The Author(s) 2023
A. G. Ramirez, E. J. Trapido (eds.), *Advancing the Science of Cancer in Latinos*, https://doi.org/10.1007/978-3-031-14436-3_16

clinical research, elevate patient-centric development, and enrich the quality of clinical information available in the development of personalized healthcare.

Advancing Inclusive Research

Genentech is deeply committed to addressing health disparities and believes all patients should have access to the best care and treatment available. As a founder of the biotech industry, Genentech envisions a world where all individuals can experience the full potential for their health and well-being while enabling a future of science that is more diverse, inclusive, and equitable.

To deliver on this vision, Genentech developed Advancing Inclusive Research, a US-focused and cross-organizational initiative to ensure clinical trial participants are representative of broader patient populations so that everyone with serious and life-threatening diseases has the opportunity to benefit from investigational medicines and enrich understanding of clinical and genomic data to inform science and personalized healthcare. As a Latina who is passionate about addressing cancer disparities impacting my community, my family, and future generations of Latinos, Advancing Inclusive Research is more to me than just an initiative. It is a moral obligation and a scientific imperative.

Insights into Action

Advancing Inclusive Research is grounded by three strategic pillars. First and foremost, Genentech's clinical development strategy is to expand inclusion of diverse patient populations. Second, we aim to generate insights from meaningful data. Third, we are committed to working with others and positioning Genentech and Roche as a trusted external partner.

Clinical Trial Strategy and Operations

Over the last 2 years, Genentech has reevaluated its clinical development strategy to determine how we could enable more clinical research participation. We began by selecting specific disease areas to pilot research based on needs in the respective therapeutic areas, the presence of known disparities, and where we believed we could have the greatest impact. While still in the early phases of these learnings, best practices will be applied to additional therapeutic areas.

Our clinical development strategy has also led to internal structural changes across the company, including a Chief Diversity Office and a health equity population and science team to elevate awareness across all internal clinical study teams in early- and late-stage development. We are educating clinical study teams on inclusive research principles, with the goal of reflecting real-world populations in Genentech's clinical trial enrollment.

Additionally, we are expanding our site networks to include some smaller, newer sites with more diverse catchment areas. As part of this process, we are asking clinical trial site investigators and research staff to be deliberate about recruiting diverse patients and to help us identify barriers to participation so that we can support needed services such as transportation and child care during clinical trial appointments. We are currently working to implement a technology in all possible trials that would enable real-time and automated payments to patients in order to cover their out-of-pocket expenses.

Through these collective efforts, we are now poised to deliver clinical trials across our pipeline portfolio that imbed inclusive research principles, as well as innovative new studies that address health disparities specifically in communities of color.

Scientific Insights and Personalized Healthcare

The concept of personalized healthcare is evolving into more individualized care. Today's model of care delivery is still grounded in the idea of evaluating one patient segment, identifying one biomarker, and developing one treatment or therapy. The paradigm of the future will be built around a single patient and creating a comprehensive profile of that person to deliver truly individualized care. Two key components that we plan to implement are leveraging key partnerships and identifying strategies to address the lack of diversity in genomic material available to scientific researchers.

To bring us closer to this reality, we aim to leverage Roche's unique partnerships with Foundation Medicine (FMI) and Flatiron to provide data insights that can help us answer scientific questions, aid with trial recruitment, and engage diverse communities to improve access to diagnostics and treatment.

Through genomic research, we can begin to identify those molecular drivers that can predict disease susceptibility, efficacy, or safety differences in response to treatments in specific patient populations. For example, a 2014 genomic study of Latina women led to the discovery of a novel variant with protective effects that lowers the risk of breast cancer (for those with more Indigenous American ancestry) [6].

We realize that the benefits of genomic testing and genomic research will require education and building trust with communities of color. We aim to continue to identify trusted partners within the community to engage patients on these complex topics.

External Partnerships

To move the inclusive research discussion from theory to an actionable path forward, Genentech formed an interdisciplinary council focused solely on addressing disparities in clinical research. Founded in 2018, Genentech's External Council on Advancing Inclusive Research has been instrumental in helping to develop strategies to address disparities in research. The group is composed of physician thought leaders, academic researchers, specialty CRO executives, and patient advocates with expertise in oncology, ophthalmology, and neuroscience clinical care, research, and genomics. As subject matter experts who are uniquely positioned to affect strategy, execution, and healthcare policies, they bring valuable insight from their collaborations with patient organizations, data-driven firms, research centers, regulators, and other stakeholders.

Key outcomes informed by Genentech's External Council on Advancing Inclusive Research include the following:

- Development of an internal guidance document for study teams
- Revision of contract language to encourage inclusion of underrepresented patients
- Update of inclusion/exclusion criteria to be more inclusive of patients with diverse ethnicity

These efforts have been instrumental in implementing changes across our clinical development teams.

Patient and Advocacy Communities Patient engagement has and continues to be a critical factor in the success of Advancing Inclusive Research. Genentech has a long history of partnering with patients and advocacy groups across oncology, ophthalmology, neurology, and PHC, in the United States and globally. Genentech's work with patient advocacy groups helps to build trust in the healthcare ecosystem, and it deepens the company's understanding of a patient's journey.

Policymakers and Regulatory Agencies Advancing Inclusive Research also relies on collaboration with policymakers and regulatory agencies. Genentech is an active participant in key discussions around policies that address obstacles that have previously prevented communities of color from participating in clinical research, such as out-of-pocket costs.

Conclusion

Our goal at Genentech is for all people to achieve a future of personalized healthcare. In order to deliver on the promise of precision medicine, we must provide the right treatment, to the right patient, at the right time.

Reflecting on the emergence of COVID-19, we see the entire industry working together to quickly innovate and develop the best possible treatments. We know that measurable progress is possible. Now imagine what is possible, if we, the trailblazers of biotech, patient advocacy, and medicine, bring that same mindset and urgency to addressing the systemic barriers that prevent Hispanic patients from clinical research participation. Imagine a world where the most vulnerable receive optimal care and enjoy better health outcomes. It is good for them. It is good for us. It is good for society at large.

Much has been accomplished over the years, and yet there is much more to do for our communities of color. To fully realize our vision—personalized healthcare for everyone—we must innovate frequently, collaborate often, and challenge outdated ideas until all people, including Latinos, help to make the promise of precision medicine a reality.

References

1. Vespa J, Armstrong DM, Medina L. Demographic turning points for the United States: population projections for 2020 to 2060. Current population reports. Washington, DC: U.S. Census Bureau; 2018. p. 25–1144.
2. Fisher JA, Kilbaugh CA. Challenging assumptions about minority participation in U.S. clinical research. Am J Public Health. 2011;101(12):2217–22.
3. US Bureau of Labor Statistics. Labor force statistics from the current population survey. https://www.bls.gov/web/empsit/cpsee_e16.htm. Accessed 7 Aug 2020.
4. Artiga S, Orgera K, Damico A. Changes in health coverage by race and ethnicity since the ACA, 2010–2018. KFF. https://www.kff.org/disparities-policy/issue-brief/changes-in-health-coverage-by-race-and-ethnicity-since-the-aca-2010-2018/. Accessed 21 July 2020.
5. Centers for Disease Control and Prevention. Covid-19 hospitalization and death by race/ethnicity. https://www.cdc.gov/coronavirus/2019-ncov/covid-data/investigations-discovery/hospitalization-death-by-race-ethnicity.html. Accessed 25 Feb 2021.
6. Fejerman L, Ahmadiyeh N, Hu D, Huntsman S, Beckman KB, Caswell JL, et al. Genome-wide association study of breast cancer in Latinas identifies novel protective variants on 6q25. Nat Commun. 2014;5:5260. https://doi.org/10.1038/ncomms6260. PMID: 25327703.

Open Access   This chapter is licensed under the terms of the Creative Commons Attribution 4.0 International License (http://creativecommons.org/licenses/by/4.0/), which permits use, sharing, adaptation, distribution and reproduction in any medium or format, as long as you give appropriate credit to the original author(s) and the source, provide a link to the Creative Commons license and indicate if changes were made.

The images or other third party material in this chapter are included in the chapter's Creative Commons license, unless indicated otherwise in a credit line to the material. If material is not included in the chapter's Creative Commons license and your intended use is not permitted by statutory regulation or exceeds the permitted use, you will need to obtain permission directly from the copyright holder.

Part XI
HPV Vaccination for Cancer Prevention

Chapter 17
The Road to Cervical Cancer Elimination

Anna R. Giuliano

Introduction

An estimated 34,800 cancers in the United States were caused by HPV between 2012 and 2016. Among those cancers (cervical, vulvar, vaginal, anal, oropharyngeal, and penile), the overwhelming majority can be prevented with vaccination and cervical cancer screening and treatment. While the incidence of cervical cancer has significantly declined in all populations in the United States since 1975, Hispanic women continue to have significantly higher rates of cervical cancer than non-Hispanic White and Black women.

A large community internationally has acknowledged for some time that we have the tools to prevent cervical cancer, but what is needed is to make elimination of cervical cancer an agenda. Between 2014 and 2018, two fortuitous events occurred—FDA approval of the vaccine Gardasil 9 and a strategic initiative from the World Health Organization (WHO). In 2018, the newly elected WHO Director-General (DG) announced a call to action to eliminate cervical cancer worldwide, which was critical in defining a path forward and engaging with partners and member states to overcome challenges and scale-up cost-effective interventions. The WHO DG recognized that several countries and UN agencies had already moved forward under the UN Global Joint Programme on Cervical Cancer Prevention and Control; however, to succeed, our partnerships must be expanded to include everyone who can help us reach our goal. In addition to reaching out to new partners, a key message of this call to action was that this work should be carried out in a more coordinated manner globally to accelerate progress in eliminating cervical cancer.

A. R. Giuliano (✉)
Center for Immunization and Infection Research in Cancer, Moffit Cancer Center, Tampa, FL, USA
e-mail: anna.giuliano@moffitt.org

© The Author(s) 2023
A. G. Ramirez, E. J. Trapido (eds.), *Advancing the Science of Cancer in Latinos*, https://doi.org/10.1007/978-3-031-14436-3_17

Cervical Cancer Elimination

It is possible to make cervical cancer and other HPV-related cancers a thing of the past, but we need more research. There are still knowledge gaps to be filled; and for Hispanic populations, this is especially true with cervical cancer. However, we already have the tools to make cervical cancer elimination a reality. The national strategy for eliminating cervical cancer is like the legs of a three-legged stool—vaccine (e.g., Gardasil and Gardasil 9), cervical cancer screening, and treatment. Why are there still high cervical cancer incidence rates in the Hispanic population? One answer may be that treatment, the third leg of the stool, tends to be left off of our national goals. The message is that we should screen 93% of women for cervical cancer, but what is not conveyed is to ensure that those who are diagnosed with precancerous lesions are actually treated.

Disease Control, Elimination, and Eradication: A Continuum

Disease reduction can be thought of as a continuum from control to elimination to eradication, and it is important in our communications that we use these terms correctly [1, 2].

- *Control* is a reduction in incidence, prevalence, morbidity, or mortality to a locally acceptable level.
- *Elimination of disease* is a reduction to zero in incidence in a defined geographical area as a result of deliberate efforts (e.g., measles in the Americas). *Elimination of infection* caused by a specific agent is a reduction to zero in a defined geographical area as a result of deliberate efforts (e.g., Chagas). *Elimination of a public health problem* is a reduction to low disease incidence, but not zero; this term should only be used if clear target definitions are commonly agreed upon (e.g., neonatal tetanus).
- Note that disease control and elimination both require continued intervention measures.
- *Eradication* is a permanent reduction to zero of the worldwide incidence of infection (e.g., smallpox); it no longer requires intervention measures. For example, we no longer continue to vaccinate for smallpox because the virus has been successfully eradicated.

So, our first goal is to eliminate cervical cancer (not eradicate); we will likely have to continue the interventions of the three-legged stool for quite some time, eliminating cervical cancer one geographic region at a time. When we eliminate cervical cancer worldwide, it will then finally be eradicated.

A World Without Cervical Cancer

The World Health Organization has a vision of a world without cervical cancer, and though their strategy to eliminate the disease is slightly different from the United States (Healthy People 2020), the components of the strategies are very similar. The WHO threshold for elimination of cervical cancer is an incidence of less than four cases per 100,000 women-years—something that is achievable for the United States. The 2030 control targets for WHO are: 90% of girls fully vaccinated against HPV by the age of 15; 70% of women screened with a high precision test at age 35 and 45; and 90% of women identified with cervical disease receive treatment and care.

The Pan American Health Organization (PAHO), the health agency for the Americas, also has a strategy for eliminating cervical cancer which predates the WHO call to action. PAHO has a strong history of eliminating immune vaccine preventable diseases; the region under their purview was the first to eliminate smallpox and polio. All of the elements are in place for them to also be the first region in the world to eliminate cervical cancer, and it is imperative that Hispanics in the United States benefit from these interventions. The PAHO plan of action for cervical cancer prevention and control aims to reduce the number of new cases and deaths from cervical cancer 30% by 2030. Their four strategic lines of action include program organization; primary prevention (vaccination); screening and treatment; and access to services.

Evidence for Achievability

Is the WHO threshold of elimination of cervical cancer achievable? To answer this question, an international team of researchers used comparative modelling to project how long it would take to eliminate cervical cancer in the United States [3]. One simulation model under status quo assumptions for vaccination and screening predicted that reaching the WHO incidence threshold of less than four cases per 100,000 women-years could be achieved by 2038 [3]. In another scenario with the assumption of screening, scale-up to 90% predicts cervical cancer elimination by 2028. Interestingly, a third scenario with the assumption of 90% vaccination coverage predicted cervical cancer elimination at about the same time as the status quo scenario. So, this suggests that the most effective intervention and fastest way for the United States to achieve the goal of cervical cancer elimination is to scale up screening and treatment, especially focusing on the underscreened and undertreated [3].

Real-World Evidence for the Effectiveness of the HPV Vaccine

What is the evidence that the vaccine will work? While the HPV vaccine is only one part of the three-legged stool, when it is added to screening and treatment, it reduces infection in the population. In sequence over time, this reduction in infection is followed by a reduction in genital warts, reduction in cervical intraepithelial neoplasia (CIN), and there is evidence that after some decades there is also a reduction in cervical cancer.

Reduction in Infection There is evidence from multiple countries to support a reduction in HPV infection after the vaccine is rolled out into public health practice. One study comparing HPV prevalence among Australian women aged 18–24 pre- and post-vaccination found a large reduction in the four types of HPV that Gardasil protects against. The prevalence was 22.7% (n = 88) pre-vaccination in the years 2005–2007; and the post-vaccination prevalence dropped to 7.3% (n = 688) from 2010 to 2012 and to 1.5% (n = 200) in 2015 [4].

Reduction in Genital Warts In the United States, even with a relatively low vaccine dissemination, there are significant reductions in genital wart incidence, pointing to the potential benefits in public health. Flagg and Torrone observed decreases in the prevalence of genital warts in young women likely to be affected by HPV several years after licensure of the HPV vaccine [5]. For example, in 2009 when only 27% of woman were vaccinated, the prevalence of genital warts in women aged 20–24 was 5.5 per thousand person-years; in 2009 when about 40% of women were vaccinated, the prevalence had decreased to 2.7 [5].

Reduction in CIN 2 Similar to the incidence pattern for genital warts, CIN 2 incidence has declined in the United States despite the low dissemination of vaccine. To evaluate the impact of HPV vaccination on the reduction of cervical precancers, McClung et al. examined archived specimens from women aged 18–39 with CIN 2+. They found that between the years 2008 and 2014, the proportion of CIN 2+ cases decreased from 51.0% to 47.3% (P = 0.03) among unvaccinated women and decreased 55.2–33.3% (P < 0.0001) among vaccinated women (n = 1065). The authors concluded that the greater decline in CIN 2+ among vaccinated women provides support for the effectiveness of vaccine and the smaller decline among unvaccinated women may be the result of herd protection [6].

Reduction in Cervical Cancer Population-based national cancer registry data from the United States show that cervical cancer declined throughout the time period 1999–2015 among all age groups and that the incidence rates declined to <1/100,000 in the youngest age cohorts [Cervical cancer incidence trends by age. There were <6 cases for the group aged 15–20 in 2015, so trends were calculated by combining the last 2 years of data for this age group (2013–2014)] (unpublished graph from Mona Saraiya, MD, MPH; CDC). The total number of cases during this period was 54,770; approximately 1% of cases were among females aged 15–20.

Greatest rate declines were among females aged <21 years who were most likely to be affected by the relatively recent introduction of the HPV vaccine; among females aged 15–20 years, cervical cancer rate decreased 6.6% per year during 1999–2014. Over time, as vaccination continues and more data are collected, the expectation is that there will be a spread with significant reductions in each of the successive birth cohorts (21–24; 25–29; 30–34; 35–39 years).

A large study in Sweden demonstrated that the HPV quadrivalent vaccine is not only efficacious and effective against HPV infection, genital warts, and high-grade cervical lesions, but is also associated with a major reduction in the incidence of cervical cancer. Using nationwide registry data from 2006 to 2017, the Swedish study followed an open population of girls and women 10–30 years of age ($n = 1,145,112$ unvaccinated; $527,871$ vaccinated). The age-adjusted incidence rate ratio comparing the vaccinated population with the unvaccinated was .51 (95%CI, 0.32–0.82). Interestingly, the authors found the greatest risk reduction (88% lower than unvaccinated women) occurred among those who were vaccinated before 17 years of age [7].

Reduction in Oral HPV Finally, there is evidence that oral HPV infection is also declining as a consequence of vaccination. One study in the United Kingdom examined the effect of HPV vaccination on the prevalence of oropharyngeal HPV-16 infection among girls and young adult women and compared infection levels with those in unvaccinated young males of similar age [8]. They found that the UK female-only vaccination program was associated with a significantly lower oral HPV-16 prevalence among vaccinated females compared to unvaccinated females (0.5% vs. 5.6%, $P = .04$). The HPV prevalence in unvaccinated males was similar to vaccinated females, and the authors proposed that vaccination of females may confer benefits of herd immunity to unvaccinated males of the same age.

Cervical Cancer Elimination Among Hispanics in the United States

The good news is that the incidence of cervical cancer has been declining in all populations over time; the bad news is that Hispanics consistently have a higher incidence of cervical cancer and their gains may not have been as great [9].

Age at Diagnosis

Examination of cervical cancer incidence by age group points to the populations that should be targeted the most for screening and treatment. For all races and for non-Hispanic whites, peak incidences occur in the 40s and then start to decline, but for African Americans and Hispanics, the incidence continues to increase with increasing age [9]. This disparity probably reflects poor utilization of health services; once women are in the post-reproductive age group, they may not be accessing screening as much, or they are accessing screening but failing to get needed treatment. More study and research are needed.

Vaccine Uptake

The Healthy People 2020 goal is for 80% of adolescents aged 13–15 to receive the full recommended dose of HPV vaccine. Unlike the disparities experienced by Hispanics in screening, treatment, and access to health care, vaccination uptake is as high or higher for Hispanic populations than for other populations. In 2018, 75.5% of Hispanic females and males aged 13–17 had received ≥1 dose and 56.6% were up to date, an uptake rate higher than non-Hispanic White (47.8%) and Black (53.3%) adolescents [10]. However, Hispanics who are older than adolescents have a lower rate of uptake than other populations [11].

Pap Smear Screening

Based on national data, the Hispanic population has lower rates of Pap smear screening; however, there is no national measurement of the percentage of women who are diagnosed with an abnormal smear who are Hispanic and who have not received adequate medical treatment. This issue requires more research, especially if the rate of Pap smear screening is actually going down for Hispanic women. If the goal is to achieve cervical cancer elimination, we must be promoting the three-legged stool—vaccination, screening, and timely and appropriate treatment for any abnormal dysplasia that requires treatment.

Progress to Date

There is a movement here in the United States. We worked closely with several of the large cancer centers to get all 70 NCI-designated cancer centers to sign on to the goal of eliminating HPV-related cancers. This was followed in 2019 with a congressional briefing and in 2021 with a congressional filing of the Prevent HPV Cancers Act. Filed by US Representative, Kathy Castor (FL 14), this act is intended to help bolster both the CDC and the NCI's effort to actually achieve elimination of HPV-related cancers. The current US incidence rate is 8/100,000; not too far down the road, we could meet the WHO goal of 4/100,000 by 2030 if we accelerate our interventions. If we continue those efforts, we can probably go further to true elimination of HPV-related cancer, which is an incidence rate of less than 1/100,000.

Conflict of Interest Disclosure   Dr. Giuliano reported receiving grants from Merck & Co, Inc., Kenilworth, NJ, USA. She is also a member of the v503 scientific advisory board for Merck & Co, Inc.; the Global Advisory Board for Merck & Co, Inc.; and the Advisory Board for Immunomic Therapeutics.

References

 1. Dowdle WR. The principles of disease elimination and eradication. Bull World Health Organ. 1998;76(Suppl 2):22–5.
 2. Heymann DL. Control, elimination, eradication and re-emergence of infectious diseases: getting the message right. Bull World Health Organ. 2006;84(2):82. https://doi.org/10.2471/blt.05.029512.
 3. Burger EA, Smith MA, Killen J, Sy S, Simms KT, Canfell K, et al. Projected time to elimination of cervical cancer in the USA: a comparative modelling study. Lancet Public Health. 2020;5(4):e213–e22. https://doi.org/10.1016/S2468-2667(20)30006-2.
 4. Machalek DA, Garland SM, Brotherton JML, Bateson D, McNamee K, Stewart M, et al. Very low prevalence of vaccine human papillomavirus types among 18- to 35-year old Australian women 9 years following implementation of vaccination. J Infect Dis. 2018;217(10):1590–600. https://doi.org/10.1093/infdis/jiy075.
 5. Flagg EW, Torrone EA. Declines in anogenital warts among age groups most likely to be impacted by human papillomavirus vaccination, United States, 2006–2014. Am J Public Health. 2018;108(1):112–9. https://doi.org/10.2105/ajph.2017.304119.
 6. McClung NM, Gargano JW, Bennett NM, Niccolai LM, Abdullah N, Griffin MR, et al. Trends in human papillomavirus vaccine types 16 and 18 in cervical precancers, 2008–2014. Cancer Epidemiol Biomarkers Prev. 2019;28(3):602–9. https://doi.org/10.1158/1055-9965. Epi-18-0885.
 7. Lei J, Ploner A, Elfström KM, Wang J, Roth A, Fang F, et al. HPV vaccination and the risk of invasive cervical cancer. N Engl J Med. 2020;383(14):1340–8. https://doi.org/10.1056/NEJMoa1917338.
 8. Mehanna H, Bryant TS, Babrah J, Louie K, Bryant JL, Spruce RJ, et al. Human papillomavirus (HPV) vaccine effectiveness and potential herd immunity for reducing oncogenic oropharyngeal HPV-16 prevalence in the United Kingdom: a cross-sectional study. Clin Infect Dis. 2019;69(8):1296–302. https://doi.org/10.1093/cid/ciy1081.
 9. Howlader N, Noone AM, Krapcho M, Miller D, Brest A, Yu M, et al., editors. SEER cancer statistics review, 1975–2016. Bethesda: National Cancer Institute. https://seer.cancer.gov/csr/1975_2016/, based on November 2018 SEER data submission, posted to the SEER web site, April 2019.
10. US Department of Health and Human Services (DHHS). National Center for Immunization and Respiratory Diseases. The 2018 national immunization survey – teen. Atlanta: Centers for Disease Control and Prevention; 2020.
11. Boersma P, Black LI. Human papillomavirus vaccination among adults aged 18–26, 2013–2018. NCHS Data Brief, no 354. Hyattsville: National Center for Health Statistics; 2020.

Open Access   This chapter is licensed under the terms of the Creative Commons Attribution 4.0 International License (http://creativecommons.org/licenses/by/4.0/), which permits use, sharing, adaptation, distribution and reproduction in any medium or format, as long as you give appropriate credit to the original author(s) and the source, provide a link to the Creative Commons license and indicate if changes were made.

The images or other third party material in this chapter are included in the chapter's Creative Commons license, unless indicated otherwise in a credit line to the material. If material is not included in the chapter's Creative Commons license and your intended use is not permitted by statutory regulation or exceeds the permitted use, you will need to obtain permission directly from the copyright holder.

Part XII
Latino Cancer Health Disparities: Moving Forward

Chapter 18
Looking Forward: Continuing Collaboration for Action

Amelie G. Ramirez and Edward J. Trapido

Introduction

The second ASCL conference was held in February 2020, about 1 month after the first case of coronavirus disease 2019 (COVID-19) was documented in the United States and before evidence of community spread. Since then, COVID-19 has become a global pandemic that has disproportionately infected, hospitalized, and killed ethnic and racial minorities in the United States [1–4]. According to a report of provisional life expectancy estimates from the National Center for Health Statistics, the life expectancy for US Hispanics decreased 3 years (81.8–78.8) between 2019 and 2020. As a result, the life expectancy advantage held by Hispanics over non-Hispanic whites narrowed by 60%, suggesting poorer health and mortality outcomes for the US Hispanic population. It is estimated that 90% of this decline in the life expectancy gap is the result of mortality caused by COVID-19 [5]. Some speculate that this disease disparity exists because Hispanics and other underrepresented groups receive the greatest exposure to the virus. They are more likely to live in densely populated areas and multigenerational households; use public transportation; and have essential public-facing jobs in the service and healthcare sectors, where working from home is not an option [4, 6, 7]. If infected, they are also more likely to experience severe symptoms of COVID-19 because of comorbidities such as diabetes, obesity, cardiovascular disease, asthma, and other chronic conditions [6].

The pandemic's disproportionate burden of disease on Hispanics and other vulnerable populations highlights health inequities in the United States, including

A. G. Ramirez (✉)
Department of Population Health Sciences, Institute for Health Promotion Research,
UT Health San Antonio, San Antonio, TX, USA
e-mail: ramirezag@uthscsa.edu

E. J. Trapido
Epidemiology Program, LSU Health Sciences Center, School of Public Health,
New Orleans, LA, USA

© The Author(s) 2023
A. G. Ramirez, E. J. Trapido (eds.), *Advancing the Science of Cancer in Latinos*, https://doi.org/10.1007/978-3-031-14436-3_18

cancer disparities. Worrisome effects of the pandemic have been delays along the cancer care continuum and increased barriers to healthcare access, which exacerbate disparities already experienced by Hispanics and other racial/ethnic groups. Early in the pandemic, the healthcare system was mobilized to care for the surge of COVID-19 patients and to prevent further spread of the disease. Non-urgent healthcare, including elective surgeries, preventive care, and cancer screening were postponed, and it is feared that delays in cancer screening will result in later-stage diagnosis and poorer outcome down the road [4]. Further, cancer patients already in treatment may have experienced less than optimal treatment because of delays in cancer surgery, chemotherapy, and radiation therapy [4, 7, 8].

Hispanic and other disparity populations are likely to experience additional pandemic-related delays in cancer screening, diagnosis, and treatment because of inequities in social determinants that create barriers to healthcare access. For example, the COVID-19 pandemic has caused economic hardship through the loss of employment and employer-based health insurance, leaving many under- and uninsured. The resulting lack of insurance and increased poverty may lead some to delay or forgo cancer care to pay for food or housing [4, 6, 7]. Secondly, health providers have turned to virtual care through telemedicine to minimize exposure to coronavirus; however, ethnic and racial barriers to the access of telemedicine put vulnerable disparity populations at risk of receiving interrupted care or of being lost to follow-up [4, 7, 9, 10]. A recent multicenter, prospective cohort study examined the effects of COVID-19 on the delivery of cancer care. While they found no significant changes in in-person visits by ethnicity or race, they found Hispanic (aOR 0.71; 95% CI, 0.51–0.98) and non-Hispanic black (aOR 0.69; 95% CI, 0.50–0.94) patients were less likely than other groups to use telemedicine during the pandemic [9]. Further, they found that Hispanic patients were more likely to experience treatment delays (aOR 1.53; 95% CI, 1.03–2.26) than non-Hispanic white patients.

The COVID-19 pandemic has worsened existing cancer disparities, so advancing the science of cancer in Latinos is now a tougher challenge. Going forward, how can we mitigate the detrimental effects of COVID-19 on cancer care? The most urgent needs are to address near-term consequences of the pandemic, such as postponements in screening and subsequent delays in diagnosis; delays and interruptions in treatment; loss to follow-up; financial hardship from job and insurance loss; and increased barriers to healthcare access. This will require redoubling outreach efforts and bolstering pre-pandemic community infrastructure and relationships, encouraging their continued partnerships with health providers, researchers, and healthcare systems (Chap. 15: Torrez-Ruiz et al.). While the pandemic's mid- and long-term consequences on Latino cancer disparities are still unknown, future research should document and evaluate these changes as they unfold [11]. The next ASCL conference in 2022 will provide an opportunity for collaboration and identification of new research opportunities to address Latino cancer disparities in the face of the COVID-19 pandemic and beyond.

Vulnerable Populations and Health Threats in the Latino Community

One aim of the ASCL conference was to identify opportunities for future research that will advance the science of cancer in Latinos. The authors made recommendations in their papers that are excerpted and offered as a resource in this and the following two sections.

- *Investigate the adverse effects of treatment for acute lymphoblastic leukemia (ALL) in Latino children.* CNS-directed ALL therapy causes acute and subacute neurotoxicity and may cause long-term neurocognitive impairment, profoundly affecting quality of life in survivors. Latino pediatric patients with ALL experience these neurotoxic events at a rate far exceeding their non-Latino counterparts, and yet current research on neurotoxicity of pediatric ALL therapy largely neglects Latino populations. There is a need for well-designed studies that account for factors linked to disparities in cognitive performance, such as SES, acculturation, inherited genetic variation, clinical characteristics, and sociocultural differences. The association between local Native American genetic ancestry and neurotoxic effects of methotrexate should be examined, and novel approaches such as admixture mapping could identify susceptibility loci responsible for ethnic disparities in the risk of neurotoxic effects of CNS-directed therapy. (Chap. 4: Brown et al.)
- *Revise the Patient Protection and Affordable Care Act (ACA) to be more inclusive of vulnerable Latino subgroups.* The ACA has improved insurance coverage and primary healthcare access and utilization across all racial and ethnic groups in the United States. Disparities remain, however, especially for Latinos in states that have not expanded Medicaid; for Mexican and Central American subgroups; and for non-citizen and undocumented immigrants. Revisions in implementing the ACA must address these disparities and include non-citizens who have been in the country for less than 5 years and undocumented immigrants (Chap. 3: Ortega).
- *Implement food insecurity screening and prevention programs in community oncology practice.* Cancer-related financial hardship and food insecurity disproportionately affects Hispanic cancer survivors, and thus there is a need for food insecurity screening and prevention programs in community oncology practice. Strategies to address food insecurity will benefit from community-based approaches that seek to understand the lived experience of food insecurity in Hispanic households. The strong relationship between food insecurity and access to cancer care points to the need for further research to address this social determinant of health and to achieve health equity (Chap. 11: McDougall et al.).

Disparities Research Along the Cancer Control Continuum

Cancer Prevention and Screening

- *Develop behavioral cancer interventions that capitalize on the strengths of Latinx culture.* US Latinos overall have a lower cancer burden than other groups; however, as Latinos become acculturated to the United States, their health behavior changes and their risk for cancer rises. Studying the cultural and behavioral patterns of recent immigrants may help identify protective behavioral practices and explain the better-than-expected health outcomes in this community. The negative change in cancer risk associated with acculturation might be mitigated by promoting healthy protective behaviors through culturally appropriate interventions that leverage aspects of Latino culture, such as collectivism, *personalismo*, and *familismo*. Research studies should integrate cultural beliefs and values to increase relevancy for Latino participants and contribute to compliance and long-term participation for improved population health (Chap. 15: Torrez-Ruiz et al.).

- *To eliminate cervical cancer, promote three existing and effective tools—HPV vaccination, Pap smear screening, and timely treatment for abnormal cervical dysplasia.* Most cancers caused by HPV (cervical, vulvar, vaginal, anal, oropharyngeal, and penile) can be prevented with these three existing tools. Even though cervical cancer incidence has declined in the United States since 1975, Hispanic women continue to have significantly higher rates of cervical cancer than non-Hispanic white and black women. The fastest way to achieve the goal of cervical cancer elimination is to screen at least 93% of age-eligible women. Only 80% now follow this recommendation, with lower percentages among Hispanic women (70–78%). Health providers must deliver strong and linguistically/culturally relevant recommendations for both HPV vaccination and cancer screening and ensure that those who are diagnosed with precancerous lesions are actually treated (Chap. 17: Giuliano).

Cancer Treatment

- *Identify and assess determinants of delays in breast cancer treatment among ethnic and racial populations.* Breast cancer incidence among Hispanic women is lower than non-Hispanic white women, but Hispanic women are more likely to be diagnosed with more aggressive disease and to experience treatment delays that contribute to worse outcome. Disparities in social determinants contribute to this outcome disparity; therefore, to improve cancer care delivery and long-term breast cancer outcomes, we must expand culturally effective health education programs and social assistance alongside research of biological differences in Hispanic tumor characteristics. Future research should focus on expanding breast cancer patient narratives to enrich qualitative understanding of treatment delays among racial and ethnic populations to develop a culturally effective framework for reducing health disparities (Chap. 6: Malinowski and Chavez Mac Gregor).

Genetic Ancestry and Precision Medicine Approaches

* *Improve understanding of subtype-specific breast cancer risk in admixed minority populations.* Hispanic women have a higher risk than non-Hispanic white women of developing ER–/PR– HER2+ and ER–/PR– HER2– breast cancer—intrinsic subtypes that have fewer treatment options and poorer prognosis than others. Research suggests there are associations between degree of Indigenous American ancestry and HER2+ tumors and between degree of African Ancestry and ER– tumors. Only a few breast cancer studies have analyzed the correlation between individual genetic ancestry proportion and tumor subtype in Hispanics. Thus, further studies are needed to find more precise tumor subtype-specific risk assessment, treatment efficacy, and outcome prognosis in US Hispanics/Latinas and Latin American women (Chap. 7: Tamayo et al.).
* *Develop novel risk-stratification strategies and targeted therapies for lung cancer that consider genetic admixture and health disparities among Latin(x) populations.* Genetic admixture creates a broad spectrum of lung cancer susceptibility among Latin(x) subgroups, and a large component of African ancestry is associated with worse clinical outcome. Targeted approaches must consider these differences in susceptibility to increase the number of lung cancer patients who may benefit from precision therapies. Lung cancer in all racial/ethnic groups is often diagnosed too late for curative surgical intervention; thus, there is a need for precise identification of individuals who are at risk for lung malignancy, such as those with chronic obstructive pulmonary disease. Development of non-invasive, early biomarkers of lung cancer is also needed, as is research to uncover molecular pathways of malignant conversion that can be targeted for therapeutic intervention (Chap. 8: Ramos, Guerra, and El-Zein).

Outcomes and Survivorship

* *Investigate how genetic ancestry,* **obesity** *phenotypes, and related comorbidities affect aggressive breast cancer presentation, treatment, and survivorship by race/ethnicity.* Hispanics are a genetically admixed population with European, Indigenous American, and African ancestry, and there is a need to collect data on Hispanic breast cancer survivors to determine if the way breast cancer affects patient-reported outcomes and prognosis differs by Hispanic subgroup. Among Hispanic and black populations, genetic ancestry has been correlated with adiposity and obesity-related physiologic measurements (e.g., BMI and waist-to-hip

ratio) and comorbidities (e.g., diabetes and hypertension). Hispanic breast cancer survivors are a growing and vulnerable population; to address their needs, we must have a better understanding of the complex interactions between race/ethnicity, culture, and ancestry (Chap. 14: Bandera, Hong and Qin).

- *Address the unique supportive-care needs of Hispanic men cancer survivors.* Hispanic men not only experience disproportionate cancer disparities, but they also have unique supportive care needs as cancer survivors. To reduce their illness burden, researchers should develop culturally competent care delivery; transcreate existing interventions that engage and meet psychosocial needs; and disseminate research findings to the Latino community, providing health information to survivors and their families. Further, new interventions should build on the strengths of the Latino community and help survivors connect with one another, relieving the burden of isolation frequently experienced by this population (Chap. 5: Martinez Tyson and Ruiz).

- *Develop and assess e-health interventions tailored for Hispanic breast cancer survivors.* Hispanic breast cancer survivors experience worse health-related quality of life (HRQOL) and symptom burden than non-Hispanics, and their highest expressed unmet needs exist in the psychosocial domain. E-health interventions such as smartphone applications can deliver accessible, culturally tailored psychosocial interventions that may improve patient engagement and patient-reported outcomes. Future studies should include a social networking component to fulfill the desire for social support and should integrate evidence-based, patient-centered tools into electronic health records. Given the multiple components of psychosocial interventions, the effect of each component should be separately evaluated to identify the most effective elements on study outcomes (Chap. 13: Baik et al.).

Cross-Cutting Research and the Future of Cancer Care

- *Engage the Latino community in cancer research.* The lack of Latinos and other racial/ethnic groups in clinical trials hinders the development of precision medicine that can benefit these vulnerable populations. There is thus a need to optimize Latino participation in research so that researchers can develop tailored therapeutics and deliver more effective public health educational interventions. One recommendation is to use community-based participatory research approaches in designing studies to optimize Latino participation and retention. Recommended communication strategies are to: (1) transfer knowledge to the community in a timely way with messages designed for different levels of acculturation and language preference; (2) deliver information using preferred social media platforms, Spanish language TV, and radio; and (3) include traditional written formats and interpersonal communication, which work well in the Latino community. To engage stakeholders in responsive communication and consultation efforts, researchers can develop community advisory boards, patient advocates, and citizen scientists. They can also widen the net of partners by collaborating and developing coalitions with community opinion leaders (Chap. 9: Baezconde-Garbanati et al.).

- *Make clinical trials more inclusive to overcome research disparities.* Clinical research should reflect demography to capture differences among underrepresented populations, making personalized healthcare available to everyone. Hispanics are underrepresented in clinical trials, so many Hispanic communities do not have equal opportunities to access investigational medicines and contribute to medical progress. Strategic priorities for the biotechnology industry are to develop more inclusive practices, increasing the amount of genomic data and scientific insights from underrepresented populations. Improving health outcomes for vulnerable communities must be a coordinated effort; the entire healthcare ecosystem must work together to increase participation of underrepresented groups in clinical trials, improve patient access to clinical research, elevate patient-centric development, and enrich the quality of clinical information available in the development of personalized healthcare (Chap. 16: Gonzales).
- *Use an exposome-wide approach to study Latino cancer disparities.* The underlying causes of Latino cancer disparities are varied and complex, and conducting exposome-wide association studies can provide the conceptual framework to help explain the role of multiple environmental exposures in the etiology and progression of cancer among Latinos. Further, much remains unknown about how social determinants in the Latino community actually cause cancer and lead to disparate outcomes; the exposome can be a model for understanding the biological mechanisms and pathways through which non-chemical stressors, such as social factors, can lead to cancer. Using prognostic and diagnostic biomarkers based on "omics" technologies holds the promise of linking measured environmental exposures to biochemical and molecular changes. Also, much of cancer disparities research does not account for subgroup heterogeneity among Latinos; an added advantage to the trans-omics approach is that it has the potential to yield robust information addressing variation among this genetically admixed group (Chap. 2: Juarez et al.).
- *Use implementation science to bridge the research to practice gap.* Translating recent research evidence into adopted medical practice often takes too long, especially for Latino populations. To ensure that new cancer discoveries reduce the cancer burden for Latinos, researchers must focus not only on *what* evidence-based interventions improve outcomes but also on *how* those interventions can be adopted, implemented, and sustained. To ensure that new and effective evidence-based interventions can be adopted, researchers should: (1) determine whether the intervention is feasible for the relevant populations; (2) train practitioners to deliver the intervention; (3) provide support and technical help to trained practitioners to offer the intervention through their routine practice; and (4) ensure the intervention can potentially reach any patient who could benefit (Chap. 12: Neta).

- *Revise public healthcare policy to reflect the predicted shift in the demography of cancer resulting from Latino population growth.* Latinos account for the majority of growth in the United States today and will in the coming decades. Even though Latinos have lower age-adjusted cancer incidence and death rates than other groups, their disproportionate growth is likely to contribute to the shifting demography of cancer and have implications for public policy. Because of the growing presence of Latinos, cancer researchers and healthcare providers must better understand the diversity that characterizes this population. It is also expected that inequities in access to affordable healthcare and lack of health insurance will increase the risk of Latinos having cancer and of dying from the disease. Finally, public policy that discourages migration from Mexico to the United States could erode Latino morbidity and mortality advantages that have existed for decades (Chap. 10: Sáenz).

Conclusion

The second ASCL conference brought together over 250 participants from 25 states and Puerto Rico to collaborate on the science of Latino cancer disparities. The papers published in this volume showcase the breadth of topics presented and describe research dedicated to improve the understanding of cancer in the Latino population. Recommendations from the conference participants provide direction for future research that will advance science and eventually save lives. Given the scope and urgency of the problem, we must work together throughout the cancer continuum to reach populations with needed screening, treatment, and improved quality of life for cancer survivors to improve long-standing inequities and reduce the cancer burden among Latinos.

References

1. Jacobson M, Chang TY, Shah M, Pramanik R, Shah SB. Racial and ethnic disparities in SARS-CoV-2 testing and COVID-19 outcomes in a Medicaid managed care cohort. Am J Prev Med. 2021;61(5):644–51. https://doi.org/10.1016/j.amepre.2021.05.015.
2. Moore JT, Ricaldi JN, Rose CE, Fuld J, Parise M, Kang GJ, et al. Disparities in incidence of COVID-19 among underrepresented racial/ethnic groups in counties identified as hotspots during June 5–18, 2020 — 22 States, February–June 2020. MMWR Morb Mortal Wkly Rep. 2020;69:1122–6. https://doi.org/10.15585/mmwr.mm6933e1.
3. Shiels MS, Haque AT, Haozous EA, Albert PS, Almeida JS, García-Closas M, et al. Racial and ethnic disparities in excess deaths during the COVID-19 pandemic, March to December 2020. Ann Intern Med. 2021. https://doi.org/10.7326/m21-2134.
4. American Cancer Society. Cancer facts & figures 2021. Atlanta: American Cancer Society; 2021.
5. Arias E, Tejada-Vera B, Ahmad F, Kochanek KD. Provisional life expectancy estimates for 2020. Hyattsville: National Center for Health Statistics; 2021.

6. Hooper MW, Nápoles AM, Pérez-Stable EJ. COVID-19 and racial/ethnic disparities. JAMA. 2020;323(24):2466–7. https://doi.org/10.1001/jama.2020.8598.
7. Balogun OD, Bea VJ, Phillips E. Disparities in cancer outcomes due to COVID-19—a tale of 2 cities. JAMA Oncol. 2020;6(10):1531–2. https://doi.org/10.1001/jamaoncol.2020.3327.
8. Cancino RS, Su Z, Mesa R, Tomlinson GE, Wang J. The impact of COVID-19 on cancer screening: challenges and opportunities. JMIR Cancer. 2020;6(2):e21697. https://doi.org/10.2196/21697.
9. Schmidt AL, Bakouny Z, Bhalla S, Steinharter JA, Tremblay DA, Awad MM, et al. Cancer care disparities during the COVID-19 pandemic: COVID-19 and cancer outcomes study. Cancer Cell. 2020;38(6):769–70. https://doi.org/10.1016/j.ccell.2020.10.023.
10. Asan O, Cooper IF, Nagavally S, Walker RJ, Williams JS, Ozieh MN, et al. Preferences for health information technologies among US adults: analysis of Health Information National Trends Survey. J Med Internet Res. 2018;20(10):e277. https://doi.org/10.2196/jmir.9436.
11. Miller KD, Ortiz AP, Pinheiro PS, Bandi P, Minihan A, Fuchs HE, et al. Cancer statistics for the US Hispanic/Latino population, 2021. CA Cancer J Clin. 2021;71(6):466–87. https://doi.org/10.3322/caac.21695.

Open Access   This chapter is licensed under the terms of the Creative Commons Attribution 4.0 International License (http://creativecommons.org/licenses/by/4.0/), which permits use, sharing, adaptation, distribution and reproduction in any medium or format, as long as you give appropriate credit to the original author(s) and the source, provide a link to the Creative Commons license and indicate if changes were made.

The images or other third party material in this chapter are included in the chapter's Creative Commons license, unless indicated otherwise in a credit line to the material. If material is not included in the chapter's Creative Commons license and your intended use is not permitted by statutory regulation or exceeds the permitted use, you will need to obtain permission directly from the copyright holder.

Appendix A: Advances in Biology and Treatment of Cancer

Harnessing iNKT Cells to Generate an Anti-Tumor Response Through the Administration of Dual-Compound Nanoparticles

Shute, T.[1]; Lai, A[1]; Salas, B.H.[1]; Vincent, B.K.[2]; Angel, D.[2]; Nash, K.L.[2]; Leadbetter, E.A.[1*]

[1]UT Health San Antonio, School of Medicine, Department of Microbiology, Immunology and Molecular Genetics, San Antonio, TX USA

[2]The University of Texas at San Antonio, Department of Physics and Astronomy, San Antonio, TX USA

Invariant natural killer T cells (iNKT) have a well-documented role in anti-tumor immunity through their release of proinflammatory cytokines and cytotoxic compounds. As iNKT cells can have direct and indirect killing effects on tumor cells, we propose a novel strategy for activating iNKT cells, via a nanoparticle delivery platform, to promote anti-tumor immune responses. An iNKT cell glycolipid agonist, alpha-galactosylceramide (αGalCer), and a tumor associated antigen can be simultaneously loaded into poly-lactic-co-glycolic acid (PLGA) nanoparticles. In an in vivo model of melanoma, using B16F10-OVA cells, prophylactic administration of nanoparticles containing αGalCer and ovalbumin (OVA) led to decreased tumor cell growth and increased survival. In addition, an immunogenic peptide from the naturally expressed melanocyte protein glycoprotein 100, gp100 25–33, can also be loaded into αGalCer containing PLGA nanoparticles. Through the use of nanoparticles labelled with Rhodamine B, a fluorescent dye, we confirmed nanoparticle uptake by antigen presenting cells by 15 minutes post subcutaneous injection. Testing the nanoparticles as a therapeutic against established B16F10 tumors is currently underway. This novel delivery system shows the potential for harnessing iNKT cells for cancer immunotherapy purposes and as part of combinational therapies with other approaches such as checkpoint inhibitors.

© The Editor(s) (if applicable) and The Author(s) 2023
A. G. Ramirez, E. J. Trapido (eds.), *Advancing the Science of Cancer in Latinos*, https://doi.org/10.1007/978-3-031-14436-3

STEAP2 Is Upregulated and Necessary for Hepatocellular Carcinoma Progression Via Increased Copper Levels and Stress-Activated MAP Kinase Activity

Easley A[1], Zeballos C[1], Bouamar H[1], Chiu Y-C[2], Chen Y[2,3], Cigarroa F[4], Sun L-Z[1*]

[1]Department of Cell Systems & Anatomy, University of Texas Health Science Center at San Antonio, TX, USA

[2]Department of Epidemiology and Statistics, University of Texas Health Science Center at San Antonio, TX USA

[3]Greehey Children's Cancer Research Institute, University of Texas Health Science Center at San Antonio, TX USA

[4]Transplant Center, University of Texas Health Science Center at San Antonio, TX USA

Background: Analysis of the differentially expressed genes in samples from paired adjacent non-tumor (ANT) liver and hepatocellular carcinoma (HCC) tissues of local Hispanic patients (LHP) revealed significant alteration in oxidation reduction. STEAP2 is a metalloreductase that plays a role in this process by promoting the reduction and uptake of iron and copper ions into a cell. Because hepatic copper overload associated with Wilson's disease is a known risk factor for HCC, we hypothesize that STEAP2 upregulation and copper accumulation may contribute to HCC progression.

Methods: Paired HCC and ANT tissues were collected from LHP for RNA sequencing, metal ion measurement, and determination of STEAP2 RNA and protein levels. Public datasets were queried for STEAP2 expression in HCC. Mechanistic studies including activation of MAP kinases, cell proliferation, migration, and tumor growth in vivo were assessed in HCC cell lines with knockdown (KD) or overexpression (OE) of STEAP2.

Results: STEAP2 is upregulated in various HCC gene expression datasets. Consistently, the levels of copper in the HCC tissues were higher compared to the ANT tissues. KD of STEAP2 decreased HCC cell growth, migration, invasion, and xenograft tumor growth, while STEAP2 OE showed opposite effects. KD of STEAP2 also reduced intracellular copper levels and activities of MAP kinases, p38 and JNK. Conversely, copper supplementation rescued cell migration and activation of p38 and JNK, while p38 or JNK inhibitors impaired cell migration.

Conclusion: STEAP2 appears to play a malignant-promoting role in HCC by driving migration and invasion via increased copper levels and MAP kinase activities. Our study uncovered a novel molecular mechanism contributing to HCC malignancy and a potential therapeutic target for HCC treatment.

Breast Cancer Antiestrogen Resistance 3 (BCAR3) Mediates Tumorigenesis in Triple Negative Breast Cancer

Janet Arras[1], Keena Thomas[1], Amare Osei[1], Mira Sridharan[1], Allison Cross[2], Amy Bouton[1]*

[1]Department of Microbiology, Immunology & Cancer Biology, University of Virginia School of Medicine, Charlottesville, VA, USA.

[2]National Cancer Institute (NCI)/National Institutes of Health (NIH), Bethesda, MD, USA.

Triple Negative Breast Cancers (TNBCs) constitute roughly 10–20% of breast cancers and are associated with poor clinical outcomes. TNBCs are characterized as lacking estrogen receptor (ER), progesterone receptor (PR), as well as human epidermal growth factor receptor 2 (HER2). The molecular mechanisms driving TNBCs remain largely unknown, leading to challenges in chemotherapeutic and targeted treatment strategies. Previous work from our laboratory has determined that the cytoplasmic adaptor protein Breast Cancer Antiestrogen Resistance 3 (BCAR3) is a potent activator of Src protein tyrosine kinase activity and is required for tumor growth in a triple negative orthotopic xenograft model. In addition, our laboratory has determined that BCAR3 regulates cell adhesion and motility through interaction with the adaptor molecule Cas. Preliminary data from patient-derived triple-negative breast cancer tumor samples show that BCAR3 protein levels are increased in TNBC compared to normal mammary tissue. Growth assays performed using MDA-MB-231 vector-controlled and shBCAR3 TNBC cells demonstrate that cells with reduced BCAR3 exhibit decreased growth compared to control. In addition, MDA-MB-231 breast cancer cells exhibit reduced epidermal growth factor receptor (EGFR) expression under conditions of BCAR3 knockdown. To identify signaling networks regulated by BCAR3, we performed RNA sequencing on TNBC cell lines with stable BCAR3 knockdown cultured in 2D (plastic) or 3D (matrigel) conditions, as well as on mammary organoids generated from wild-type and BCAR3 knockout mice. Using pathway analysis along with genetic and biochemical strategies, future studies are designed to identify molecular mechanisms by which BCAR3 drives TNBC tumor growth and progression.

Patient Derived Xenograft Facility for the Study of Hispanic Children and Adolescents with Cancer

Gail Tomlinson*[1], Anna Rogogina[1], Abhik Bandyopadhyay[1], Luz Perez Prado[1], Allison Grimes[1], Myron Ignatius[1], Rashaun Kurmasheva[1], Erin Butler[2], Laura Klesse[2], Dinesh Rakheja[2], Stephen Skapek[2], Peter Houghton[1]

Clinical contributors: Christine Aguilar[1], Chatchawin Assanasen[1], Greg Aune[1], Melissa Frei-Jones[1], Anne-Marie Langevin[1], Shafqat Shah[1], Aaron Sugalski[1], Rajiv

Rajani[1], Izabela Tarasiewicz,[1] Francisco Cigarroa[1], Jaime Estrada[3], Maria Falcon-Cantrill[3], Jose Esquilin[3], Vinod Gidvani-Diaz[3]
  [1]UT Health San Antonio, San Antonio TX, USA
  [2]UT Southwestern, Dallas TX, USA
  [3]Methodist Children's Hospital, San Antonio, TX, USA

Background: The South Texas Health Status Review reveals that the incidence of childhood leukemia in South Texas in 2000–2009 was 53.5 cases/million, higher than that in Texas overall (46.0/million) and higher than the nation overall (44.9/million). Similar data from California demonstrates an increased incidence in Hispanics. Toxicity and response to therapy also differ among ethnic groups and Hispanic children have a less favorable outcome. The biological reasons behind these disparities are poorly understood necessitating further study. Few preclinical patient derived xenograft (PDX) model systems exist from Hispanic children with leukemia and other cancers.

Methods: In 2016, researchers at the Greehey Children's Cancer Research Institute embarked on a systematic process to develop PDX models as a renewable resource that can be used to test new therapies that can ultimately be tested in Hispanic children including the most vulnerable group of older adolescents and young adults (AYAs).

Results: Of 64 patient-derived acute leukemia PDXs, 40 (62%) were derived from Hispanic children and AYAs. Eight of these PDXs were derived from AYAs over the age of 18, most of which were highly refractory or of high-risk phenotype. Of 40 PDXs derived from patients with solid tumors, 20 (50%) were from Hispanic children. Tumor types from Hispanic children consisted of osteosarcomas (5), germ cell tumors (4), hepatoblastoma (3), Wilms (2), soft tissue sarcomas (2), and one each neuroblastoma, medulloblastoma, glioblastoma, and adenocarcinoma.

Conclusion: Together these models, enriched for Hispanic ethnicity, comprise a highly unique resource for the study of cancer in children.

Different Patient, Different Tumor, and Different Consequence: The Systemic Implications of Pancreatic Cancer Are Diverse and Wide-Ranging in Latinos

Miles E. Cameron[1,2], Andrea N. Riner[1], Michael U. Maduka[1], Patrick W. Underwood[1], Andrew R. Judge[2], Jose G. Trevino[1]*
  [1]Department of Surgery, University of Florida Health Sciences Center, Gainesville, FL, USA
  [2]Department of Physical Therapy, University of Florida Health Sciences Center, Gainesville, FL, USA

Background: Pancreatic cancer (PC) is the deadliest of all common cancers with a five-year survival below 9%. Mortality rates are worse for certain ethnic populations, but we have shown that Latinos have the best outcomes of all groups in the United States. Cancer cachexia, the systemic wasting of muscle and fat associated with cancer, is experienced by roughly 80% of all patients with PC and directly increases morbidity and mortality. Owing to the heterogeneity of Latino identity, we hypothesize that Latinos with PC display a range of systemic sequelae consequent of cachexia not seen in other patient populations.

Methods: Patients were classified as Latino, non-Latino white (NLW), and non-Latino black (NLB) and matched by sex, age, and disease burden. Body composition was analyzed through computed tomography (CT) with sliceOmatic™ (Tomovision).

Results: 101 patients were identified, and 70% of patients had severe muscle wasting or cachexia. Latinos had the highest muscle mass (SMI), followed by NLB and NLW (49.84 cm^2/m^2, 43.91 cm^2/m^2, 41.54 cm^2/m^2, $p = 0.05$). Muscle density (radiation attenuation) correlated to SMI in NLW (Pearson's $R = 0.67$, $p < 0.05$) but not in Latinos ($R = -0.064$, $p = 0.86$). In spite of higher muscle mass, Latinos and NHB had higher intermuscular adipose deposition than NLW (7.8% vs. 4.6%, $p < 0.05$).

Conclusion: Latinos have distinct qualitative changes to muscle ultra-structure and radiodensity that are indicative of metabolic changes. Intermuscular fat is higher than expected. This may be due to the wide diversity in Latino ethnicity associated with better clinical outcomes.

Appendix B: Cancer Epidemiology and Prevention

Is Ethnicity Related to the Distribution of Lymphomas by Subtype in a Majority – Minority Hispanic Community?

Juan Francisco Garza[1*], Michelle Janania[1], Prathibha Surapaneni[1], Tyler Snedden[1], Jeremy Rollins[1], Snegha Ananth[1], David Gregorio[1], Enrique Diaz[1]

[1]Mays Cancer Center, UT Health San Antonio. MD Anderson Cancer Center, San Antonio, TX, USA

Introduction: Cancer continues to be one of the leading causes of death in the USA, only second to heart disease. Non-Hodgkin Lymphoma (NHL) is in the top 10 of all cancer related deaths. Diffuse Large B Cell Lymphoma (DLBCL) is the most common lymphoma reported in the USA and worldwide. Discrepancies exist among world regions in lymphoma subtype incidence, with a percentage of DLBCL being higher in Latin America versus Nordic countries.

Methods: This is an observational study, we retrospectively analyzed patients with diagnosis of Lymphoma (HL and NHL), at UT Health San Antonio, between 2008-2018. Key variables included age, gender, race/ethnicity, stage, bone marrow involvement, treatment received, vitality at 3 and 5 years and vitality status in 2018.

Primary end point was to characterize distribution of HL and NHL by subtypes in our Cancer Center and compare to North American and overall global distribution.

Results: 676 patients with lymphoma were identified. NHL subtypes; DLBCL was the most common identified ($n = 209$, 31%), Follicular Lymphoma was the most common indolent lymphoma among all demographic groups ($n = 123$, 26%), followed by HL ($n = 116$, 17%), it was more common among non-Hispanic subgroup ($n = 73$, 63% vs $n = 42$, 36%), Marginal Zone extranodal lymphoma was the second most common indolent subtype ($n = 41$, 6%).

© The Editor(s) (if applicable) and The Author(s) 2023
A. G. Ramirez, E. J. Trapido (eds.), *Advancing the Science of Cancer in Latinos*, https://doi.org/10.1007/978-3-031-14436-3

Conclusion: From the results described, within our Hispanic Serving Academic Institution, our population and distribution of lymphoma subtypes are similar to global and USA data.

Raising Awareness of Sugar Consumption and Cancer Risk: Applying Lessons Learned from Tobacco Countermarketing Campaigns to Prevent Cancer Among Latinas

A. Susana Ramírez[1*], Deepti Chittamuru[1], Kimberly Arellano Carmona[1]
[1]University of California – Merced, Merced, CA, USA

Introduction: Sugar-sweetened beverages (SSB) account for many of the excess calories consumed by Latinos, contributing to high rates of chronic disease and cancer risk. Latinos' high SSB-consumption is the result of targeting by the soda industry; parallels among SSB-consumption and tobacco use have previously been made. The dramatic 30-year decline in smoking was the result of multilevel interventions, including countermarketing campaigns, taxation, and environmental policies. A critical first step was ensuring sufficient awareness of the harms of tobacco and raising awareness of targeted marketing as a social justice issue.

Aim: Evaluate a countermarketing approach to nutrition communication, integrating culturally-relevant values with education about social determinants of health.

Methods: Participants ($N = 433$ Latinas aged 18–29) were randomly assigned to view countermarketing or a traditional fear-appeal about individual harms of SSB. Logistic-regression models and difference-in-proportion tests of hypotheses that countermarketing messages are more effective than fear-appeals at increasing public health literacy and knowledge of SSB-consumption and cancer risk.

Results: Participants were more receptive to ($p < .001$) and accepting of ($p < .01$) countermarketing messages compared with fear-appeal. Countermarketing messages increased SSB media literacy ($p < .05$), and perceived efficacy of civic actions including boycotting ($p < .05$) and social media advocacy ($p < .001$) more than fear-appeal but public health literacy and knowledge of SSB and cancer risk increased in both conditions. Countermarketing messages engender identification ($p < .001$) and activate social justice values ($p < .05$).

Conclusion: Modeled on successful tobacco control messaging, values-based countermarketing messages that raise awareness of predatory marketing tactics of soda companies hold considerable promise for Latino cancer prevention.

Disparities in Gastric Cancer and Its Precursors in South Texas: A Secondary Analysis of Electronic Health Data

Dorothy Long Parma*, Eric E. Moffett, Ariel Morales, Amelie G. Ramirez
   Department of Population Health Sciences, University of Texas Health Science Center at San Antonio, San Antonio, TX, USA.

Introduction: Gastric cancer (GC) disparities in Latinos vs non-Hispanic whites (NHWs), particularly in South Texas, may be linked to differences in diagnosis and management of precursor conditions, including chronic *Helicobacter pylori* infection (HP), gastric ulcer (GU) and atrophic gastritis (AG). This study aimed to identify differences among Latino and NHW patients at two affiliated health systems.

Methods: Aggregate data were compiled from an electronic health record dataset. Diagnoses included precursor conditions and gastric adenocarcinoma (GCA); non-Hodgkin's lymphoma (GL); and mucosa lymphoid tissue (MALT) lymphoma. Rate ratios (RR) were analyzed using STATA v. 15.1 (StataCorp, 2017). Odds ratios (OR) of all GCs combined were determined by logistic regression by covariates age, gender, ethnicity, site and insurance type using SAS.

Results: Over 845,000 records, 54.6% female, were analyzed. Over 60% of all diagnoses were HP-positive. There were no site differences in diagnosis rates. Latinos had ≥ 4 times higher rates than NHWs ($p < 0.05$), except for GU (NHW RR = 1.78 at one site); and MALT (no ethnic difference). Latinas were twice as likely to have GCA (RR range 1.87–2.20; $p < 0.001$) as NHW women, and almost three times as likely to have HP-positive AG (2.47–2.95; $p \leq 0.03$). Predictors of all GCs combined included age (OR = 1.04), male gender (2.78), site (15.99) and insurance (Medicare, Medicaid, and VA; 1.93) (all $p \leq 0.002$), but not ethnicity. UTMed providers prescribed more bismuth quadruple *H. pylori* therapy (RR 5.09).

Conclusions: HP rates were higher than national and state estimates. The roles of ethnicity, female gender and socioeconomic status require further exploration.

HPV Vaccination Rates Among Childhood Cancer Survivors in a Predominantly Hispanic Population

Meera Gurung[1], Aubree Shay[2], Leanne Embry[1], Christine Aguilar[1], Allison Grimes[1]
   [1]University of Texas Health Science Center at San Antonio, TX, USA
   [2]The UT Health School of Public Health at San Antonio, TX, USA

Introduction: Human papillomavirus (HPV) causes most cervical, anal, and oropharyngeal cancers. Compared to the U.S. general population, childhood cancer survivors (CCS) experience significantly higher rates of HPV-related malignancies.

Despite these increased risks, CCS have low HPV vaccination rates. In border regions of Texas where the population is predominately Hispanic, most CCS receive their treatment at the Texas Pediatric Minority Underserved NCI Community Oncology Research Program (TPMU NCORP) sites, comprised of five separate treatment facilities. Our project goal is to increase HPV vaccination rates among eligible CCS within the TPMU NCORP.

Method: At five TPMU NCORP sites across the state of Texas, we delivered an evidence-based HPV provider and staff education program focused on unique risks and needs of CCS. We also implemented practice-level changes to build a vaccine-friendly culture and begin to offer on-site delivery of the HPV vaccine to eligible CCS.

Results: Of 338 eligible CCS who had a clinic visit over the past six months, 304 (90%) received HPV vaccine recommendations from their provider. Of these, 235 (77%) accepted the vaccine and initiated the series (1-dose) and 87 (29%) completed the series (3-dose).

Discussion: Despite the increased vulnerability of CCS to secondary HPV-related cancers, this population has largely been neglected in research, education, and large-scale HPV vaccine initiatives. With the rising incidence of HPV-related cancers in Texas, low uptake of HPV vaccination in this region, and increased susceptibility of CCS to HPV-related disease, targeting this population within the oncology follow-up setting is both novel and risk-directed.

Barriers to Completing HPV Vaccination Schedule Among Latinas: Examining the Results of a Community Intercept Survey in Los Angeles, California

Bibiana Martinez[1*], Carol Ochoa[1], Rosa Barahona[1], CarolLina Aristizabal[1], Yaneth L. Rodriguez[1], Sheila Murphy[2], Lourdes Baezconde-Garbanati[1]

[1]Department of Preventive Medicine, Keck School of Medicine, University of Southern California, Los Angeles, CA, USA.

[2]Annenberg School for Communication and Journalism, University of Southern California, Los Angeles, CA, USA.

Introduction: While cervical cancer rates have decreased substantially over the past 40 years, disparities in cervical cancer burden and mortality persist among Latinas in the United States. Vaccination against Human Papillomavirus (HPV) is the most effective strategy for preventing cervical cancer. Current guidelines for HPV vaccination call for three doses for children who receive their first dose after their 15th birthday. It is fundamental that we understand the barriers that prevent women in general and Latinas in particular from receiving the full HPV vaccination schedule for themselves and their children.

Methods: We administered community intercept surveys in Los Angeles, California to assess knowledge, attitude, and beliefs related to HPV vaccination and cervical cancer. A total of 92 women identifying as Latina aged 21+ years responded to the survey between July and September of 2019. The survey included questions related to cervical cancer, HPV vaccination and perceived barriers to completing the HPV vaccination schedule. Descriptive statistics will be used to explore perceived barriers to full HPV vaccination; multivariable regression modeling will be performed to determine factors associated with these barriers, including age, nativity and insurance status.

Results: Data management is currently underway; results will be available in time for the Conference.

Conclusion: To eliminate disparities in cervical cancer outcomes we must address barriers to all effective prevention strategies, including completing the HPV vaccination schedule. Our results will help clarify opportunities for policies and interventions that can guide prevention efforts at the community, local, state and national levels.

The Effectiveness of Two Films in Educating, Changing Attitudes and Intentions About the Uptake of the HPV Vaccine Among Spanish Speaking Mexican American Women

Carol Y. Ochoa*[1], Bibiana Martinez[1], Sheila T. Murphy[2], Lauren B. Frank[3], Lourdes A. Baezconde-Garbanati[1]

[1]Department of Preventive Medicine, University of Southern California, Los Angeles, CA, USA

[2]Annenberg School for Communication and Journalism, University of Southern California, Los Angeles, CA, USA

[3]Department of Communication, Portland State University, Portland, OR, USA

Background: Hispanics have lower rates of initiation and completion of the Human Papillomavirus (HPV) vaccine series; and have higher rates of HPV-associated cervical cancer than non-Hispanic women.

Methods: A randomized controlled telephone trial compared the effectiveness of two HPV educational films in Los Angeles County. Both films were 11 minutes; one used a fictional narrative (Tamale Lesson/Conversando entre Tamales) and the other used a more traditional nonnarrative film (It's Time/Es Tiempo) to describe information on HPV and the HPV vaccine. Data was collected at baseline, two weeks, and six months after viewing either film. Analysis of covariance will be conducted to examine any main effects on HPV-related knowledge, attitudes towards HPV vaccine, and intention to vaccinate daughters against Human Papillomavirus based on the film watched.

Results: 109 Spanish-speaking Mexican-origin women aged 25–45 completed the three surveys. The majority of women reported having less than high school education, limited English proficiency, and being lower income. At baseline, women assigned to the narrative film, were less likely to have heard of HPV (54% vs 78%, $p = 0.008$) but more likely to know that the HPV vaccine was for both males and females (66.1% vs 48.9%, $p = 0.08$), compared to women assigned to the nonnarrative film.

Conclusion: Our findings suggest a lack of awareness and knowledge of HPV and the HPV vaccine among Hispanic women. It is important to evaluate the effectiveness of health education delivery methods among lower income and less acculturated Hispanic women, in order to help change health behaviors and save lives.

Analysis of *TP53* Gene Mutations Demonstrates that Aflatoxin Is a Risk Factor for Hepatocellular Carcinoma in Guatemala

Christian S. Alvarez[1*], Jeremy Ortiz[2], Giovanna Bendfeldt-Avila[3], Yi Xie[1], Mingyi Wang[4], Dongjing Wu[4], Herb Higson[4], Elisa Lee[4], Kedest Teshome[4], Joaquin Barnoya[5], David E. Kleiner[6], John Groopman[7,8], Roberto Orozco[9], Katherine A. McGlynn[1], Eduardo Gharzouzi[5], Michael Dean[1]

[1]Division of Cancer Epidemiology and Genetics, National Cancer Institute, Bethesda, MD, USA

[2]Instituto de Cancerología/INCAN, Guatemala City, Guatemala

[3]Hospital Centro Médico Militar, Guatemala City, Guatemala

[4]Cancer Genetics Research Laboratory, Division of Cancer Epidemiology and Genetics, Leidos Biomedical Research Inc.; Frederick National Laboratory for Cancer Research, Gaithersburg, MD, USA

[5]Integra Cancer Institute, Guatemala City, Guatemala

[6]Laboratory of Pathology, Center for Cancer Research, NCI, NIH, Bethesda, MD, USA

[7]Department of Environmental Health and Engineering, Bloomberg School of Public Health, Johns Hopkins University, Baltimore, MD, USA

[8]Department of Epidemiology, Bloomberg School of Public Health, Johns Hopkins, University, Baltimore, MD, USA

[9]Department of Pathology, Hospital General San Juan de Dios, Guatemala City, Guatemala

Introduction: Guatemala has the highest incidence of hepatocellular carcinoma (HCC), the dominant type of liver cancer, in the Western Hemisphere. The major risk factors in Guatemala are not well-characterized, but the prevalence of hepatitis B (HBV) and hepatitis C virus (HCV) appear to be low, while the prevalence of aflatoxin (AFB_1) exposure appears to be high. To examine whether AFB_1 could be a risk factor for HCC in Guatemala, this study examined the frequency of the AFB_1-signature mutation in the *TP53* gene (R249S) as well as other somatic mutations.

Methods: Ninety-one formalin-fixed, paraffin-embedded (FFPE) HCC tissues were obtained from three hospitals in Guatemala City. An additional, eighteen tumor tissues preserved in RNAlater were also obtained. Targeted sequencing of *TP53* was successfully performed in 89 of the FFPE samples, and a panel of 245 genes were sequenced in the RNAlater samples.

Results: Overall, 47% of HCCs had a *TP53* mutation. The AFB_1-signature R249S mutation was present in 24%. Among the RNAlater samples, 44% had any *TP53* mutation and 33% had the R249S mutation. Other somatic mutations were identified in known HCC driver genes such as *ARID1A*, *ARID2*, and *CTNNB1*.

Conclusions: The presence of the *TP53* R249S mutation indicates that AFB_1 is a risk factor for HCC in Guatemala. The proportion of HBV positive tumors was low, suggesting that AFB_1 is associated with HCC in the absence of concomitant HBV infection. To decrease the risk of HCC in Guatemala, AFB_1 abatements efforts are warranted.

Awareness of Vaccination Availability for the Human Papillomavirus: Implications for Latino and Non-Latino Black Adults from the 2018 Health Information National Trends Survey

Derek Falk[1*], Carla Strom[2], Kelsey Shore[2], Karen Marie Winkfield[2,3], Kathryn E. Weaver[1,2]

[1]Department of Social Sciences & Health Policy, Wake Forest University School of Medicine, Winston-Salem, NC, USA.
[2]Office of Cancer Health Equity, Wake Forest Baptist Health Comprehensive Cancer Center, Winston-Salem, NC, USA.
[3]Department of Radiation Oncology, Wake Forest Baptist Medical Center, Winston-Salem, NC, USA.

Introduction: FDA approval for vaccination against the human papillomavirus (HPV) was originally approved for individuals aged 9–26, but in 2018, the FDA expanded approval to include men and women aged 27–45. Current vaccination rates are 49.5% for adolescent females and 37.5% for adolescent males; no studies have assessed HPV vaccine awareness for newly eligible adults.

Methods: Using data collected through the 2018 Health Information National Trends Survey, a weighted logistic regression model evaluated the odds of adults aged 18–45 being aware of the HPV vaccine. Covariates included age, sex, race/ethnicity, including Latino, non-Latino black (NLB), and non-Latino white (NLW), education, insurance status, and general health status. Interactions between sex and race/ethnicity were also specified, and stratified models examined the results by sex.

Results: Prevalence rates of vaccine awareness were higher in older adults (74%) and females (80%) versus younger adults (67%) and males (57%). In the adjusted model, there were main effects for race/ethnicity, education level, and a significant interaction between sex and race/ethnicity. Latina (OR: 0.22, CI: 0.10–0.50) and NLB (OR: 0.25, CI 0.04–0.68) women had lower odds of HPV vaccine awareness compared to NLW women. Adults with a high school education or less (OR: 0.15, CI: 0.07–0.31) were less likely to be aware compared to their counterparts.

Conclusion: Overall, rates of HPV vaccine awareness among younger adults and males were low. If recommendations expand to include slightly older adults, the results indicate the need for greater HPV vaccination education for Latina and NLB women and lower educated individuals.

The Interaction of Alcohol and Smoking Rate in Relation to Cigarette Dependence, Perceived Barriers for Quitting, and Expectancies for Smoking Among Spanish-Speaking Latinx Smokers

Ruben Rodriguez-Cano[1,2*], Janice A. Blalock[1], Jafar Bakhshaie[3], Lorra Garey[2], Justin M. Shepherd[2], Michael J. Zvolensky[1,2,4]

[1]Department of Behavioral Science, The University of Texas MD Anderson Cancer Center, Houston, TX, USA.
[2]Department of Psychology, University of Houston, Houston, TX, USA.
[3]Menninger Department of Psychiatry and Behavioral Sciences, Baylor College of Medicine, Houston, TX, USA.
[4]HEALTH Institute, University of Houston, Houston, TX, USA.

Introduction: Although smoking and alcohol use are the leading preventable causes of cancer among Latinx, no studies have evaluated their interactive effects in terms of cigarette dependence, and cognitive-based smoking processes. It is possible that the greater frequency of alcohol use and smoking rate may synergistically affect those smoking variables. The present study explored the interactive effects of frequency of alcohol use and smoking rate in terms of cigarette dependence, perceptions of barriers for quitting smoking and expectancies about smoking among Spanish-speaking Latinx adult smokers.

Methods: Participants ($n = 362$, *mean age* = 33.30, 58.8% women) were Spanish-Speaking Latinx daily smokers. Participants were recruited through an on-line panel system via Qualtrics that has shown to yield valid and reliable data. Spanish-language measures were employed and included instruments focused on alcohol usage, smoking rate, cigarette dependence, smoking expectancies, and perceptions about quitting.

Results: There was a significant interaction ($p < .05$) for alcohol use and smoking rate for perceived barriers for quitting smoking ($B = -0.08$, standard error [SE] = 0.03), negative reinforcement expectancies ($B = -0.11$, SE = 0.03), and appetitive-weight control expectancies ($B = -0.07$, SE = 0.03). Particularly, the lower smoking rate per day, the higher a greater alcohol use was related to higher rates with barriers for quitting, negative reinforcement expectancies, and appetitive-weight control expectancies.

Conclusion: The current findings suggest that there is interplay between alcohol consumption and smoking rate in terms of some cognitive-based smoking processes. The reduction of alcohol use in Latinx daily smokers who smoke a lower quantity of cigarettes might help to reduce the cognitive based smoking processes related to smoking maintenance.

Never Too Young: Retrospective Study on Age and Racial Disparity in the Outcome of Primary CNS Lymphoma in South Texas

Snegha Ananth[1], Michelle Janania Martinez[1], Prathibha Surapaneni[1], Juan F. Garza[1], Tyler W. Snedden[1], David J. Gregorio[1], Sushanth Kakarla[1], Jeremy A. Rawlings[1], Joel E. Michalek[1], Qianqian Liu[1], Enrique Diaz Duque[1]*

[1]UT Heath San Antonio, Mays Cancer Center, Department of Hemato-Oncology, San Antonio, TX, USA

Introduction: Primary CNS lymphoma (PCNSL) is a rare malignancy, comprising only 2% of primary CNS tumors in the United States. The purpose of this study was to describe differences in clinical characteristics and survival by Hispanic ethnicity in PCNSL.

Methods: This is a retrospective study, where we identified patients who were diagnosed and treated for PCNSL at UT Health San Antonio, between January 2008 and December 2018. The epidemiology, therapeutic measures, and clinical characteristics were listed as descriptive statistics.

Results and Discussion: During 2008–2018, a total of 29 patients of PCNSL were included. Among those, 62% were HI (Hispanic) and the remaining 38% were NH (Non-Hispanic). The median age at diagnosis was 61 years (58 years in HI and 70 years in NH). 55% were below 65 years and 45% were older than 65 years. Everyone received chemotherapy (89% received R-MPV (DeAngelis protocol) and 9% received other high dose methotrexate containing regimens). However, in terms of receiving Whole Brain Radiation Therapy (WBRT), the patients in the younger group were more likely to receive it than were those in the elderly group (68% versus 23% respectively). Overall Survival (OS) rate at 3 years was 41% in HI and 33% in NH ($p = 0.08$) and at 5 years was 41% in HI and 25% in NH ($p = 0.03$).

Conclusion: While there is increasing data on higher incidence of non-HIV PCNSL in elderly population >65 years, HI in our population had a significantly lower median age at diagnosis with better survival and outcomes.

U.S.-MX. Border Health CBPR: HPV Cancer Prevention – El Paso, TX

Moya, E., M.[1*], Cordero, J., I.[2,3], Zamore, C.[4], Ramirez, M[1], Munoz, R.[1] Aragones, A.[4]

[1]Department of Social Work, College of Health Sciences, University of Texas at El Paso, El Paso, TX, USA.

[2]Border Biomedical Research Center (BBRC), University of Texas at El Paso at El Paso, El Paso, TX, USA.

[3]Department of Health Promotion and Behavioral Sciences, The University of Texas Health Science Center at Houston, School of Public Health, El Paso, TX, USA.

[4]Department of Psychiatry & Behavioral Sciences, Memorial Sloan Kettering Cancer Center, Immigrant Health & Cancer Disparities Service, New York, NY, USA.

Introduction: Human papillomavirus (HPV) associated cancers exhibit disparities among Hispanics, with cervical cancer rates significantly higher in this population among others. El Paso (80% Hispanic), designated Medically Underserved Area (MUA), shows high rates of HPV-associated cancers (2012–2016) compare to overall Texas and U.S. (cervical: 10.4, 9.2, 8.0), (oropharyngeal: 7.0, 11.0, 12.0). *Approach*-Community approach using tailored education to increase HPV vaccination. *Hypothesis*-Latino participants exposed to culturally and demographically tailored interventions will be receptive to education regarding HPV vaccination for child(ren) in El Paso, TX.

Objectives-(1) develop community-informed, bi-lingual educational tools in collaboration with community partners; (2) target parents of CDC recommended age-groups 11–17 years; (3) navigate parental decision-making in obtaining the vaccine. *Goals*-(1) increase HPV awareness, its relationship to cancer, and vaccine access;

(2) increase positive perceptions of vaccine among parents; (3) encourage parents to request child vaccination. PURPOSE-To cultivate an interdisciplinary team science, community-based participatory approach preventing HPV-associated cancers in El Paso.

Methods: Development of educational tools (YR1); recruitment of adult parents/caregivers (n = 200) in El Paso (YR2–4). Participants receive (1) educational and baseline components on first contact, (2) receive navigation/follow-up 1-year post-baseline.

Results: Preliminary findings include tools and data specific to El Paso demographics

- Adult low health insurance access (28%); higher access to regular care (52%)
- HPV awareness among adults of Mexican-origin
- Mexico refusal to administer vaccine to males

Discussion: Current findings will inform policy and future prevention efforts among interdisciplinary team science approaches of effective methods to increase vaccine completion among a diverse U.S.-Mexico border region; with preceding large-scale cancer bio-genetic-behavioral U54 project launching in El Paso.

Association of Variants in *MSH2* and *PMS2* Genes with Colorectal Cancer in Mexican Patients

González-Mercado A[1], Rico Méndez MA[2], Moreno Ortiz JM[1], Ramírez Ramírez R[2], Ayala Madrigal ML[1], González-Mercado MG[4], Centeno Flores MW[5], Gutiérrez Angulo M[3*]
[1]Universidad de Guadalajara CUCS, Guadalajara, Jalisco, México
[2]Universidad de Guadalajara CUCBA, Guadalajara, Jalisco, México
[3]Universidad de Guadalajara CUALTOS, Tepatitlán, Jalisco, México
[4]Tecnológico de Monterrey campus Guadalajara, Guadalajara, Jalisco, México
[5]Hospital Civil "Juan I. Menchaca", Guadalajara, Jalisco, México

Introduction: Colorectal cancer (CRC) represents a group of molecular and heterogeneous diseases with a range of genetic and epigenetic alterations. It is the third most common type of cancer in Mexico and in the world. The MSH2 and PMS2 genes encoded for proteins involved in DNA mismatch repair. The objective was to estimate the association of rs2303426 (c.211+9C>G) and rs10179950 (c.211+811C>T) of MSH2 gene and rs2286681 (c.804−164T>G) and rs62456178 (c.989−701C>T) of PMS2 gene with CRC in Mexican patients.

Material and Methods: DNA samples of 143 CRC patients and 146 reference population were included. Peripheral blood DNA was extracted by CTAB-DTAB method and genotyping was performed by TaqMan® SNP Genotyping Assays. Genotypic and allelic frequencies were determined by direct counting. The association was evaluated by odds ratio. All participants signed an informed consent letter.

Results: The alleles rs2303426C, rs10179950C, rs2286681T and rs62456178C were more frequently in both groups (between 53–66%). The association analysis showed no association of the variants with CRC ($p > 0.05$).

Discussion: The genotypic and allelic frequencies of the SNPs between both groups did not show differences ($p > 0.05$); the allelic frequencies of the reference group are similar to those of the population of Los Angeles CA with Mexican ancestry ($p > 0.05$) and different from those of the world population ($p < 0.001$) reported in 1000 genomes.

Conclusion: The frequencies of these variants are reported for the first time in Mexican population and it is suggested that it do not have an important role in the development of CRC in our population.

Methylation Analysis of *MLH1* Gene in Tumor Tissue of Mexican Patients with Colorectal Cancer

Moreno-Ortiz JM[1], Jiménez-García J[1, 2], Ayala-Madrigal ML[1], González-Mercado A[1], Ramírez-Ramírez R[3], Ramírez-Plascencia H[1], Alvizo-Rodríguez CR[1], Flores-López BA[1], Hernández-Sandoval A[1], Macias-Gutiérrez VM[4], Gutiérrez-Angulo M[2*]
[1]Centro Universitario de Ciencias de la Salud, Universidad de Guadalajara
[2]Centro Universitario de los Altos, Universidad de Guadalajara
[3]Centro Universitario de Ciencia Biológicas y Agropecuarias, Universidad de Guadalajara
[4]Hospital Civil "Dr. Juan I. Menchaca. Guadalajara, Jalisco, México.

Introduction: *MLH1* gene encodes a protein that participates in DNA mismatch repair. Its promoter contains a CpG island of 1128 bp (chr3:37034229-37035356) involved in gene regulation. This island is divided in four regions: A (located at -711 to -577), B (-552 to -266), C (-248 to -178) and D (-109 to $+5$). The aim of this work was to analyze the methylation of the CpG island in A, B and C regions in colorectal cancer (CRC) patients.

Material and Methods: Previous informed consent, 101 samples of tumor tissue were obtained from Mexican patients with histopathological diagnosis of CRC. All the patients were derived from the Civil Hospital "Dr. Juan I. Menchaca". The methylation status was evaluated by methylation specific-PCR.

Results: The methylation analysis showed 22% of CRC patients were positive for methylation in any region and only 4% had all the regions methylated (A, B and C). A and B regions had the higher frequency of methylation.

Discussion: As described by Deng *et al*, 2001 and Miyakura *et al,* 2014., methylation of regions C and D have a determining role in protein expression in patients with CRC, but in this work, regions A and B had a higher percentage of methylation than region C.

Conclusion: Regions A and B of *MLH1* had a higher frequency of methylation. Although the C region is related with gene expression in CRC, it would be necessary to analyze the methylation role of A and B regions associated to CRC in Mexican patients.

Admixture Mapping with Genome-Wide Association Analyses Identifies Potential Risk Variants for HER2+ Breast Cancer in Latinas

Valentina Zavala[1], Tatiana Vidaurre[2], Katie Marker[3], Jeannie Vásquez[2], L. Tamayo[4], Sandro Casavilca[2], M. Calderon[2], J. Abugattas[2], H. Gómez[5], H. Fuentes[2], C. Monge-Pimentel[2],Jovanny Zabaleta[6], Laura Fejerman*[1]
[1]University of California San Francisco, San Francisco, CA, USA
[2]Instituto Nacional de Enfermedades Neoplasicas, Peru
[3]University of California Berkeley, CA, USA
[4]University of Chicago, IL, USA
[5]Instituto Nacional de Enfermedades Neoplasicas, Peru
[6]Louisiana State University Health Sciences Center, New Orleans, LA, USA

Introduction: Human Epidermal Growth Factor Receptor 2 positive (HER2+) breast cancer (BC) incidence is higher in Latinas. Our preliminary analyses showed an association between Indigenous American (IA) ancestry and HER2 status. We hypothesize that population-specific germline variants predispose Latinas with IA ancestry to develop HER2+ tumors. We aim to discover germline variants associated with ancestry and HER2+ BC in patients with high IA ancestry.

Methods: We genotyped 1,312 BC patients recruited at the Instituto Nacional de Enfermedades Neoplasicas in Lima, Peru. We infered locus-specific ancestry and estimated global ancestry. Admixture mapping analysis was conducted using logistic regression with HER2+ patients as cases and HER2- as controls. Fine mapping within regions of interest was performed using imputed genotypes. RNA was extracted from 47 tumor samples from this same cohort and exome sequencing was conducted with the Illumina-NextSeq500 system. Gene expression for genes within suggestive regions was compared between HER2+ and HER2- tumors.

Results: Admixture mapping results are suggestive for two different chromosomal regions: 2q11–2q12 and 3p14. Fine mapping within these regions showed novel suggestive variants in the 2q11–2q12 region near genes such as MAP 4K4 and genes from the interleukin 1 receptor family, with known roles in BC development. Within the 3p14 region, we found differential expression for the FLNB gene with higher expression among HER2-patients.

Conclusion: Combining Admixture mapping with genome-wide association analyses and transcriptomics is a promising approach to discover population-specific variants associated with subtype-specific BC risk. We will replicate suggestive findings and expand sample size to increase power.

The Role of Social Deprivation on Smoking Assessment and Smoking Status Among Latino Adolescents in Community Health Centers

John Heintzman*[1,3], Miguel Marino[1,2*], Katie Fankhauser[1], Jon Puro[3], Sophia Giebultowicz[3], David Ezekiel-Herrera[1], Jennifer Lucas[1], Steffani Bailey[1]

[1]Department of Family Medicine, Oregon Health and Science University, Portland, OR, USA

[2]Biostatistics Group, OHSU-PSU School of Public Health, Portland, OR, USA

[3]OCHIN, Inc., Portland, OR, USA

Introduction: Assessment of smoking status is a recommended cancer prevention service in adolescents, but it is unknown if community deprivation affects the likelihood of smoking assessment in Latino/a adolescents compared to non-Hispanic whites.

Methods: We utilized an electronic health record (EHR) dataset, serving community health center (CHC) patients nationally, linked to neighborhood-level social deprivation data, to assess the differences in smoking assessment at any visit (yes vs. no) and use (current vs. never smoker) among 10–17 year-olds. We compared three groups: 1) Latino Spanish-language preferred, 2) Latino English-language preferred, 3) non-Hispanic white, assessing if ethnicity/language disparities were moderated by neighborhood social deprivation, controlling for important confounders (e.g. healthcare utilization, insurance, household income, etc.).

Results: Our study included 124,314 adolescents across 15 states, 53.4% of whom were non-Hispanic white, 32.0% Spanish-preferring Latinos and 14.6% English-preferring Latinos. Among neighborhoods with the highest deprivation, the likelihood of being assessed for smoking was ~88% for all ethnicity/language groups. Among neighborhoods with the lowest deprivation levels, Spanish-preferring Latinos had similar likelihood of being screened for smoking (88.0%, 95%

CI = 85.9–90.5%) as English-preferring Latinos but showed a higher likelihood compared to non-Hispanic whites (83.5%, 95% CI = 81.1–85.9%). Spanish-preferring Latinos had the lowest prevalence of smoking (0.4%), followed by English-preferring Latinos (1.6%) and non-Hispanic whites (3.1%), which did not differ by social deprivation levels.

Conclusion: In CHCs, smoking assessment of Latino adolescents was frequent and equivalent across patients residing in socially deprived neighborhoods. CHC models of care may be strategic objects of further study to deliver equitable cancer prevention.

Evaluation of a Provider-Directed HCV Education Intervention to Improve HCV Screening

Bertha E. Flores[1*], Wang, CP[2], Fernandez, A[1], Rochat, A[2], Bobadilla, R[2], Hernandez, L[2], Turner, BJ[2]

[1]UT Health San Antonio, School of Nursing, San Antonio, TX, USA.
[2]UT Health San Antonio, ReACH Center, San Antonio, TX, USA

Introduction: The incidence of cirrhosis and liver cancer is increasing in the U.S., with Hispanics in South Texas especially affected. Expert guidelines endorse one-time Hepatitis C virus (HCV) screening of baby-boomers (born 1945–1965) but limited education about HCV is a barrier to screening in primary care. We developed an educational program for clinicians and staff about HCV epidemiology, screening, and basic management of chronic HCV. This program was implemented in practices serving low income, Hispanic majority communities.

Methods: The program was delivered to primary care clinicians and staff in 6 practices. The pre-test and post-test asked 12 questions. Change between pre- and post-test scores were compared using McNemar and likelihood ratio test (LRT) for binary and Likert scales, respectively.

Results: The intervention was associated with significantly improved percent change in pre- and post-test scores for questions addressing chronic HCV infection (45% improvement for both clinicians and staff), vaccine recommendations (8% and 23% improvement), and diagnostic tests (32% and 29% improvement). Significant improvement was also observed for items measuring attitudes about screening and care including feasibility of HCV testing (0.30 and 0.39 improvement), feasibility of linking HCV patients to care (0.54 and 0.49 improvement), and importance of HCV (0.51 and 0.52 improvement).

Conclusion: Provider/staff educational program improved knowledge about HCV epidemiology, screening and management in both clinicians and staff. This program underpins a comprehensive implementation program to deliver screening for HCV in baby boomers and to evaluate and manage chronic HCV to reduce the threat of HCV in at-risk Hispanics.

Alcohol Use, Physical Activity and Body Mass Index in the Mexican American Mano a Mano Cohort

Natalia I. Heredia[1*], Qiong Dong[1], Shine Chang[1], and Lorna H. McNeill[1]
[1]The University of Texas MD Anderson Cancer Center, Houston, TX, USA

Introduction: Hispanics have the highest rates of liver cancer in the U.S. Alcohol use, lack of physical activity (PA), and obesity are liver cancer risk factors. Although studies indicate PA is positively associated and alcohol consumption is negatively associated with body mass index (BMI), these relationships remain elusive for Hispanics. This study assessed the association of PA and alcohol use with BMI, stratified by gender in Mexican-origin adults.

Methods: Secondary data analysis using interviewer-administered questionnaire data, including self-reported PA, alcohol consumption, and demographics; trained staff measured height and weight. Linear regression assessed the association between PA and alcohol consumption with BMI controlling for key variables.

Results: Among 3,897 participants, average age was 49; individuals were mostly women, had not attained a high school degree, obese (60%), and never drinkers (67%). Current drinkers had a higher proportion of individuals achieving high PA (32%) than either never (26%) or former drinkers (24%). We found an inverse relationship between high PA and BMI in females only (Beta = -1.48, 95% C1: -2.12, -0.84, $p < .001$). An inverse relationship between current drinking and BMI was identified in the full sample (Beta = -0.88, 95% CI: -1.51, -0.25, $p < .01$) and across sexes and acculturation groups. Among male never drinkers, high PA was associated with increased BMI (Beta = 2.48, 95% CI: 0.82, 4.14, $p < .01$).

Conclusions: High PA and current drinking were independently protective against obesity. Differences seen between independent and interaction results illustrate the importance of evaluating multiple risk behaviors together and by gender to inform cancer prevention efforts in Mexican-origin adults.

Acculturation and Differences in Breast Cancer Screening Behaviors of Immigrant Women in the U.S.

Federico Ghirimoldi[1], Susanne Schmidt[1*]

[1]UT Health San Antonio, San Antonio, TX, USA

Background: Despite reduced breast cancer mortality in the U.S., disparities among minority and immigrant women remain. We examine disparities in cancer screening behaviors of immigrant women from different regions of birth, by estimating the influence of acculturation and a family history of cancer.

Methods: Using National Health Interview Survey data and multilevel logistic regression models, we examine the determinants of breast screening behaviors among immigrant women ($n = 8,662$), half of who were from Mexico/Central America/the Caribbean or South America.

Results: In multilevel models, women without a family history of cancer (Odds Ratio = 0.63, $p < 0.001$) and unacculturated women (Odds Ratio = 0.48, $p < 0.001$) were less likely to have ever had a physical breast exam. Further, significant variation in having had a breast exam exist by region of birth. Although this variation was reduced after adjusting for sociodemographic characteristics, acculturation, and family history of cancer, it remained statistically significant across models.

Conclusion: This paper improves our understanding of factors related to the adoption of cancer screening behaviors among U.S. immigrants from around the world, including the role of acculturation and increased awareness of cancer risk due to a family history of cancer. Breast cancer advocates should consider both the extent of language-related barriers and the regional and cultural differences among the immigrant groups within the population that they serve. Addressing personal and cultural barriers in health education programs and cancer awareness campaigns can help reduce disparities and increase cancer screening uptake among difficult to reach immigrant women.

Impact of a Community-Based Educational Intervention on Prostate Cancer Among Hispanic and African American Community/Patient Advocates and Promotores de Salud

Carolina Aristizabal[1*], Linda Behar-Horenstein[2], Yingwei Yao[2], Sandra Suther[3], Angela Adams[2], Nissa Askins[2], Folakemi Odedina[2], Mariana C. Stern[1], Lourdes Baezconde-Garbanati[1]

[1]Florida-California Cancer Research, Education and Engagement Health Equity (CaRE[2]) Center, University of Southern California, Los Angeles, CA, USA

[2]CaRE[2] Center, University of Florida, Gainesville, FL, USA

[3]CaRE[2] Center, Florida Agricultural and Mechanical University, Tallahassee, FL, USA

Presenter and corresponding author: Carolina Aristizabal, MD, MPH, CHES® (caristiz@usc.edu)

Introduction: Blacks are disproportionately impacted by prostate cancer (PCa) compared to other racial/ethnic groups. While the burden of PCa in Hispanics is low, there is limited understanding of the disparities in subpopulations of Hispanics. We developed, culturally adapted, translated, implemented and evaluated a Prostate Cancer Advocacy Training (PCAT).

Methods: Culturally and language specific content on PCa cause, risk factors, epidemiology, detection, diagnosis and treatment was delivered through a workshop and simultaneously broadcasted in Spanish in Los Angeles County ($n = 29$) and in English in Tallahassee, Florida ($n = 9$). Pre- and post-test surveys assessed impact.

Results: The following pre vs. post differences were statistically significant ($p < 0.05$), in knowledge (5.0 ± 1.6 vs 6.3 ± 1.1) and advocacy intentions (3.9 ± 0.9 vs 4.3 ± 0.8). On correctly identifying warning signs for PCa (50% vs 87%), intent to inform and educate patients, family, and friends about PCa within the next three months, (69% vs 95%), to ensure that high quality research is sensitive to the priorities of patients (63% vs 84%), to help increase patient recruitment, compliance and retention for clinical trials within the next month (62% vs 84%), intent to engage in PCa patient education within the next three months, (67% vs 92%); and in engaging in PCa community outreach within the next three months, (67% vs 94%). There were no significant differences due to race/ethnicity.

Conclusion: The PCAT led to increased knowledge, awareness, and intention to engage in advocacy regarding PCa in the next three months. Results suggest that delivering culturally and language specific educational information increases engagement of Hispanic and African American patient/community advocates.

Preliminary Findings of a Cancer Risk Cohort Study in a Predominately Hispanic Border Region

Crystal Costa[1*], Jennifer Salinas[3], Adam Alomari[2], Alok Dwivedi, PhD[3], Navkiran Shokar[2]

[1]The University of Texas at El Paso, El Paso, TX, United States

[2]Texas Tech University Health Sciences Center El Paso School of Medicine, Department of Family & Community Medicine, El Paso, TX, United States

[3]Texas Tech University Health Sciences Center El Paso School of Medicine, Department of Molecular & Translational Medicine, El Paso, TX, United States

Introduction: Cancer, the leading cause of death among US Hispanics, will increase its burden as this relatively young group ages and acculturates. It is important therefore to understand biological and behavioral risk factors and prevention behavior in this group. Despite ongoing efforts, Hispanics remain underrepresented in oncology studies.

Methods: The Hispanics of El Paso Cancer Cohort (HELP-CC) study was established as a longitudinal community-based cohort, in order to identify cancer risk factors (environmental, personal and biological), medical history and cancer screening behaviors relevant to cancer outcomes within a predominantly Mexican-American population. Recruitment was community–based and stratified by gender and SES. Variables collected included self-reported medical history, risk factors and screening behaviors, anthropometric measurements and collection of biological specimens. Consent was obtained for obtaining medical records and linkage to clinical information through the Texas Cancer Registry. Descriptive analysis of data was conducted among a sample of 195 adult males and females.

Results: Mean age was 59.82 (SD 8.994), 97.4% were Hispanic, 47.2% were uninsured. HELP-CC compared to the US general population for disease prevalence was: cardiovascular disease (46.2% vs 35.4%) and diabetes (23.1% vs 20.6%). For cancer risk factors obesity prevalence was (53.8% vs 39.6%) and current smoking status (9.7% vs 24.7%). Up to date cancer screening behaviors were: colorectal (27.1% vs 62.4%), cervical (20.8% vs 83.0%) and breast (71.2% vs 71.5%).

Conclusions: The HELP-CC profile was similar for disease prevalence and different for both cancer risk factors and cancer screening behaviors as compared to the adult US general population.

Investigating Disparities in Pancreatic Ductal Adenocarcinoma – The Significance of Latino Ethnicity on Clinical Outcomes

Andrea N. Riner[1], Patrick W. Underwood[1], Kai Yang[2], Kelly M. Herremans[1], Miles E. Cameron[1,3], Srikar Chamala[4], Peihua Qiu[2], Thomas J. George[5], Jennifer B. Permuth[6], Nipun B. Merchant[7], and Jose G. Trevino*[1]

[1]Department of Biostatistics, University of Florida College of Medicine, Gainesville, FL, USA

[2]Department of Physical Therapy, University of Florida College of Medicine, Gainesville, FL, USA

[3]Department of Pathology, Immunology and Laboratory Medicine, University of Florida College of Medicine, Gainesville, FL, USA

[4]Division of Hematology and Oncology, Department of Medicine, University of Florida College of Medicine, Gainesville, FL, USA

[5]Departments of Cancer Epidemiology and Gastrointestinal Oncology, Moffitt Cancer Center and Research Institute, Tampa, FL, USA

[6]Department of Surgery, University of Miami College of Medicine, Miami, FL, USA

Introduction: Disparities exist among patients with pancreatic ductal adenocarcinoma (PDAC). Non-White race is regarded as a negative predictor of expected treatment and overall survival. Data suggest Academic Research Programs (ARP) provide better outcomes for minorities, but ethnic/minority outcomes are underreported. We sought to determine if outcomes among diverse racial/ethnic patients with PDAC are influenced by treatment facility, with a focus on Hispanic subgroups.

Methods: The National Cancer Database identifies Latinos as Hispanics. NCDB identified 170,327 patients diagnosed with PDAC (2004–2015), including 8,341 Hispanics. Cox proportional-hazard regression was used to compare survival between race/ethnic groups across facilities.

Results: In unadjusted models, compared to Non-Hispanic Whites (NHW), Non-Hispanic Blacks (NHB) had the worst overall survival (HR = 1.05, 95% CI:1.03–1.06, $p < 0.001$) and Hispanics had the best overall survival (HR = 0.92, 95% CI:0.90–0.94, $p < 0.001$). After controlling for covariates, NHB (HR = 0.95, 95% CI:0.93–0.96, $p < 0.001$) had better overall survival compared to NHW, and Hispanics continued to have the best comparative outcomes (HR = 0.84, 95% CI:0.82–0.86, $p < 0.001$). Amongst Hispanics, Dominicans and South/Central Americans lived the longest, at 10.25 and 9.82 months, respectively. The improved survival in Hispanics was most pronounced at ARP (HR = 0.80, 95% CI:0.77–0.84, $p < 0.001$) and Integrated Network Cancer Programs (HR = 0.78, 95% CI:0.73–0.84, $p < 0.001$).

Conclusion: Hispanics with PDAC have better overall survival compared to Non-Hispanics at all treatment facilities. The most profound survival benefit amongst Hispanics is at ARP and INCP. Dominicans and South/Central Americans have the best comparative survival outcomes. Subtle differences in Hispanic patients' genome, microbiome, cultural, and psychosocial factors may alter the disease phenotype through the inflammatory response and tumor biology.

Racial and Ethnic Differences in Tobacco Product Use Patterns Among U.S. Adults: Findings from the National Adult Tobacco Survey, 2009–2014

Saida Coreas[1], Kristyn Kamke[2], Eliseo J. Pérez-Stable[1], Sherine El-Toukhy[2*]

[1]Division of Intramural Research, National Heart, Lung, and Blood Institute, National Institutes of Health Bethesda, MD, USA.

[2]Division of Intramural Research, National Institute on Minority Health and Health Disparities, National Institutes of Health Bethesda, MD, USA.

Introduction: With an evolving tobacco landscape, little is known about tobacco use patterns throughout adulthood, particularly in light of differential preferences of tobacco products by race and ethnicity that are established during adolescence.

Methods: Data came from 3 waves of the National Adult Tobacco Survey, 2009–2014. We used time-varying effect modeling on a nationally representative sample of adults ($N = 254,006$; age 18–65 years) to examine tobacco product use patterns (TPUPs) over age by race and ethnicity. TPUPs classify tobacco use based on number (single, dual, poly) and categories (cigarettes, noncigarette combustible (NCC), noncombustible (NC)) of tobacco products used, resulting in five mutually exclusive use patterns: cigarettes, NCCs, NCs, dual use and poly use. Regression coefficients were estimated for each TPUP among racial/ethnic groups as a non-parametric function of age.

Results: Between 2009 and 2014, cigarette use ranged from 12.1% to 13.4%, NC use from 1.9% to 2.6%, and cigarette and NC dual use from 0.8% to 2.4%. Compared to Whites, Latinos were less likely to be users of any TPUP throughout adulthood. Blacks were more likely than Whites to be NCC users in early adulthood (18 to 29), cigarette users by age 40, and poly users by age 50.

Conclusion: Despite their susceptibility to smoking during adolescence, Latino adults exhibited decreased prevalence of all TPUPs. Blacks exhibited elevated prevalence of cigarette, NCC use, and poly use. Tracking trends in TPUPs over age allows a timely implementation of tobacco product-specific cessation interventions to reduce cancer and non-cancer risks especially among minorities.

Latino Patients with Pancreatic Neuroendocrine Tumors: A Survival Analysis in the National Cancer Database

Patrick W. Underwood[1], Andrea N. Riner[1], Miles E. Cameron[1], Michael U. Maduka[1], Jose G. Trevino[1*]

[1]Department of Surgery, University of Florida College of Medicine, Gainesville, FL, USA

Introduction: Pancreatic neuroendocrine tumors (PNET) represent a rare, deadly form of pancreatic cancer. Health disparities have not been well described in this patient population. Latinos have been excluded from previous analyses. We hypothesize that health disparities exist in patients with PNETs.

Methods: The National Cancer Database (NCDB) defines Latino and Hispanic as equivalent. Hispanic will be used for consistency with the NCDB. Patients treated for PNETs were identified in the NCDB for the years 2004–2015. Kaplan-Meier analysis and Cox proportional hazards models were used to assess overall survival and covariates of survival, respectively.

Results: There were high rates of uninsured among Hispanic White (HW) and Hispanic Black (HB) patients compared to non-Hispanic, White (NHW) patients

($p < 0.001$). HW and HB were more often from zip codes with median income of <\$47,999 and >21% of the population without a high school degree compared to NHW ($p < 0.001$). Despite these differences, there was no significant difference in median survival between races. On multivariate analysis, greater age, male sex, lack of insurance, residence in a zip code with lower median income and lower percentage with high school degree, no surgical treatment, and higher stage were associated with worse survival. Race was not associated with survival.

Conclusion: Socioeconomic factors, but not race, are associated with survival in patients with PNETs. Latino patients represent a growing population in the United States and should be included in all analyses of health disparities.

Process Evaluation of a Culturally Targeted Video for Latinas About Hereditary Breast and Ovarian Cancer

Alejandra Hurtado-de-Mendoza*[1,2], Kristi Graves[1,2], Sara Gómez-Trillos[1,2], Pilar Carrera[3], Lyndsay Anderson[4], Claudia Campos[5], Beth N. Peshkin[1,2], Marc Schwartz[1,2], Paula Cupertino[6], George Luta,[1] Nathaly Gonzales[7], Andrés Gronda[1], Halyn Orellana,[1] Vanessa B. Sheppard[8]

[1]Department of Oncology, Georgetown University Medical Center, Washington, DC, USA

[2]Jess and Mildred Fisher Center for Hereditary Cancer and Clinical Cancer Genomics, Washington, DC, USA

[3]Department of Social Psychology and Methodology, Universidad Autónoma de Madrid, Ciudad Universitaria de Cantoblanco, Madrid, Spain

[4]College of Health and Human Services, School of Nursing, California State University, Sacramento, CA, USA

[5]Nueva Vida, DC Office, Alexandria, VA, USA

[6]Cancer Prevention and Control Program, John Theurer Cancer Center, Hackensack University Medical Center, Hackensack, NJ, USA

[7]Capital Breast Cancer Center, Washington, DC, USA

[8]Department of Health Behavior Policy, Virginia Commonwealth University, Richmond, VA, USA

Introduction: Genetic counseling and testing (GCT) can give life-saving information to individuals at risk for hereditary breast and ovarian cancer (HBOC). Latinas at risk HBOC have low awareness and low GCT uptake compared to non-Hispanic Whites (NHW). Few interventions address disparities for at-risk Latinas. Narratives are an effective method to communicate complex information for low literate populations. Transportation, identification with characters, and emotions are three mechanisms associated with the persuasive influence of narratives. The goal of this study was to evaluate the acceptability of a culturally targeted video about HBOC and

GCT as well as participants' transportation, identification with characters, and emotions elicited by the video.

Methods: 40 Latina immigrants at risk for HBOC watched the culturally targeted video. Using mixed methods, we assessed acceptability, transportation, identification with characters, and emotions using validated surveys and a semi-structured interview.

Results: Participants were 47 years old in average. The acceptability of the video was high ($M = 9.82$; SD = .41). Participants felt transported to the story ($M = 5.01$, SD = 0.91), felt highly identified with the main character ($M = 8.34$, SD = 1.74) and felt positive emotions ($M = 8.73$, SD = 1.48). Interviews revealed that participants liked the video, gained knowledge, felt empowered by the information learned, and would share it with family and friends. One participant said: "*It is something educational that also brings us peace of mind and helps us make decisions and prevent it.*"

Conclusions: The culturally targeted video is an acceptable intervention that can be easily disseminated and has the potential to reduce GCT disparities.

Examining the Knowledge of Tobacco Regulations and Tobacco Retail Practices Among Latino Independent Tobacco Retailers

Robert García[1]*, Patricia Escobedo[2], Rosa Barahona[2], Yaneth Rodriguez[2], Lourdes Baezconde-Garbanati[2]

[1]Texas A&M University, School of Public Health, College Station, TX, USA
[2]University of Southern California, Keck School of Medicine, Los Angeles, CA, USA

Introduction: The retail environment has been identified as an area that contributes to tobacco use disparities which also exacerbate the current burden of tobacco related cancers. Given the variability and complexity of tobacco regulations it can be expected that independent retailers are not knowledgeable of the new regulatory role of the Food and Drug Administration (FDA).

Methods: This project used community health workers to recruit 200 independent tobacco retailers from Latino communities in Los Angeles, CA. The participating retailers were interviewed and the CHW's also conducted store observations. The retailer interview addressed their knowledge of the FDA and tobacco policies, attitudes towards the FDA, and their perceived benefits of selling tobacco products. The observation addressed product availability and placement, presence of promotions, exterior ads, and regulatory materials.

Results: Less than half of the retailers were aware of the FDA's role in tobacco regulation. Nearly half of the retailers viewed cigarettes and cigarillos and financially beneficial to their store compared to only 7% for e-cigarettes. A little less than half of the retailers (47.5%) knew the regulatory role of the FDA but 66.3% believed they had the right to regulate tobacco products. A third of the retailers reported receiving regulatory information from the FDA. 23% of the retailers displayed price promotions for cigarettes and 20.3% displayed such promotions for menthol cigarettes.

Conclusions: The retail environment contributes to continued disparities in tobacco use. Outreach with racial/ethnic communities will be essential to increase retailers' and community buy-in to work towards reducing the burden of tobacco related cancers in linguistically and culturally diverse communities.

Delineate Disparity in Prostate Cancer Mortality Associated with Hispanic Ethnicity

Wang, Chen-Pin*[1], Schmidt Susanne[1], MacCarthy[1], Liss Michael[2]

[1]Department of Population Health Science, University Texas Health San Antonio, San Antonio, TX, USA

[2]Department of Urology, University Texas Health San Antonio, San Antonio, TX, USA

Introduction: Disparity in prostate cancer mortality that is attributed to Hispanic ethnicity remains understudied. This study identified significant risk factors underlying disparity in prostate cancer mortality associated with Hispanic ethnicity.

Methods: We identified a cohort of 129,100 nonBlack men diagnosed with prostate cancer at age of <65 years in the 2007–2014 Surveillance, Epidemiology, and End Results database. These data were linked to neighborhood socioeconomic variables from the American Community Survey and lifestyle variables from the Behavioral Risk Factor Surveillance System. A series of inverse propensity scores weights (IPSW) were incorporated in Cox regression analyses to allow varying adjustments for imbalances by Hispanic ethnicity regarding age at diagnosis, PSA level, Gleason score, stage, treatment, insurance, socioeconomic and behavioral variables.

Results: All-cause mortality (ACM) and prostate cancer mortality (PCM) rates were 5.5% and 3.1% for Hispanics, and 4.7% and 2.1% for non-Hispanics. Under fully-adjusted IPSW, there was no ethnic difference in ACM (HR = 0.98, $p = 0.34$); ethnic difference in treatment along with insurance or stage attributed to 7.1–8.2% increased ACM (HRs = 1.05–1.06, $p < 0.01$); ethnic difference in treatment, insurance, and stage jointly attributed to 26.5% increased ACM (HR = 1.24, $p < 0.001$).

Hispanic ethnicity was associated with 6% increase in PCM under fully-adjusted IPSW (HR = 1.06, p = 0.023). Age, treatment, stage, and insurance each individually or jointly attributed to 17–19% increased PCM disparity (HRs: 1.19–1.21, p < 0.001); socioeconomic and behavioral risk factors jointly attributed to additional 27% increase in PCM disparity (HR = 1.54, p < 0.001).

Conclusion: Disproportional prostate cancer mortality in Hispanics could be alleviated via access to health insurance, care, and lifestyle interventions.

Design and Development of a Bilingual Facebook Messenger Chat for Smoking Cessation

Patricia Chalela,[1] Alfred McAlister,[1] Edgar Muñoz,[1] Cliff Despres,[1] Sukumaran Pramod,[1] Illeana Tiemann,[1] Sahak Kaghyan,[2] David Akopian,[2] Amelie G. Ramirez[1]*
[1]University of Texas Health Science Center at San Antonio, San Antonio, TX, USA.
[2]University of Texas at San Antonio, San Antonio, TX, USA.

Introduction: Quitxt is a mobile phone texting system for smoking cessation promoted in via social media advertising. Quitxt results found a 21% cessation rate at 7 months, confirming that a text and mobile media service specifically designed for young adults provides a feasible, potentially cost-effective approach to promoting cessation. Quitxt is now being expanded to reach Latino, non-Latino white and African American young smokers.

Objective: We present the design and development process of a theory-based, bilingual, interactive Facebook Chat to promote smoking cessation among young adults.

Methods: We conducted focus groups (3) and an online survey (200 young adult smokers) to assess images, video testimonials, and messages for social media and updated webpages linked to in Quitxt text messages. Results informed the development of the Chat prototype, which is now active for recruitment.

Results: Formative research participants positively reviewed the images, messages, and videos, within the Quitxt mobile program, with the suggested addition of more information on negative consequences of smoking. Suggestions to improve the linked-to web content included adding more color and logos for credibility. Facebook was the most popular social media platform, making the Messenger Chat a viable, appropriate way to offer the program. This platform also enabled additional graphic content (gifs and memes) to make the messages more appealing to young adults.

Conclusions: We followed an iterative design process to develop a bilingual, culturally tailored and interactive Chat prototype to deliver our Quitxt smoking cessation program. The anticipated outcome is a scalable, evidence-based, easily disseminated smoking cessation intervention.

Bladder Cancer Incidence and Survival in the United States and Texas Non-Hispanic Whites and Hispanics

Shenghui Wu[1]*, Edgar Munoz[1]
[1]Department of Population Health Sciences, University of Texas Health San Antonio, San Antonio, TX, USA; *Corresponding author

Background: Bladder cancer (BC) poses an enormous burden on health care systems. Not included in the Surveillance, Epidemiology, and End Results (SEER) Program, Texas (TX) Hispanics make up one-fifth of the U.S. Hispanic population. No studies have examined the BC difference between TX and the U.S. for non-Hispanic Whites (NHW) and Hispanics. This study determined whether BC incidence and survival differ among U.S., Texas and South TX Hispanics and NHW.

Methods: Data were collected from the U.S. SEER Program, Texas Cancer Registry and Texas Department of State Health Services. Annual age-specific and age-adjusted BC incidence rates, annual incidence percent changes and 95% confidence intervals, and annual 5-year relative survival were calculated.

Results: Of the three Hispanic groups compared, South Texas Hispanics had the lowest and SEER Hispanics had the highest age-adjusted BC incidence rates. Of the three NHW groups compared, Texas NHW had the lowest and SEER NHW had the highest age-adjusted BC incidence rates. BC incidence significantly decreased over time among Hispanics and NHW in all three geographic groups. In contrast, South Texas Hispanics had the lowest and SEER Hispanics had the highest BC 5-year relative survival rates. Texas NHW had the lowest and SEER NHW had the highest BC 5-year relative survival rates.

Conclusion: South TX Hispanics had a lower BC incidence rate but a worse survival than TX and US SEER Hispanics. TX NHW had a lower BC incidence rate but a worse survival than South TX and US SEER NHW. The findings indicate future research directions.

Incidence of Hepatocellular Carcinoma (HCC) in Latinos in Texas, 2010–2015: A Follow-Up

Pramod Sukumaran[1], Edgar Munoz[1], Dimpy Shah[1], Aron Mathews[1], Patricia Chalela[1], Amelie G. Ramirez[1]

[1]Institute for Health Promotion Research, Department of Population Health Sciences, UT Health San Antonio, San Antonio, TX, USA

Our previous studies showed Hepatocellular Carcinoma (HCC) rates to be higher among Hispanic/Latinos in Texas and highest among South Texas Latinos compared to other non-Hispanic whites (NHW) and other Latinos in the United States (U.S.) (1,2). HCC age-adjusted incidence rates have almost tripled in U.S over the past 20 years (3). We used more recent data to assess trends in HCC among Texas Latinos and to reassess the elevated HCC incidence rate in Latinos in Texas and South Texas. We used data from the U.S. SEER Program and the Texas Cancer Registry. To calculate annual moving average age-specific and age-adjusted HCC incidence rates, annual percent changes (APCs), and their corresponding 95% confidence intervals for Latinos and NHW in the U.S., Texas and South Texas. We also used age-period-cohort models to identify patterns in cancer incidence in the region. The result suggested Texas Latino male and female incidence rates were 2.1 and 2.6 times higher than their NHW counterparts in SEER regions. Latino males and females in South Texas had the highest rates of HCC incidence overall; rate ratios were 2.6 and 2.5 times higher than their NHW counterparts. There are statistically significant increases in HCC incidence rates in all groups (Texas and South Texas Latinos and NHW groups) and across all age groups. The elevated HCC rates in Texas Latinos are consistent over the 2010–2015 period.

Appendix C: Emerging Latinos in Research Across the Cancer Continuum

Translation and Validation of the Pediatric Nausea Assessment Tool (PeNAT) for Use by Spanish-Speaking Children and Adolescents Receiving Chemotherapy

Erica Garcia Frausto[1,7]; Araby Sivananthan[2]; Carla Golden[3,8]; Molly Szuminski[3,8]; Luz Nereida, Perez Prado[4]; Mercedes Paloma Lopez[6]; Virginia Diaz[4,7]; Dominica Nieto[4,7]; Anne-Marie Langevin[4,7]*; L. Lee Dupuis[2,5]

[1]Methodist Hospital of South Texas, San Antonio, TX, USA
[2]Research Institute, SickKids, Toronto, ON, Canada
[3]Children's Hospital and Research Center at Oakland, Oakland, CA, USA
[4]UT Health San Antonio, San Antonio, TX, USA
[5]University of Toronto, Toronto, ON, Canada
[6]SWOG Cancer Research Network, Operations Office, San Antonio, TX, USA
[7]Texas Pediatric Minority Underserved NCORP
[8]Bay Area Tumor Institute NCORP

Background: The lack of a Spanish-validated Pediatric Nausea Assessment Tool (PeNAT) excluded Spanish-speaking children from antiemetics clinical trials.

Objective: Create a Spanish-language PeNAT with face validity among Hispanic-American children.

Methods: *Translation*: Forward and backward translations of the PeNAT documents (script, diary, and instructions) were performed. A bilingual panel verified the accuracy of all translated and back-translated documents. Four mono-lingual, Spanish-speaking dyads (child/parent) and 4 bilingual dyads piloted the Spanish-language PeNAT documents. Four additional bilingual dyads read both document versions and completed a diary page using their preferred version. Completed diary pages were reviewed for errors due to misunderstanding. *Face validity testing*: Children aged 4–18 yrs who spoke Spanish at home, were about to receive

© The Editor(s) (if applicable) and The Author(s) 2023
A. G. Ramirez, E. J. Trapido (eds.), *Advancing the Science of Cancer in Latinos*, https://doi.org/10.1007/978-3-031-14436-3

chemotherapy and were without impairments precluding PeNAT use were eligible. Participants used the Spanish-language PeNAT during a chemotherapy block. A co-investigator administered a standardized questionnaire to parents for feedback on the PeNAT documents (readability, clarity and ease of use). Recruitment continued in sets of 5 until at least 10 consecutive participants offered no substantive suggestions for revision.

Results: The panel changed the documents to improve cultural sensitivity. All child/parent dyads completed diary pages without errors attributable to misunderstanding. The Spanish-language PeNAT was preferred by 3 of 4 bilingual dyads. Ten patients (mean age: 10.6 yrs) used the Spanish-language PeNAT. All parents felt their child understood the PeNAT and none felt the documents were hard or very hard to use. Questionnaire responses led to no changes.

Conclusion: The Spanish-language PeNAT documents have face validity among Hispanic-American children.

First Hispanic/Latino Community Cancer Advisory Board for the Penn State Cancer Institute – Addressing Cancer Needs in Central Pennsylvania

Sol Rodríguez-Colón[1]*; Eugene J. Lengerich[1]; Marcela Diaz-Myers[2]
[1]Penn State Cancer Institute, Hershey, PA, US.
[2]WellSpan Community Health, York, PA, US.

Background: Though central Pennsylvania (PA) is not often recognized for a large Hispanic/Latino population, the number of Hispanic/Latinos increased 24% from 2010 (297,000) to 2017 (373,000). To reduce cancer burden, the Penn State Cancer Institute (PSCI), through the Office for Cancer Health Equity, established in 2018 the Hispanic/Latino Community Cancer Advisory Board (CAB).

Methods: Composed of 15 active community members, the CAB follows a bidirectional engagement approach co-chaired by a community and an academic member. The CAB's mission is to advise the PSCI on cancer or risk factors affecting Hispanic/Latinos; improve the care and health outcomes among Hispanic/Latinos; promote culturally appropriate care; help conduct outreach and education in the community; review PSCI's research protocols addressing the Hispanic/Latino community; and promote the participation of Hispanic/Latinos in research.

Results: In 2019, the CAB reviewed research grant submissions, facilitated the inclusion of Spanish-speakers in research, and modified and promoted the PSCI Community Health Assessment (CHA). The CAB also convened Hispanic/Latino-serving organizations to a June 2019 meeting to review cancer incidence and mortality among Hispanics/Latinos; learn about cancer-related research involving Hispanics/Latinos; review preliminary data the first 200 Hispanic/Latino CHA respondents; and set priorities for cancer prevention and control among Hispanics/ Latinos. In the concluding session, participants provided strong support and specific strategies for two community-based initiatives promoting cancer education, physical activity, and nutrition among Hispanic/Latinos.

Conclusions: The CAB is a bidirectional, community-based strategy with a strong potential to develop and disseminate initiatives to measurably reduce the burden of cancer among Hispanics/Latinos in central PA.

A Closer Look at Hispanics with Follicular Lymphoma: The UT Health San Antonio Experience

Michelle Janania Martinez[1], Tyler W Snedden[1], Juan F Garza[1], Prathibha Surapaneni[1], Snegha Ananth[2], Jeremy Rawlings[2], David J Gregorio[2], Sushanth Kakarla[1], Qianqian Liu[3], Joel E Michalek[3], Adolfo E Diaz[1]*

[1]Hematology-Oncology Division, Mays Cancer Center UT Health San Antonio MD Anderson, San Antonio, TX, USA

[2]Department of Internal Medicine, University of Texas Health San Antonio, San Antonio, TX, USA

[3]Department of Epidemiology and Biostatistics, University of Texas Health at San Antonio, San Antonio, TX, USA

Background: Follicular Lymphoma (FL) is the most common indolent non-Hodgkin-lymphoma (NHL); usually diagnosed in non-Hispanic (NH) and well characterized in this population. Hispanics (HI) are underrepresented with little data available. Our objective was to determine demographics/clinical characteristics of FL patients, comparing outcomes between HI/NH.

Methods: Identified 616 Lymphoma patients; retrospectively analyzed 123 FL (seen 2008–2018). Continuously distributed outcomes were summarized with mean/standard deviation; categorical outcomes with frequencies/percentages. One-way-ANOVA assessed significance of mean variation with disease category; Pearson's Chi Square or Fisher's Exact test assessed significance of categorical outcome associations.

Results: Identified 123 FL, 71-HI (58%), 49-NH (40%), 3-unspecified (2%). 88% Caucasian, 5% African American, 4% Asian, 3% other. Median age 56.31. Females 56%, males 44%. Funding: commercial $N = 55$ (45%), Medicare $N = 40$ (33%), hospital-payment-plan $N = 20$ (16%), unfunded $N = 5$ (4%), Medicaid $N = 3$ (2%). Prevalent co-morbidities HTN $N = 49$ (40%) and diabetes mellitus $N = 24$ (20%); 40% no co-morbidities ($N = 49$). ECOG 0–1 in 116 (94%); 21 Stage-I (17%), 19

Stage-II (15%), 40 Stage-III (33%), 43 Stage-IV (35%). FLIPI 0–1 in 43 (35%), 2 in 32 (26%), 3 in 23 (19%).

Median PFS 1287.10. At 3 years: complete/partial response in 40-HI (76%) vs 27-NH (84%); progression 10 (19%) vs 4 (13%); death 3 (6%) vs 1 (3%), respectively (p-value = 0.739). At 5-years: complete/partial response in 32 HI (76%) vs 25 (86%); disease progression in 6 (14%) vs 3 (10%); death 4 (10%) vs 1 (3%), respectively (p-value = 0.62). At end of 2018, 44-HI (88%) were alive vs 36-NH (95%), [p-value = 0.457].

Conclusion: Within limitation of sample, in our prevalently HI population, HI with FL have no statistically significant difference in outcome compared to NH. To our knowledge this is the largest cohort of FL from a single institution serving primarily HI.

State of Recent Literature on Communication About Cancer Genetic Testing Among Latinx Populations

Daniel Chavez-Yenter[1,2*], Kimberly Kaphingst[1,2]
[1]University of Utah, Department of Communication, Salt Lake City, UT, USA
[2]Huntsman Cancer Institute, Cancer Control & Population Science, Salt Lake City, UT, USA

Background: Cancer Genetic Testing (CGT) among Latinx communities is notably lower than White counterparts, and approaches to address this disparity are needed. Communication about CGT may affect differences in utilization of these technologies. This project was to examine the recent research on communication about CGT among Latinx populations.

Methods: A comprehensive literature review of six databases identified English-language articles related to communication about CGT published between January 2010 and January 2017. Broad search terms included cancer, genetic/genomic communication, provider/direct-to-consumer, and patient/public. A total of 513 manuscripts were identified; for the current study, only studies with over 50% Latinx representation were assessed.

Results: 13 of the 513 papers (2.5%) had over 50% Latinx representation; in nine of these (69.2%) had fully Latinx comprised study cohorts. The majority of identified studies ($n = 9$) were conducted to assess knowledge and attitudes regarding CGT. Qualitative and quantitative designs were used equally, with 5 studies having a mixed method design. Most of the studies ($n = 9$) examined psychosocial outcomes. Only 4 studies used existing theoretical frameworks in designing their studies.

Conclusion: There is a critical need for Latinx representation within research on communication about CGT. We also found a need to incorporate theory into future studies. While a few studies did incorporate theoretical frameworks into their design, none elected to develop their own theory specific to Latinx communities. These findings therefore highlight substantial gaps in the literature on communication about CGT and opportunities for future research.

Sociocultural Factors of Cancer Clinical Trial Recruitment and Multidisciplinary Team Recruitment of Latin-American Patients in Mexico, Peru and Colombia

David Isla[1*], Robert Krouse[2*], Alejandro Mohar[1], Alberto Leon[1*], Marco Sanchez[3], Oscar Guevara[4], Mercedes Lopez[5], Gabriela Mora[1], Ninoska Macavilca[3], Carolina Carrillo[4]

[1]Instituto Nacional de Cancerología (INCan), Mexico City, Mexico
[2]University of Pennsylvania, Philadelphia, PA, USA
[3]Instituto Nacional de Enfermedades Neoplasicas (INEN), Lima, Perú
[4]Instituto Nacional de Cancerologia, Bogotá, Colombia
[5]SWOG Operations Office, San Antonio, TX, USA

Background: Protocol SWOG S1316: PROSPECTIVE COMPARATIVE EFFECTIVENESS TRIAL FOR MALIGNANT BOWEL OBSTRUCTION is currently active and recruiting patients to their randomized arm in three Latin-American sites; Mexico, Peru and Colombia. The patient recruitment to the protocol has uncovered important differences in patient accrual patterns. Aside from regulatory barriers to participation, sociocultural factors have played a two-fold role in patient recruitment in Latin-America.

Purpose: Identify the main factors that determine this difference. Cultural, social and economic factors can be observed in all three sites. The economic support of patients when included in protocols and the integration of the research staff have also been important factors to note in this process.

Methods: Metrics include: accounting of patients recruited by the before mentioned institutions, description of process during the integration of the research staff, comparison in cultural differences, socioeconomic levels and factors surrounding the patients, access to the type of medical care (private, by insurance, by own means, by the government), process for obtaining the informed written consent for participation. From these data, we can have the proportion of patients randomized versus not randomized by institute and country, as well as the main differences which could influence in these results.

Results: The protocol has reached 96% of the planned accrual. All Latin-American patients have opted for randomization. Mexico recruited 8 randomized patients; Peru has recruited 6 randomized patients and Colombia registered their first patient recently. All sites continue to recruit successfully and have a multidisciplinary mechanism in place to reach accrual goals.

HPV/Cervical Cancer Health Disparities Among South Texas Hispanics

Andrew Olguin[1], Bertha Flores[1*], Martha Martinez[1], Lyda Arrevalo-Flechas[1,3]
[1]University of Texas Health San Antonio, San Antonio, TX
[2]University of Texas at Austin, Austin, TX, USA
[3]South Texas Veterans Health Care System/Geriatrics and Extended Care Service, San Antonio, TX, USA

Introduction: The human papillomavirus (HPV) is the most common sexually transmitted infection (STI) in the United States, with over 80 million Americans infected and 15 million new cases each year. HPV is known to cause cervical, oropharyngeal, anal, penile, vaginal, and vulvar cancers. Though, through the use of the HPV vaccine, cervical cancer can be essentially eradicated as it has a near 100% effectiveness against the strains of HPV that cause it. However, there is a significant lack of HPV vaccinations and cervical cancer screenings among the South Texas Hispanic population.

Aim: This study's aim is to investigate the links between language, culture, location, financial stipulations, and HPV vaccinations and cervical cancer screenings among the Hispanic population in the South Texas community.

Methods: Qualitative and quantitative data was collected through the use of focus groups and surveys in South Texas. This mixed method study is beneficial to gaining a wider perspective on the disparities for this unique population.

Conclusion: Many participants report there was difficulty navigating scientific knowledge and expected Hispanic cultural norms. Typical Hispanic gender identities, such as machismo and marianismo, were noted to contribute to the lack of knowledge regarding this health concern. Suggestions for promoting education throughout the local community include involving multi-generational education, including males in cervical cancer prevention education, providing incentives to the community to participate in educational programs, and beginning prevention education at an earlier age. The researchers intend to gather more data and work with community health workers to create a new intergenerational family-oriented educational program for the South Texas Hispanic population.

Feasibility and Reliability of a Self-Administered Geriatric Assessment Tool for Spanish-Speaking Older Women with Breast Cancer

Jessica Vazquez[1*], Enrique Soto-Perez-de-Celis[1,2], Heeyoung Kim[1], Canlan Sun[1], Yuan Yuan[1], James Waisman[1], George Somlo[1], Joanne Mortimer[1], Lesley Taylor[1], Laura Kruper[1], Niki Patel[1], Jeanine Moreno[1], Kemeberly Charles[1], Elsa Roberts[1], Ashley Celis[1], Jennifer Liu[1], Carolina Uranga[1], Vani Katheria[1], Dale Mitani[1], Daneng Li[1], William Dale[1], Arti Hurria[1,] Mina S. Sedrak[1]

[1]City of Hope Comprehensive Cancer Center, Duarte, CA USA

[2]Instituto Nacional de Ciencias Medicinas y Nutricion Salvador Zubiran, Mexico City, Mexico

Background: By 2060, 25% of older adults in the US will identify as Hispanic/Latino. The geriatric assessment (GA) developed by Hurria and colleagues has demonstrated success in predicting cancer treatment toxicity and survival of older adults, however, the feasibility and reliability of administering this tool among Spanish-speaking older adults with cancer has not been tested.

Methods: Spanish-speaking women with breast cancer $\geq$ 65 years completed the validated Spanish GA twice on the same day. Completion rate, average completion time, rating of difficulty, and proportion of patients needing assistance were used as indicators of feasibility. Spearman's correlation coefficient was used to assess for test-retest reliability.

Results: Of the 211 patients approached, 86% ($n = 181$) agreed to participate. 177 participants completed the GA at least once. Median age was 70 y (range 65–95) and 54% had $\leq$8th grade education. 41% ($n = 73$) were unable to complete the GA on their own; median completion time was 28 min (range 8–90); and 23% ($n = 41$) rated the GA as difficult/very difficult. The most common reason for needing assistance was difficulty understanding questions (37%). Patients with $\leq$8th grade education took longer to complete the GA (median 30 vs 25 min, $p = 0.0036$), and needed more assistance (59% vs 19%, $p < 0.001$) than those with $\geq$9th grade education. Test–retest reliability was high ($r \geq 0.81$) for all scales except social activity (0.73).

Conclusion: Delivering the GA among Spanish-speaking older adults is feasible and reliable. Low educational level may be a predictor for a patient requiring assistance to complete the GA.

Potential Meets Opportunity: Capacity Building Through *ÉXITO*

Cordero, J., I.[1,2*] Moya, E., M.[3], Ramirez, A., G.[4], Aragones, A.[5]

[1]Border Biomedical Research Center (BBRC), University of Texas at El Paso at El Paso, El Paso, TX, USA

[2]Department of Health Promotion and Behavioral Sciences, The University of Texas Health Science Center at Houston, School of Public Health, El Paso, TX, USA

[3]Department of Social Work, College of Health Sciences, University of Texas at El Paso, El Paso, TX, USA

[4]Institute for Health Promotion Research, Mays Cancer Center, University of Texas Health San Antonio, San Antonio, TX, USA

[5]Department of Psychiatry & Behavioral Sciences, Memorial Sloan Kettering Cancer Center, Immigrant Health & Cancer Disparities Service, New York, NY, USA

Background: Éxito! Latino Cancer Research Leadership Training program engages Latinos in academia-based cancer control research, the only Latino training program focused on doctoral-level preparation in population sciences. *Approach*-Éxito supported an alumni's Human papillomavirus (HPV)-associated cancer prevention research internship in El Paso, TX. Hypothesis-Project will enhance current and future HPV prevention initiatives in the region through engagement in academia-based community cancer research (ABCCR). Objectives-(1) contribute to current initiatives of EdTech-HPV project; (2) contribute to future HPV prevention efforts as team member on U54 interdisciplinary grant submission; (3) provide research/impact report of project informed by community-based participatory research (CBPR) framework. Goals-(1) further establish partnerships and understanding among local university students/alumni and faculty; (2) collaborate with community organizations currently engaged in cancer prevention efforts; (3) lessen disparities associated with acquiring an HPV infection through ABCCR. PURPOSE-To engage in CBPR using culturally appropriate empowerment interventions targeting cancer prevention, sexual and reproductive health, and health services navigation.

Methods: Mix-methods CBPR data collected from internship (June–November 2018) through community engagement, program reporting, and translational research efforts on parent grant contributions.

Results: EdTech-HPV – recruitment efforts increased (141%); follow-ups increased (778%) over 3-month span

- U54 grant – submission (November 2018); grant awarded (7/2019); BBRC PhD Research Associate (2019–2024)
- Éxito report – completed (December 2018); doctoral application (12/2018); acceptance (2/2019)

Discussion: ABCCR provides a pipeline to engage students, faculty, community with similar goals to collectively engage in sustainable community health protection efforts.

- Results from this project are expected to enhance current capacity-building initiatives to engage and support minority researchers by illustrating possible opportunities and challenges when engaging in academia-based research.

Familismo and *Espíritu*: Protective Cultural Values for Latino/a Adolescents and Young Adults Coping with Parental Cancer

Amanda M. Marín-Chollom
    Central Connecticut State University, New Britain, CT, USA

Background: Parental cancer has a strong influence on the psychological well-being of children at all ages. Children from the U.S. Latino/a population may face additional challenges, such as, discrimination, that compounds the stress of having a parent with cancer. At the same time, facets of the Latino/a culture may play a crucial role in how Latino/a adolescents adapt to parental cancer, specifically the Latino/a cultural values of *familismo* (familism), and *espíritu* (spirit).

Methods: This cross-sectional study examined the relation of Latino/a cultural values to coping and psychological adjustment among 38 adolescents and young adults (AYAs) whose mother had breast cancer. AYAs completed questionnaires in-person or by mail.

Results: Results from Generalized Estimating Equation (GEE) analyses demonstrated that stress appraisals and the coping responses of secondary control and disengagement were positively correlated with symptoms of depression and anxiety. A protective pattern of the Latino/a values (*familismo* and *espíritu*) against symptoms of anxiety and depression was evident from the interaction of the values with stress appraisals and coping responses.

Conclusions: The findings suggest that Latino/a AYAs whose parents have cancer experience significant psychological distress, but those with higher levels of *familismo* and *espíritu* may fare better than those with lower levels. The findings suggest that psychosocial interventions for Latino/a AYAs with parental cancer should incorporate or strengthen these values.

Health Literacy Among Spanish-Language Preferring Latino Patients Enrolled in a Colorectal Cancer Screening Pilot Randomized Controlled Trial

Shannon M. Christy[1,2*], Steven K. Sutton[1,2], Enmanuel A. Chavarria[3], Rania Abdulla[1], Julian Sanchez,[1,2] Diana Lopez,[4] Clement K. Gwede[1,2], & Cathy D. Meade[1,2]

[1]H. Lee Moffitt Cancer Center and Research Institute, Tampa, FL, USA
[2]University of South Florida, Tampa, FL, USA
[3]University of Texas Health Science Center at Houston, Brownsville Regional Campus, Brownsville, TX, USA
[4]Suncoast Community Health Centers, Inc., Brandon, FL, USA

Background: Cultural background, language, and literacy are factors that may impact access, healthcare utilization, and cancer screening behaviors. This study examined associations between health literacy (HL) and health beliefs among patients receiving care at federally-qualified health care centers in Southwest Florida.

Methods: Participants ($N = 76$) self-identified as Hispanic/Latino, preferred health information in Spanish, were 50–75 years old, at average colorectal cancer (CRC) risk, not up-to-date with CRC screening, and enrolled in a CRC screening trial. Sociodemographic characteristics, health beliefs, and HL were assessed at baseline. HL was measured with two self-report items, assessing confidence in completing health forms and frequency of difficulty reading written materials. HL responses were dichotomized (very confident vs. less than very confident and always difficult vs. not always difficult, respectively).

Results: Most participants were female (67.1%), born outside of the U.S. (93.4%), and had less than a high school education (61.8%). The majority (52.6%) reported difficulty with written health information and 25% reported low confidence with completing health forms. Difficulty in understanding written materials was significantly associated with higher cancer worry ($p = .02$) and higher religious beliefs ($p = .03$). None of the health beliefs were significantly associated with confidence in completing health forms, although religious beliefs was marginally significant ($p = .09$).

Conclusion: Findings highlight the importance of delivering clear health information through multiple methods and in preferred language. Difficulty in understanding written health information was associated with multiple health beliefs, which informs content, language, and design features of future CRC screening interventions.

E-Cigarette Perceptions, Marketing and Availability Among Tobacco Retailers in Low-Income Communities in California

Patricia Escobedo[1]*, Robert Garcia[2], Claradina Soto[1], Yaneth Rodriguez[1], Rosa Barahona[1], Lourdes Baezconde-Garbanati[1]

[1]Department of Preventive Medicine, University of Southern California, Los Angeles, CA, USA

[2]Health Science Center School of Public Health, Texas A&M University College Station, College Station, TX, USA

Background: Given the recent surge in e-cigarette use among adolescents and adults, it is imperative to assess tobacco retailer awareness of e-cigarette products and examine e-cigarette availability and marketing within vulnerable, lower-income ethnic communities.

Methods: Retail stores on American Indian (AI) Tribal lands in California and retail stores in low-income African American (AA), Hispanic/Latino (H/L), Korean (K), Non-Hispanic White (NHW) communities in Southern California were recruited to complete 800 in-person retailer interviews and 775 store observations from January 2016 to January 2017. Retailer interviews and store observations were conducted by community health workers and promotores de salud who reflected the ethnicity of each ethnic community.

Results: Interview findings indicate that retailers in NHW communities were most likely to be asked to sell e-cigarette products (50%), were most likely to report that e-cigarettes were safer than combustible cigarettes (20%) and were most likely to sell e-cigarette products (70%). The lowest priced e-cigarette products ($1.99) were found in the NHW and AA communities. Retail stores in NHW (17%) and AI (14%) were most likely to sell e-cigarette products placed within 12 inches of toys and candy, while retailers in NHW (16%) communities had were more likely to have storefront e-cigarette advertising.

Conclusions: Findings indicate differences in e-cigarette perceptions, availability and marketing by ethnic community. In addition, placement of products and marketing that expose youth to e-cigarettes within the retail environment should be restricted and regulated by tobacco regulatory agencies to reduce the burden of cancer and other tobacco-related diseases among vulnerable populations.

Central American Immigrant Parents' Awareness of the HPV Vaccine and Interest in Participating in HPV-Related Cancer Education and Prevention Research: A Study Conducted in Two New England States

Joanna Pineda[1*], Madelyne J. Valdez[1*], Sherrie F. Wallington[2], Ana Cristina Lindsay[1]

[1]University of Massachusetts–Boston, College of Nursing and Health Sciences, Boston, MA, USA.

[2]George Washington University School of Nursing and Milken Institute School of Public Health, Washington, DC, USA.

Objective: Despite increasing interest in understanding factors influencing awareness and acceptability of the human papilloma virus (HPV) vaccine among Latinx parents, to date limited information is available specific to Central American (CA) immigrant parents living in the United States (U.S.).

Methods: Cross-sectional survey assessing CA parents' awareness of the HPV infection and the HPV vaccine, HPV information sources, and interest in participating in HPV-related cancer education and prevention research.

Results: Fifty-three CA, majority immigrant (94%; $n = 51$) parents completed the survey in Spanish (100%, $n = 53$). Approximately 45% ($n = 26$) were from El Salvador, 27.5% ($n = 14$) from Guatemala, 23.5% ($n = 12$) from Honduras, and 2% ($n = 1$) from Panama. Approximately 55% ($n = 29$) of the sample was female, approximately 77% ($n = 41$) was married, and parents' mean age was 43.2 years (SD = 6.4). Although the majority of the parents reported being aware of the HPV infection (81.1%, $n = 43$), only about 70% ($n = 37$) reported being aware of the HPV vaccine, and only about 64% ($n = 34$) reported their son or daughter aged 11–19 years of age receiving at least one dose of the HPV vaccination. Fewer fathers than mothers were aware of the HPV vaccine (58.3%; $n = 14$ vs. 79.4%, $n = 23$; $p = 0.45$). Of those parents who were aware of the HPV vaccine ($n = 36$), only about 67% ($n = 24$) reported hearing about the HPV vaccine from their child's physician. Additionally, about 90% ($n = 48$) reported interest in participating in a future HPV-related cancer prevention research.

Conclusion: Findings indicate parents' low to moderate awareness of the HPV vaccine, and high interest in participating in HPV-related cancer prevention and education research. These findings serve as a valuable first step toward building a knowledge foundation needed for developing future studies and interventions targeting CA immigrant parents living in the U.S.

Understanding the Cancer Prevention Needs of the Western New York Puerto Rican Hispanic Community: The Puentes (Bridges) Study

Elisa M. Rodriguez*, Melany Garcia, Isnory Colon, Jomary Colon
  Roswell Park Comprehensive Cancer Center, Buffalo, NY, USA

Puerto Ricans (PR) demonstrate a more marked cancer burden in comparison to other Hispanic subgroups and are the second largest Hispanic subgroup in the U.S. residing predominantly in the Northeast. In Western New York (WNY) two-thirds of the Hispanic population is of PR birth or parentage, and resides in urban as well as rural areas bordering part of Appalachia. The focus of this pilot-study was to conduct a community-based assessment to define the cancer health education needs and concerns among the PRs in WNY to inform, develop, and aide in the implementation and dissemination of relevant cancer-related education, services, interventions, and research opportunities using preferred communication platforms. A mixed-methods design including standardized survey items and semi-structured questions was used to gain a deeper understanding. Univariate analyses were used to describe and summarize quantitative data and identify patterns. The analytic sample comprised 60 participants and approximately 88% were born in Puerto Rico. Overall, 57% reported Spanish as the language spoken at home and an income <$20,000. Over 80% are overweight or obese and >60% indicated liking to eat at fast food restaurants. Close to 73% have not discussed their cancer risk with a doctor and 42% perceive their cancer risk to be the same as others. Most own a smart phone (90%) and have internet access on their cell phone or mobile device. Survey results demonstrate high cell phone usage suggesting potential feasibility and opportunity to disseminate targeted information to increase awareness of cancer-related services and research among this at-risk group.

Florida Pancreas Collaborative: Addressing the Underrepresented Needs for Latinos with Pancreatic Cancer

Michael U. Maduka[1], Patrick W. Underwood[1], Andrea N. Riner[1], Miles E. Cameron[1], Shraddha Vyas[2], Kaleena B. Dezsi[2], Nipun B. Merchant[3], Jennifer B. Permuth[2], Jose G. Trevino[1]*
  [1]University of Florida College of Medicine, Gainesville, FL, USA
  [2]Moffitt Cancer Center and Research Institute, Tampa, FL, USA
  [3]University of Miami College of Medicine, Miami, FL, USA

Background: Health disparities in pancreatic cancer (PC) exist and Latino patients are often underrepresented in these studies. Florida is one of the most diverse states in the country and is home to 8% of all Latinos in the United States. We aimed to build a statewide collaborative with other institutions in the state of Florida to increase access to tissues, biofluids, images, and data from a diverse patient population for health disparities research.

Methods: The Florida Pancreas Collaborative (FPC) was established between the University of Florida, Moffitt Cancer Center, and the University of Miami to develop a centralized tissue and data bank for Florida's diverse population. Tumor, muscle, blood, images, and clinical data is centralized for the 14 participating centers. These biospecimens are used to create patient-derived cell lines and preclinical models. Muscle and adipose tissue, CT scans, and blood will be analyzed to evaluate the presence and severity of cancer cachexia.

Results: The FPC has recruited 14 institutions from around the state, with several sites expected to primarily enroll Latino patients. To date, 175 patients have been enrolled. Of 29 Latino patients that were approached, 29 met inclusion/exclusion criteria and 28 ultimately enrolled in this study (96.5% participation rate). Biospecimens and clinical data have been collected for the majority of these cases.

Conclusion: The FPC has successfully established infrastructure to aid in studying cancer health disparities. The large and centralized tissue bank will help improve understanding of biological mechanisms that may lead to racial disparities in PC.

The SWOG Latin America Initiative Is a Long-Standing Effort to Achieve Latino Inclusion to Cancer Clinical Trials and Building a Culture for Research in Latin America

John Crowley[1]*, Curt Malloy[1], Alejandro Mohar[2]*, Gabriela Mora[2], Mercedes Lopez[3], Sarah Basse[4]
[1]SWOG Statistics and Data Management Center, Seattle, WA, USA
[2]Instituto Nacional de Cancerología, Mexico City, DF, Mexico
[3]SWOG Cancer Research Network, San Antonio, TX, USA
[4]Fred Hutchinson Cancer Research Center, Seattle, WA, USA

Background: The SWOG Latin America Initiative (SLAI) was founded in 2009. Since its founding, the cancer institutes of Mexico, Colombia, Peru, Chile and Uruguay have signed on as members, and more than 500 researchers in those countries have taken part in biostatistics and SWOG clinical trials training courses.

Purpose: Identify clinical research opportunities, particularly for cancers with a pathogenesis of infection and inflammation. Establish a long-term commitment to excellence in clinical research including best practices in study design, data collection and management amongst physician investigators, Clinical Research Associates, and Ph.D. level statisticians in Latin America; Organize and assist in development of a strong set of institutions in Latin America that can attract continuous funding for an independent and sustainable Latin American Cancer Cooperative Group.

Methods: Metrics of success for SLAI include, first and foremost, patient participation in SWOG trials. Metrics maintained by SLAI staff demonstrate our progress in increase engagement and participation, amongst both our collaborators in Latin America as well as Investigators in the United States.

Results: To date, the initiative has led to the enrollment of 621 trial participants. As members become more integrated into SWOG's network, they can open more trials at their national cancer centers. We have noted a 91% increase in US investigator interest in Latin America. Currently the SLAI Core Group is evaluating and submitting inclusions to nine viable active studies and evaluating international participation in two studies in development.

Elevated Cortisol Levels and Abnormal Stress Reactivity Among Rural Latina Breast Cancer Survivors: Nuevo Amanecer-II

Cathy Samayoa*[1,2], Jasmine Santoyo-Olsson[3], Anita L. Stewart[2,4], Leticia Márquez-Magaña[1], Anna Maria Nápoles[5]

[1]Health Equity Research Lab, Department of Biology, San Francisco State University, San Francisco, CA, USA

[2]Center for Aging in Diverse Communities, University of California San Francisco, San Francisco, CA, USA

[3]Division of General Internal Medicine, Department of Medicine, University of California San Francisco, San Francisco, CA, USA

[4]Institute for Health and Aging, University of California San Francisco, San Francisco, CA, USA

[5]National Institute on Minority Health and Health Disparities, National Institutes of Health, Bethesda, MD, USA

Background: Latinas experience breast cancer health disparities in disease free survival, health-related quality of life, and rates of depression and anxiety which may be a result of experiences of chronic stress. Chronic stress impacts the hypothalamic pituitary adrenal (HPA) axis, resulting in cortisol dysregulation that is predictive of breast cancer survival. However, cortisol profiles among rural, Spanish-speaking Latina breast cancer survivors (LBCS) are poorly characterized due to their lack of inclusion in biomedical research.

Methods: This study reports on baseline biological stress measures in rural LBCS enrolled in a RCT to test the effectiveness of a stress management intervention. Community-based participatory research methods and participant-centered recruitment and collection strategies were used to obtain biospecimens for cortisol analysis. Mean hair cortisol concentration (HCC) was used to assess chronic stress and a cortisol awakening response (CAR) measure was used to assess stress reactivity.

Results: Participants (n = 103) were recruited from two rural communities in California who participated in the parent RCT, Nuevo Amanecer-II. Mean age was 56 years, mean years since diagnosis was 2.7 years, 78% had a high school education or less, and 37% reported financial hardship. Cortisol analysis revealed an elevated mean HCC level of 362.9 pg/mg and an abnormal CAR in 37% of participants.

Conclusion: Rural Latina breast cancer survivors demonstrate high levels of biological stress and abnormal patterns of cortisol secretion, implicating these molecular mechanisms in long-term survival disparities experienced by this high-risk population. Interventions that regulate cortisol have the potential to improve disease-free survival for rural LBCS.

Qualitative Exploration of Family Influences on Physical Activity in Latino Households

John JC[*1], Heredia NI[1], McNeill LH[1], Hoelscher D[2], Schembre S[3], Lee MJ[2], Reininger B[2], Strong LL[1]
[1]The University of Texas MD Anderson Cancer Center, Houston, TX, USA
[2]The University of Texas Health Science Center, Houston, TX, USA
[3]The University of Arizona Health Sciences, Tucson, AZ, USA

Background: Given that the Latino culture strongly emphasizes the importance of the family unit, further research should explore how the family unit can support healthy physical activity (PA) habits. This qualitative study explored family influences on PA in adult Latino dyads to inform the adaptation of a family-focused intervention to promote PA in Houston Latino families.

Methods: We interviewed 20 dyads (n = 40) comprised of adult Latino family members from the same household. Interviews were audio-recorded, transcribed, and translated into English by an outside vendor. Two researchers coded text separately using NVivo 11, met to discuss findings, and reconciled differences. A general inductive approach guided the discovery of themes related to household influences on PA.

Results: Participants were mainly women (70%), from Mexico (61.5%), and from parent-child (50%) and spousal/partner (40%) dyads. The most common family-level facilitators for PA were emotional encouragement, exercising with someone, and child-driven PA, while the most frequently reported PA barriers were family negative attitudes, lack of family support, and competing household responsibilities. We observed that parent-child dyads were more likely than spousal/partner dyads to give positive examples for how their study partners could help them achieve PA. We also discovered that most women preferred instrumental support (e.g. exercising together, help with responsibilities) from their study partners, while most men thought advice/suggestions from study partners were more helpful for PA engagement.

Conclusions: Behavioral interventions should consider the role of the family environment and different types of support (emotional, instrumental and informational) in promoting healthy PA behaviors.

Cervical and Colorectal Cancer Screening Compliance in Mexican-Born and Non-Mexican-Born Hispanics

Ergueen Herrera[1], Bianca Luna-Lupercio[1,2], Yu-Chen Lin[1], Christie Y. Jeon[1], Robert W. Haile[1], Zul Surani[1*]

[1]Cedars-Sinai Medical Center, Research Center for Health Equity, Los Angeles, CA, USA

[2]University of Southern California, Dornsife College of Letters, Arts and Sciences, Los Angeles, CA, USA

Background: Colorectal cancer (CRC) and cervical cancer (CVC) are the second and seventh most common cancers in Hispanics, respectively. Hispanics are less likely to undergo CRC and CVC screening tests than non-Hispanic populations. Predominant reasons for avoiding pap test (PT) and stool-based test or colonoscopy (SBTC) are fear of results, uncomfortable sensation, and lack of knowledge. Prevention guidelines supporting CVC and CRC screening for Hispanic subpopulations are lacking and may impact screening compliance.

Methods: Participants were recruited through different churches in Los Angeles as part of the Cedars-Sinai Cancer Health and Faith Initiative. The survey was administered to Latinos, a total of 177 surveys were collected. People who reported born in the US ($n = 34$) were excluded, this report includes age eligible participants. Qualifying participants included ages 45–75 for CRC screening and women ages 21–65 for CVC screening.

Results: MBW ($n = 49$), and NMBW ($n = 38$) shared similar experiences not having PT (22%, 16% respectively). Likewise, 67% of MB ($n = 30$) participants had never received SBTC, while 50% of NMB ($n = 26$) hadn't.

Conclusion: Differences in rates for the never screened for CRC and CVC have been observed in Los Angeles among both groups. Compliance rates among the MB and NMB are about the same, however the MB has a higher never screened rate than NMB, for CRC. Among the CVC, NMBW have a higher compliance and lower for never screened rate, compared to MBW. A prospective study examining the benefit of both screening with tailored compliance guidelines for Hispanic is suggested.

Developing Bridges to Genetics Services for Latinos: Initial Outcomes of the ÁRBOLES Familiares Training Program

Katherine Lopez[1], Laura Moreno[2], Jennifer Garcia[2], Jennifer Ulloa[3], Katie Fiallos[4], and Charité Ricker[5], Alejandra Hurtado-de-Mendoza[1], Larisa Caicedo[6], Lina Jandorf[3], Susan Vadaparampil[2*] and Kristi D. Graves[1*]
[1]Lombardi Comprehensive Cancer Center, Georgetown University
[2]Moffitt Cancer Center
[3]Icahn School of Medicine at Mount Sinai
[4]Sidney Kimmel Comprehensive Cancer Center, Johns Hopkins University
[5]University of Southern California, Keck School of Medicine
[6]CS Consulting, LLC.

Introduction: Gaps exist in the use of genetics services among Latinos at high risk for hereditary breast and ovarian cancer syndrome (HBOC). Barriers include low awareness and lack of referrals and access. We developed the ÁRBOLES Familiares (Family Tree) training program to educate bilingual community outreach and education professionals about HBOC. We sought to increase knowledge; self-efficacy and skills related to identification and referral of high-risk Latinos to appropriate genetics services.

Methods: ÁRBOLES Familiares is a 4-month training program that includes a 2-day in-person workshop and 8 online learning sessions. We assessed trainee HBOC knowledge, self-efficacy and behaviors at baseline, immediately post-training, 6- and 12 months post-training.

Results: 86 trainees have completed ÁRBOLES thus far. Mean age was 42.2 years (SD 14.3), 72% were born in Latin America. To date, 16 trainees have completed the 12-month follow up (66% retention of pilot cohort). HBOC knowledge increased from baseline ($M = 6.2$, SD = 1.9) to 12 months ($M = 7.8$, SD = 1.1), $t = 2.70$, $p < .016$. Self-efficacy increased from baseline ($M = 4.5$, SD = 1.2) to 12 -months ($M = 8.2$, SD = 1.2), $t = 9.7$, $p < 0.001$). At 12 -months, 100% reported they had educated community members about HBOC, 62% had interacted with other health care professionals about HBOC and 44% had navigated one or more patients to genetics services.

Conclusions: Initial results suggest ÁRBOLES Familiares trainees exhibit increased knowledge, self-efficacy and implementation of skills related to identification and referral of Latinas at risk of HBOC. This approach holds promise as a training model to bridge the gap between Latino communities and referral and access to genetics services.

Appendix D: Living with and Beyond Cancer: Taking Action to Improve Outcomes

A Secondary Analysis on the Effectiveness of a Holistic Intervention in Latino Versus Non-Latino Cancer Survivors

Corina Zamora[1], Daniel Hughes[1], Alexis Ortiz[2], Angelika Aguilar[3], Amelie Ramirez[1]

[1]University of Texas Health -San Antonio, San Antonio, TX, USA
[2]University of Incarnate Word, San Antonio, TX, USA
[3]University of Texas at San Antonio, San Antonio, TX, USA

Background: A cancer survivor's health-related quality of life (HR-QOL) can be conceptualized as the physical, mental, and spiritual aspects that define a human being. A HR-QOL focused holistic approach has the potential to optimize outcomes for _all_ these aspects of a cancer survivor's health outcomes. Attempts to improve quality of life should work for all survivors – specifically for Latinos, the fastest growing demographic in the U.S. The purpose of this analysis is to understand differences in how a holistic intervention approach impacts HR-QOL in Latino cancer survivors as compared to non-Latino cancer survivors.

Methods: Thirty adult cancer survivors in the greater San Antonio area will complete a holistic 16-week intervention to maximize physical, mental, and spiritual outcomes. Differences in primary outcomes will be compared between Latino versus non-Latino participants.

Results: This study is undergoing final protocol review approvals. We anticipate being able to report on differences in between Latinos/non-Latino adult cancer survivors that participate in the intervention. The analysis will include group differences in primary outcome measures as well as single system analyses.

Conclusions: The growth of the cancer survivor population has led to an increasing demand for research that improves the QOL for all cancer survivors. This analysis will inform intervention strategies specific to Latino cancer survivors by

© The Editor(s) (if applicable) and The Author(s) 2023
A. G. Ramirez, E. J. Trapido (eds.), *Advancing the Science of Cancer in Latinos*, https://doi.org/10.1007/978-3-031-14436-3

273

understanding what components of a holistic approach best optimizes outcomes for Latino adult cancer survivors. We anticipate our methods will be generalizable to other cancer population and thus can improve the state of cancer survivorship as whole.

Impact of a Natural Disaster on Access to Care and Biopsychosocial Outcomes Among Hispanic/Latino Cancer Survivors

Mary Rodriguez-Rabassa[1,2], Ruthmarie Hernandez[1], Zindie Rodriguez[3], Claudia B. Colon-Echevarria[5], Lizette Maldonado[3], Nelmit Tollinchi[1], Estefania Torres[1], Adnil Mulero[1], Daniela Albors[5], Jaileene Perez-Morales[7], Idhaliz Flores[4,6], Heather Jim[8], Eida M. Castro[1,2], Guillermo N. Armaiz-Pena[3,4,5*]

[1]Clinical Psychology Program, School of Behavior and Brain Sciences, Ponce Health Sciences University, Ponce, Puerto Rico, USA

Divisions of [2]Mental Health, [3]Cancer Biology and [4]Women's Health, Ponce Research Institute, Ponce, Puerto Rico, USA

Department of Basic Sciences, Divisions of [5]Pharmacology and [6]Microbiology, School of Medicine, Ponce Health Sciences University, Ponce, Puerto Rico, USA

Departments of [7]Cancer Epidemiology and [8]Health Outcomes and Behavior, H. Lee Moffitt Cancer Center and Research Institute, Tampa, Florida, USA

Background: Cancer is the leading cause of death in Puerto Rico (PR). Hurricane Maria (HM) and its aftermath lead to widespread devastation in the island, including the collapse of the healthcare system. Medically fragile populations, such as cancer survivors, were significantly affected. The goal of this study was to assess the impact of HM on barriers to care, emotional distress, and inflammatory biomarkers among cancer survivors in PR.

Methods: This exploratory longitudinal study was conducted in health care facilities and community support groups from PR. Cancer survivors ($n = 50$) and non-cancer participants ($n = 50$) completed psychosocial questionnaires and provided blood samples that were used to assess inflammatory cytokines levels. Data were analyzed through descriptive, frequencies, correlational, and linear regression analyses.

Results: Cancer survivors that were affected by HM reported increased barriers in accessing medical care, which were directly associated with anxiety, perceived stress, and post-traumatic symptomatology. Moreover, being a cancer survivor, along with closeness in time from HM predicted more barriers to receiving health care. Several inflammatory cytokines, such as CD31, BDNF, TFF3, Serpin E-1, Vitamin D BP, VCAM-1, Osteopontin, Chitinase 3 like 1, MMP-9 and MIF were significantly upregulated in cancer survivors while BDNF, MMP9 and Osteopontin had significant positive correlations with barriers to care.

Conclusions: HM significantly impacted Puerto Ricans psychosocial well-being. Cancer survivors had significant barriers to care and showed increased serum inflammatory cytokines, but didn't show differences in anxiety, stress and post-traumatic symptoms compared to non-cancer participants.

Depression and Markers of Breast Cancer Tumor Progression: The Role of Exposure to Social-Environmental Adversity

Eida M. Castro-Figueroa*, Karina I. Acevedo, Cristina Peña, Guillermo Armaiz-Peña
Ponce Health Sicences University-Ponce Research Institute, Puerto Rico, United States

Background and Purpose: There is growing evidence that highlights inflammation as a common factor in depression, chronic psychosocial stress and tumor microenvironment. However, little is known about the role of current and past exposure to social-environmental adversity (SEA; e.g., child abuse, domestic violence) in the relationship between depression and markers of inflammation in the breast cancer (BC) tumor microenvironment.

Methods: Participants ($n = 32$) were recruited before undergoing BC tumor surgery and completed a package of surveys through interviews that included the PHQ-8, Adverse Childhood Events (ACE) questionnaire and the Trauma History Questionnaire (THQ). Regarding BC tumor samples, 10x fields were quantified for CD68 (macrophages), CD19 (B cells) and CD3 (T cells). Pearson Correlation Tests are used to explore correlation between the variables of interest.

Results: Preliminary findings ($n = 22$) reveal that the most common SEA experience were general disasters and trauma ($n = 21$), physical and sexual abuse ($n = 16$) and, crime-related trauma ($n = 13$). Out of those reporting childhood abuse experiences ($n = 16$), 6 reported exposure to more than 4 ACE experiences. Mean score of PHQ-8 symptoms were low ($M = 3.77 \pm 4.19$). The relationship between depression symptoms and inflammatory markers of tumor microenvironment (macrophages, B cells and T cells) was not statistically significant. However, there were statistically significant relationship between B cell lymphocytes and adverse childhood events ($p < 0.05$).

Conclusions: Significant correlations between ACE and B cells lymphocytes needs further exploration considering that Lymphocytes has been recognized as a new hall mark in BC treatment prognosis and outcomes.

Underrepresentation of Hispanic Advanced Cancer Patients in Quality-of-Life Randomized Behavioral Clinical Trials: A Systematic Review

Torres-Blasco, Normarie*, González Cordero, Karina, Padilla Acosta, Nicole, Castro-Figuero, Eida

Ponce Health Sicences University-Ponce Research Institute, Puerto Rico, United States

Background: Patients with advanced cancer are at higher risk of experiencing poor quality of life and Hispanic patients are at higher risk. Behavioral interventions have the potential to address this need, however, little is known about the inclusion of Hispanic patients in behavioral randomized clinical trials targeting quality of life care. The purpose of this systematic review is to characterize behavioral interventions targeting quality of life among patients with advanced cancer and identify the rate of Hispanics included in such trials.

Methodology: MEDLINE, PubMed, EBSCOhost and Google Scholar databases were searched up to the year 2018 for randomized behavioral clinical trials (RCT) aimed at improving the quality of life of patients with advanced cancer. Articles were excluded if the behavioral RCT was targeting patients receiving end of life care. Studies were graded for quality using the QualSyst quantitative checklist. Levels of evidence were ascertained by completing the National Health and Medical Research Council criteria. Results are presented under the AMSTAR guidelines.

Results: Overall, 19 RCT studies were included and 47% rated as good methodology quality. Outcome measures across studies were heterogeneous. Most interventions were delivered at hospital clinics ($n = 16$) by psychotherapists ($n = 11$). Interventions were mostly targeting female Caucasian patients (53%) and 33% of the studies included Hispanics patients in the sample; furthermore, the percentage of Hispanics included in the sample ranged from 1% to 11%.

Conclusion: Critical gaps remain regarding the underrepresentation of Hispanic patients with advanced cancer in behavioral randomized clinical trials targeting quality of life psychosocial support.

Disparity in Urinary Diversion Performed During Radical Cystectomy for Bladder Cancer in the Hispanic Population

Emily M. Rios[1], Mitchell A. Parma[2], Roman A. Fernandez[3], Timothy N. Clinton[1], Ryan M. Reyes[3], Kristy Cunningham[1], Dharam Kaushik[1], Deepak Pruthi[1], Ahmed M. Mansour[1], Jon Gelfond[3], Karen M. Wheeler[1] and Robert S. Svatek[1]*

[1]Department of Urology, University of Texas Health San Antonio, San Antonio, TX, USA

[2]School of Medicine, University of Texas Health San Antonio, San Antonio, TX, USA

[3]Department of Biostatistics, University of Texas Health San Antonio, San Antonio, TX, USA

Background: Healthcare resource use and outcomes discrepancies among ethnicities have recently become a topic of concern. Studies have shown that discrepancies in surgical options offered exist between non-Hispanic whites (NHW) and other races for pancreatic, prostate, colorectal and breast cancers, but none have explored the various quality of care metrics that are relevant for Hispanic patients with invasive bladder cancer (BC) undergoing radical cystectomy (RC). This study aimed to determine if disparities in quality of surgical care exist between Hispanics and NHW undergoing RC for BC.

Methods: We performed a retrospective review on patients who underwent RC for BC at our institution between 2005 and 2018. Data was collected on demographic, clinical, and pathological characteristics, including self-reported race and ethnicity. Univariable and multivariable logistic or linear regression were used to evaluate the association of ethnicity with quality of care outcomes, including receipt of neoadjuvant chemotherapy (NAC), utilization of laparoscopic surgery, number of lymph nodes removed and type of urinary diversion. We identified 507 patients, 136 (27%) were Hispanic and 371 (73%) were NHW. Compared to NHW, Hispanics had a higher BMI ($p = 0.006$) and lived further away from site of surgery ($p = 0.02$).

Results: Hispanics were more likely to receive an incontinent urinary diversion on multivariable analysis (OR 0.38, 95% CI 0.16–0.93, $p = 0.03$).

Conclusion: Hispanics in our region were less likely to receive a continent urinary diversion compared to NHW after adjusting for multiple clinical features. Further investigation is warranted to determine potential causes for this disparity in care delivered.

Qualitative Analyses of a Holistic Quality-of-Life Intervention for Latinos as Compared to Non-Latino Cancer Survivors.

Julissa Marin, Daniel C. Hughes[*], Amelie G. Ramirez
    Institute for Health Promotion Research, University of Texas Health - San Antonio, San Antonio, TX, USA.

Background: Latinos compared to non-Latino whites have poor outcomes for various cancers (e.g. breast cancer). The factors contributing to these differences are multi-faceted and complex. What intervention strategies optimize outcomes for Latino versus non-Latino cancer survivors? To understand these differences requires both quantitative and qualitative approach.

Methods: We examine the feasibility of a holistic approach to maximize health-related quality of life (QOL) outcomes for 30 adult cancer survivors in San Antonio, Texas. The 16-week intervention consists of group yoga-meditation, individualized exercise, diet guidance, and motivational text messages. Participants complete comprehensive assessments of QOL outcomes (body, mind and spirit) using validated instruments and semi-structured interviews to self-report current and ideal QOL. During pre (week 0), mid (week 8), post (week 16), and follow-up assessments (week 42), the interviews are recorded, transcribed, and analyzed with Atlas. ti software using theme recognition and theme endorsement. This analysis refines cultural adaptation strategies to enhance adherence for cancer prevention behaviors in future studies.

Results: This pilot study is undergoing final protocol review approvals. We anticipate completing the first half of the holistic intervention, including pre-assessments and mid-assessments, to report differences between Latinos/non-Latino adult cancer survivors.

Conclusion: First, the analysis informs of future implementation strategies. Second, holistic interventions and customized health plans for cancer survivors optimize QOL outcomes. The far-reaching potential to minimize negative effects of cancer and chronic diseases for vulnerable populations can affect the cancer survivor community. Eliminating unnecessary costs and advancing the general health of the cancer population improves a strained public health system.

Improving Patient Care for Hispanic Pediatric Oncology Patients with Limited English Proficiency

Terrie Flatt[1]*, Sara Donnelley[1], Pilar Coromina[1], Theresa Torres[2]
[1]Children's Mercy Hospital, Kansas City, MO USA
[2]All Children's Hospital, St. Petersburg, FL USA

Background: Caregivers of pediatric oncology patients with limited English proficiency face challenges as they navigate the English-speaking medical system in the US. Population and language specific clinics can improve patient outcomes and parent/patient engagement. Our objective is to present a model of clinical care for pediatric cancer patients that has improved patient care and parent satisfaction.

Methods: This is a description of a bilingual model of clinical care and the materials utilized to improve patient outcomes, compliance and parent satisfaction.

Materials and methods used to facilitate compliance and outcomes will be demonstrated.

Results: The HOPE Clinic (Clínica de Hematología y Oncología: Puente de Esperanza) a model of clinical care developed for pediatric cancer patients at the Children's Mercy Cancer Center, Kansas City, MO was established in 2012 and provides services to approximately 30 new Hispanic oncology patients annually. The provider is bilingual. Encounters are in Spanish. A dedicated language navigator is available. Parent satisfaction scores with provider and services rendered were 99% (0–100% satisfaction). Utilizing bilingual oncology specific tools and parent training programs, oral chemotherapy compliance is >95% for patients with acute lymphoblastic leukemia/lymphoma (ALL), no-show appointment rate is <0.05%, triage time to antibiotics decreased for patients with fever/neutropenia. Overall survival for Hispanic patients with ALL is 91%, which is above the national average.

Conclusions: Population specific clinics and bilingual models of care can improve access, decrease triage times, improve medication compliance and improve over-all outcomes. Patient/Parent engagement and satisfaction are improved with this model of care.

CARE-ing for Spanish-Speaking Cancer Patients: The Role of a Latino Cancer Support Group in a Safety-Net Hospital

Ana I. Velazquez[1*], Evelin Trejo[1], Aunée Tarango[2], Gabriela Quezada-Perez[1]
[1]University of San Francisco, San Francisco, CA, USA
[2]University of California San Francisco, San Francisco, CA, USA

Background: Latino cancer patients/survivors (CPS) are known to experience significantly higher levels of distress and lower quality of life compared to Non-Latino Whites. Social support resources are limited in availability and uptake among non-English speaking CPS due to language, economic, and socio-cultural barriers. Cancer Awareness, Resources, and Education (CARE) is a cancer wellness support group that offers three independent quarterly educational series in English, Cantonese, and Spanish for CPS at Zuckerberg San Francisco General Hospital (ZSFGH). We aimed to evaluate the role of Spanish CARE for Latino CPS participants.

Methods: Anonymous surveys were administered by volunteer staff to program participants. Pre-program surveys were administered during the first 3 weeks of the program and a post-program survey was administered on the final session. Surveys assessed participants demographics, perceived social support and role of the program.

Results: Among 14 Latino CPS surveyed, 26% identified getting emotional support as the main reason they attended Spanish CARE. Other common responses included talking with other patients affected by cancer (22%) and learning more about cancer from the educational presentations (24%). All participants were likely or very likely to refer the CARE program to other CPS.

Conclusions: Spanish CARE provides cultural and language concordant emotional and social support to Latino CPS while providing patient education and well-being resources. Our current efforts include the development of surveys and focus groups to evaluate the educational and wellness needs of Latino CPS, as well as their preferred delivery methods.

The Importance of Patient Engagement to Patient Satisfaction and Quality of Life Among Latina Breast Cancer Survivors

Jackie Bonilla[1], Cristian Escalera[1], Jasmine Santoyo-Olsson[2], Carmen Ortiz[3], Anita L. Stewart[4], Anna María Nápoles*[1]

[1]National Institute on Minority Health and Health Disparities, National Institutes of Health, Bethesda, MD, USA

[2]Division of General Internal Medicine, Department of Medicine, University of California San Francisco, San Francisco, CA, USA

[3]Círculo de Vida Cancer Support and Resource Center, San Francisco, CA, USA

[4]Institute for Health and Aging, University of California San Francisco, San Francisco, CA, USA

Background: Compared to their white counterparts, Latina breast cancer survivors experience poorer quality care and worse health-related quality of life (HRQOL). Limited English proficiency (LEP) and less patient engagement in cancer care could help explain these disparities. We assessed associations of LEP and difficulty engaging with clinicians with patient satisfaction and emotional and physical well-being among rural and urban Latina breast cancer survivors.

Methods: Analyses used cross-sectional baseline survey data from two studies that tested a stress management program among rural and urban Latina breast cancer survivors in California. Linear regression models examined bivariate and multivariate associations of LEP status (yes or no (reference)), difficulty engaging with physicians scale (1–4; higher score = greater difficulty), and rural versus urban (reference) site, on patient satisfaction and emotional and physical well-being, controlling for demographic and medical factors.

Results: The total sample included 304 women. Most were LEP (84.5%) and had less than a high school education (67.8%). Difficulty engaging with physicians was inversely associated with patient satisfaction ($B = -0.190$, $p = 0.014$), emotional well-being ($B = -1.866$, $p < 0.0001$), and physical well-being ($B = -1.272$, $p = 0.002$). Having LEP (vs. not; $B = 1.987$, $p = 0.040$) was independently associated with physical well-being only. Rural/urban status was not related independently to any outcome.

Conclusion: Rural and urban Latina breast cancer survivors who report greater difficulty engaging with clinicians experience worse patient satisfaction and HRQOL. Promoting greater engagement of Latina breast cancer survivors in cancer care and providing medical interpreters could improve patient outcomes. Clinicians need to proactively elicit patients' concerns and preferences among Latina breast cancer patients.

Acknowledgement of Funding: This research was supported by the California Breast Cancer Research Grants Program Office of the University of California grants number 15BB-1300, 15BB-1301 and 21OB-0135, grant number 1 P30 AG15272 from the National Institute on Aging, and the Division of Intramural Research, National Institute on Minority Health and Health Disparities, National Institutes of Health.

Cancer Metaphors "A la Carta"

Isabel María Centeno Sánchez*
    Centro de PsicoOncología y Salud Narrativa, Monterrey, NL, México

Background: We know that metaphors help us to make some sense of life challenging situations, as a cancer diagnosis could be. The battle, war and warriors against cancer has been questioned as a useful narrative resource to figure out what cancer means to each patient. Metaphors have close relation with culture and education, so it is almost impossible to find a universal metaphor to fit all cancer patients.

Methods: Based on the work of Lancaster University about Cancer Metaphors, I am developing a "Purpose resource" so health care providers can offer Mexican patients with narrative options to understand their illness. The study is being developed with breast cancer patients and in an individual interview we are reading together other persons' metaphors options to evaluate how much it resonates with their own perception. We finish each session with a brief report and a possible new metaphor that fits the patient own perception.

Results: We created a metaphors menu that is in continuous growth. It turns out that some of our patients feel very comfortable with the "battle" narrative while most of them consider that everybody else refer to them as warriors while they don't see themselves like that. Most of them mention that they don't find a real purpose in this "social narrative" as fighters against cancer.

Conclusion: Creativity and Language in the form of metaphors has shown to us that can be a helpful resource for talking and thinking about the experience of illness.

Community-Based Programs for Latina Cancer Survivors: An Evaluation Campamento Alegria

Emalyn Deak[1*], Amy Garcia [2*], Ana Gutierrez [1*], Paola Mancera[1*], Viviam Sifontes[3], Dr. Claudia Aguado Loi[2], Dr. Dinorah Martinez Tyson[1]
   [1]University of South Florida, Tampa, FL, USA
   [2]University of Tampa, Tampa, FL, USA
   [3]Latinos Unidos por un Nuevo Amanecer, Inc

Background: There are limited resources that support Latina women through the process of survivorship that is linguistically and culturally relevant. Overnight camps are one service event that can have a powerful impact on cancer survivors. However, Latina cancer survivors often report a disconnect at these camps (e.g., English-only). Camp Alegria was created to bridge this gap through culturally tailored activities (e.g., Spanish, food, music, educational content) to better support Latina cancer survivors.

Methods: We present evaluation data from the 2018 camp to assess the impact the camp had on the participants' satisfaction, the overall level of wellbeing, and support from other cancer survivors. A pre-post survey with open-ended questions was provided at the beginning of the 3-day camp. Data analysis included a paired-sample t-test via IBM SPSS v26 and applied thematic analysis techniques.

Results: Participants ($n = 55$, 83% response rate) self-reported statistically significant improvement in their emotional, spiritual, and physical health well-being ($p < 0.01$). Based on the applied thematic analysis, most participants felt the program was beneficial by promoting a sense of peace and happiness, as well as offering them the opportunity to connect and bond with other cancer survivors. Many participants were grateful for the experience, and some provided suggestions for improvement.

Discussion: Camp Alegria allows Latina cancer survivors to feel connected and supported. Our findings demonstrate the success and highlight the need for culturally and linguistically relevant community-based programs like Camp Alegria.

Keywords: survivorship, evaluation, social support, Latina, cancer.

Chronic Medical Conditions and Psychological Distress Among Undocumented Mexican Immigrants: Findings from *Proyecto Voces*

Luz M. Garcini, Kathryn E. Kanzler, Lisa Smith Kilpela
 University of Texas Health Science Center at San Antonio, San Antonio, TX, USA

Background: Undocumented immigration is often accompanied by multiple complex stressors, including limited access to healthcare. This can be particularly distressing for undocumented immigrants living with chronic medical conditions, who must rely on cash to pay for health services or neglect health care due to cost. This study is aimed at identifying the prevalence of and psychological distress related to chronic medical conditions among undocumented Mexican immigrants residing near the U.S.-Mexico border.

Methods: We used respondent-driven sampling to collect and analyze data from clinical interviews with 254 undocumented Mexican immigrants, enabling inference to a population of 22,000. Chronic medical conditions were assessed using the World Health Organization Composite International Diagnostic Interview (CIDI) Chronic Conditions Module. For all analyses, inferential statistics accounted for design effects and sample weights to produce weighted estimates. We conducted logistic regression analyses to identify vulnerabilities associated with having a chronic medical condition, as well as to identify factors associated with psychological distress among undocumented immigrants with chronic medical conditions.

Results: Approximately 52% of undocumented Mexican immigrants reported having one or more chronic medical conditions ($M = 2.36$; SD $= 1.49$), with the most prevalent conditions being chronic pain (43%), asthma (36%), gastric-related disorder (34%) and hypertension (27%). In the logistic regression model to identify factors associated with having a chronic medical condition, being older (OR $= 1.09$, 95% CI [1.05, 1.14]), arriving to the U.S. at a younger age (OR $= 1.06$, 95% CI [1.11, 1.01]), and having experienced a greater number of traumatic events (OR $= 1.12$, 95% CI [1.04, 1.21]) were significantly associated with having a chronic medical condition. Among undocumented immigrants with one or more chronic medical conditions, difficulty accessing health services (OR $= 1.39$, 95% CI [1.07, 1.81]) was the only factor significantly associated with clinical levels of psychological distress, after controlling for age, sex, income, age of arrival to the U.S., and history of trauma.

Conclusion: Our findings emphasize the magnitude of chronic medical conditions as a health concern for undocumented Mexican immigrants, with attendant public health implications. Revising policies to devise solutions grounded in evidence and developing new alternatives to facilitate access and provision of health services to these immigrants is critical, including building efforts to develop prevention programs that are context- and culture-sensitive.

Translating the *Together* Pediatric Cancer Website into Spanish: Process and Lessons Learned

Heather Chambliss[1*], Diane Roberts[1], Diana Ruggiero[2], Owen McGuire[1]

[1]Department of Medical Content Outreach, St. Jude Children's Research Hospital, Memphis, TN, USA

[2]Department of World Languages and Literatures, The University of Memphis, Memphis, TN, USA

Background: Pediatric cancer families often turn to the internet for information related to diagnosis, treatment, care, and support. Together serves as a comprehensive web-based resource for families, no matter where the child receives treatment. The next development phase includes translation of content into additional languages, beginning with Spanish (US).

Methods: Translation of the Together website followed a multistep approach. A translation service provided the initial human translation. This allowed for a linguistics team of native Spanish speakers with medical writing experience, compatible technology for digital platform integration, and translation memory for efficiency and consistency across the website. After initial translation, an unaffiliated external reviewer examined and edited content. Issues were reconciled through consultation with writers and subject matter experts.

Results: To date, 400 pages have been translated into Spanish. Translation also included captioning of 18 medical illustrations and 48 videos. An additional 12 videos were developed specifically for the Spanish-language website. The translation process took approximately 4 months. Content analysis of reviewer notes revealed that syntax, pragmatics, sociolinguistics, semiotics, medical word choice, contextual meaning, and use of abbreviations were some of the most common problems encountered.

Conclusion: Barriers to translating content range from technical writing concerns to more complex issues of cultural competence and dialect. Learnings from this translation experience, along with usability, user experience and analytics data, will help identify ways to improve the translation process and inform next steps for the Spanish-language site. These lessons will also inform the process for additional language translations for the Together website.

Latinas Cancer Survivors: A Qualitative Approach

Donaji Stelzig[1*], Vicky Suruky[2], Daniel M. Price[3]
Corresponding author and early career investigator*
[1]University of Houston – Honors College Community Health Worker Training Center, Houston, TX, USA
[2]University San Diego, CA, USA
[3]University of Houston – Honors College Community Health Worker Initiative, Houston, TX, USA

Background: Breast cancer continues to be a priority public health concern among Hispanic/Latinos survivors. Quality of life, emotional support, and relationship issues facing female survivors with heterosexual partners after cancer treatment have not been adequately studied and potential educational interventions have not been explored.

Methods: A phenomenological research approach was conducted to learn about the life experiences among ten breast cancer survivors with their heterosexual partners, living in a southeast urban city of the United States.

In-depth interviews were conducted by the first author, who is also a bilingual community health worker (CHW). Ten Latino/Hispanic breast cancer survivors agreed to at least 45 minutes of interview time. All interviews surpassed the requested initial time for at least 30 minutes. Interviews provided three main themes after conducting this research.

Results: Three main themes emerged from the interviews: (1) deciding among treatment options based on post treatment body images, (2) communicating (or not) regarding intimacy after treatment, and (3) needing education on sexuality after cancer treatment.

Conclusions: More tools and support need to be developed to serve this population. More interventional programs, including community health workers are needed to address health disparities among Latino/Hispanics women, who are breast cancer survivors. The University of Houston CHW Initiative plans to provide care coordination services to ethnic and minority groups and may be well-placed to implement appropriate interventions and trainings that would improve the quality of life outcomes for breast cancer survivors with heterosexual partners.

Active Living After Cancer: An Evidence-Based Program That Has Demonstrated Quality-of-Life Improvements Among Hispanic/Latino Cancer Survivors

Stacy Mitchell[1], Gissell Montoya[1], Leticia Gatus[2*], Karen M. Basen-Engquist[2]
University of Texas MD Anderson Cancer Center, Houston, Texas United States

Background: Physical activity is associated with improved quality of life and increased disease free survivorship in cancer survivors. Active Living After Cancer (ALAC) is a program funded by the Cancer Prevention and Research Institute of Texas to improve the quality of life among cancer survivors by increasing physical activity and providing survivorship information.

Methods: ALAC is an evidence-based program that has demonstrated effectiveness in the Hispanic/Latino community. A mixed-methods approach will be used to describe Hispanic participant graduation rates and descriptions of their social interactions. Nearly 70% of enrolled participants in ALAC identify as Hispanic/Latino. Data on graduation and completion rates were used to assess retention and adherence to the Active Living After Cancer program. Using a hybrid approach of qualitative data analysis, we will describe how Hispanic ALAC participants develop camaraderie and use of social support.

Results: Data from quantitative analysis revealed that collectively ALAC participants complete the program at a rate of 77.2%. Hispanic/Latinos graduate at a rate of 68% demonstrating that there is great interest among the Hispanic/Latino for programs like ALAC. Preliminary qualitative analysis indicate Hispanic ALAC participants develop camaraderie or find social support in their class participants, accountability partner, or ALAC Health Educator.

Conclusion: Insights gained from this analysis suggest that it is feasible to adapt the program for areas with a high Hispanic/Latino survivor population. Our quantitative analysis demonstrates that physical activity based programs like Active Living After Cancer are of interest to Hispanic/Latino populations and provide social support.

Cognitive Executive Functioning and Health in Latina Breast Cancer Survivors

Amanda M. Marin-Chollom[*1], Christiane Hale[2], Margarita Santiago-Torres[3], Pam Koch[4], Ann Ogden Gaffney[5], Wei-Yann Tsai[6], Dawn Hershman[2,6], Isobel Contento[4], Adam M. Brickman[2], Heather Greenlee[3]
[1]Central Connecticut State University, New Britain, CT, USA

[2]Columbia University Irving Medical Center, New York, NY, USA
[3]Fred Hutchinson Cancer Research Center, Seattle, WA, USA
[4]Columbia University Teachers College, New York, NY, USA
[5]Cook for Your Life, New York, NY, USA
[6]Columbia University Mailman School of Public Health, New York, NY, USA

Background: Physical activity and body composition are modifiable lifestyle factors that can affect cognitive functioning, but have been minimally studied in underserved cancer populations, such as Hispanics/Latinos. This study examined the relationship of waist to hip ratio, body mass index (BMI), and physical activity with cognitive functioning among Latina breast cancer survivors.

Methods: Participants were 65 Latina breast cancer survivors (Age $M = 55.70$, SD = 9.09) who completed the NIH Toolbox Cognition Battery via the NIH Toolbox iPad App. The cognition scores used for analysis were provided and corrected for age, gender, education, and race/ethnicity by the app. Linear regression models were used to examine six cognition domains (cognitive flexibility, inhibitory control and attention, working memory, processing speed, episodic memory, and overall fluid cognitive abilities) with waist to hip ratio, body mass index (BMI), and self-reported physical activity as assessed via the 7-Day Physical Activity Recall (PAR). The PAR classifies physical activity as moderate, hard, and very hard. Additional model covariates included time since breast cancer diagnosis and receipt of chemotherapy.

Results: Very hard physical activity was associated with faster processing speed ($B = 7.12, p = .004$), and better overall fluid abilities ($B = 4.62, p = .01$); hard physical activity was associated with better working memory ($B = 3.74, p = .02$); while moderate physical activity was not associated with any of the six domains. Waist-to hip-ratio and BMI were not associated with any of the cognition domains examined.

Conclusions: These findings show that engagement in hard or very hard physical activity are associated with better cognitive functioning among Latina breast cancer survivors. Trials are needed to determine whether increasing physical activity can improve cognitive functioning in Latina breast cancer survivor.

Psychosocial Issues Faced by Adolescent and Young Adult Latino Survivors of Pediatric Cancers: A Targeted Review

Kimberly Arellano Carmona*, A. Susana Ramírez
     University of California – Merced, Merced, CA, USA

Background: Advances in childhood cancer treatment mean that most children diagnosed with cancer survive into adulthood. Yet a growing body of research has raised concerns about the long-term challenges of pediatric cancers, including treatment sequelae and psychosocial issues associated with surviving disease. Adolescent and young adult (AYA) survivors face particular challenges as they negotiate the typical development issues with the added challenges of cancer survivorship. One-quarter of U.S. children are Latino and have higher rates of cancer incidence; although Latinos are also less likely to survive, the growing population of Latino children suggests that survivorship research must aim to understand their unique challenges. This review critically centers Latinos in examining what is known about psychosocial and quality of life outcomes for AYA survivors of pediatric cancers.

Methods: Systematic search of PubMed, PsychINFO, Google Scholar, complemented by hand-searching reference lists and citing articles to identify publications (2009 to 2019) reporting psychosocial issues facing AYA survivors diagnosed before age 15.

Results: Of 122 articles identified, ten met inclusion criteria. Psychosocial issues included anxiety and depression, and issues related to daily living, finances, educational attainment, and employment. Only one article reported results by ethnicity, in which there was not enough power to consider whether issues were different for Latinos; most studies were based on cohorts from cancer treatment centers serving primarily Caucasian patients.

Conclusion: Psychosocial issues faced uniquely by Latinos are unknown. More research is needed to understand AYA survivorship issues for the growing population of Latino children who disproportionately suffer from cancer.

Index

© The Editor(s) (if applicable) and The Author(s) 2023
A. G. Ramirez, E. J. Trapido (eds.), *Advancing the Science of Cancer in Latinos*, https://doi.org/10.1007/978-3-031-14436-3

Printed in the United States
by Baker & Taylor Publisher Services